Global Health Informatics

Global Health Informatics

Principles of eHealth and mHealth to Improve Quality of Care

edited by Leo Anthony G. Celi, Hamish S. F. Fraser, Vipan Nikore, Juan Sebastián Osorio, and Kenneth Paik

The MIT Press
Cambridge, Massachusetts
London, England

This book was set in Times Ten LT Std by Toppan Best-set Premedia Limited. Printed and bound in the United States of America.

Library of Congress Cataloging-in-Publication Data is available.

Names: Celi, Leo Anthony G., editor. | Fraser, Hamish S. F., editor. | Nikore, Vipan, editor. | Osorio, Juan Sebastián, editor. | Paik, Kenneth, editor.
Title: Global health informatics: principles of ehealth and mhealth to improve quality of care / edited by Leo Anthony G. Celi, Hamish S.F. Fraser, Vipan Nikore, Juan Sebastián Osorio, and Kenneth Paik.
Description: Cambridge, MA: The MIT Press, [2017] | Includes bibliographical references and index.
Identifiers: LCCN 2016031382 | ISBN 9780262533201 (pbk.: alk. paper)
Subjects: | MESH: Telemedicine | Global Health | Medical Informatics | Mobile Applications | Quality of Health Care
Classification: LCC R858 | NLM W 83.1 | DDC 610.285—dc23 LC record available at https://lccn.loc.gov/2016031382

10 9 8 7 6 5 4 3 2 1

Contents

Chapters available online at https://mitpress.mit.edu/books/global-health -informatics

Preface

Disease has no respect for country borders. Increased global travel has fueled the spread of infectious disease, as evidenced by the Ebola virus epidemic. Chronic diseases such as diabetes and heart disease, initially confined to the developed world, now exist side by side with malnutrition in low- and middle-income countries (LMIC). Global warming is widening the endemicity of vector-borne diseases.

One driving force that sweeps across nations even faster than disease is technology. The spread of mobile phones that bring computational power and data to our fingertips has led to new paradigms in tracking and battling disease. This book explores ways to leverage technology to combat disease and promote health, especially in resource-constrained settings.

The book was born out of the volunteer organization Sana, hosted by the Institute for Medical Engineering and Science at the Massachusetts Institute of Technology (MIT). The print version has four sections—the global health landscape, introduction to health information technology, implementing a health informatics project, and digital health applications. A fifth section, a collection of health informatics software and systems, is available as an online supplement (https://mitpress.mit.edu/books/global-health-informatics).

Sana, the group behind this book, consists of doctors, informaticians, engineers, public health practitioners, business entrepreneurs, social scientists, and others who share the goal of improving quality of health care in resource-poor settings. Sana began with the development of an open-source, cell phone—based telehealth software, but the members quickly realized that technology by itself would not transform health outcomes in the developing world. The organization then began to focus on health care quality and safety through empowerment and education using technology. This led to the group offering HST.936, a global health informatics course at MIT offered to a worldwide network of partner universities; a massive online open course, or MOOC, under MITx; and this book.

This book is targeted toward individuals interested in designing or implementing a health information and communication technology (ICT) solution in the developing world. This includes, but is not limited to, students, academic researchers, entrepreneurs, clinicians, hospital administrators, and government officials. Implementing a health information technology project requires multidisciplinary teams. Thus, with this book, we hope to bring together individuals from a variety of disciplines—computer science, medicine, engineering, public health, policy, and business. Lastly, we anticipate audiences from both the developed and the developing world who have vastly different amounts and types of resources at their disposal.

Reaching such a broad audience with different skill sets makes the design and content of this book a challenge. Most of the topics we discuss have entire books dedicated to that specific topic, but we are only able to dedicate a single chapter to it. While we cannot explore in depth the entire set of required principles, we can introduce a basic understanding of key concepts, frameworks, practical examples, and lessons learned. With vast differences in the structure, resources, and culture of health care systems, we cannot definitively state what will or will not work in every country, but we can offer lessons based on real examples of successes and failures in the field. We also encourage our readers to supplement this book with our Global Health Informatics course available on MITx.

The use of ICT in health care has lagged behind compared to other industries such as telecommunications, banking, trading, and retail merchandising, but has recently picked up, especially in LMIC. The health care industry has been slow to adopt new technologies in general, making the excitement around ICT for health in the developing world even more remarkable. The use of ICT in health care has the potential to track quality of care, address many root causes of disease, promote healthy behaviors, improve the efficiency of delivery, and reduce soaring health expenditures.

When exploring innovations in information systems in developing countries, it is important to focus not only on the technology (i.e., eHealth), but also on broader issues necessary for its success, such as quality improvement, project management, and leadership skills. Ultimately, health care delivery systems require fundamental and sound operations, such as physical infrastructure and supply-chain management, to deliver high-quality care. Technology is simply a tool to help facilitate this process.

The quality of care theme is critical to this book. The first step stakeholders in health systems should focus on prior to introducing an innovation is to establish a culture of quality improvement and patient safety. An information system can then play a facilitative role by enabling care coordination, tracking processes and outcomes, supporting decision making, and fostering learning through data analysis. But a paradigm shift is a prerequisite for all these changes to take place. An information system without an accompanying organizational transformation risks reinforcing the same failed processes. For example, using technology to improve access to care without any other quality-improvement elements will yield the same and not necessarily better results, but more of them. Innovations need to address gaps in quality and demonstrate improvement in health outcomes, otherwise they won't sustain or scale.

Unfortunately, there has been scant data on the quality of care in LMIC. One of the few pieces of quality evidence comes from a 2009 bulletin published by the World Health Organization entitled "Medicines used in primary care in developing and transitional countries," which evaluated 679 studies from 97 developing and transitional countries between 1990 and 2006. The results demonstrated poor quality of data and poor-quality prescribing for both private and public sectors. It showed that more than 50% of all medicines are prescribed, dispensed, or sold inappropriately, and half of all patients fail to take medicines correctly. Less than 30–40% were treated according to existing clinical guidelines. There is evidence that technology can improve these statistics by informing prescriber decisions, improving patient adherence, or providing better data capture, but a concurrent cultural transformation must take place to unleash technology's full potential.

The future is bright, though. Cell phones have become ubiquitous in the developing world. Smartphones and tablets are becoming more popular as they become cheaper. In fact, there are now more cell phones than people in the world. Electronic Medical Records have been rolled out to hundreds or even thousands of clinics in some LMICs. More funding is being funneled toward digital health technologies in the developing world, and young local talent is increasingly drawn toward improving health outcomes. These forces are enabling LMIC to move more quickly than those in the developed world in several key areas. In general, LMIC have fewer legacy systems and thus fewer interoperability issues to untangle, and can focus on implementing with fewer barriers. This has allowed some innovations that were developed in LMIC to be exported to high-income countries. For example, architectures such as DHIS2 and OpenMRS, initially deployed in resource-poor countries, have gained traction in Western countries, and mHealth applications to support community health care workers are now making that transition. LMIC are also beginning to accelerate developments in biometrics at a faster rate than many Western countries have been able to. This leads to the question whether the next "Silicon Valley" could be located somewhere in the developing world. It is too early to predict, but it is certainly within the realm of possibility given the enabling environment, which allows ideas and innovation to flourish. LMIC in East Africa, including Kenya, Tanzania, and Rwanda, are developing indigenous eHealth industries, for example.

Despite the promising future, scaling a successful digital health solution remains a tall task. Embedded within optimism are numerous historical examples of abandoned IT solutions despite successful feasibility studies. This has left countries demanding measurable impact—and rightfully so, as the implementation of any new solution should undergo rigorous evaluation. Health care and technology are at times in two diametrically opposed fields: one slow to respond to change, the other changing so quickly; one focused on long and rigorous randomized control trials, the other focused on rapid iteration and modification; one notorious for deep hierarchical structures, and the other known for flat organizational structures with 25-year-old CEOs. In health informatics, these worlds often collide; this book will explore these tensions and suggest a middle ground forward.

Lastly, as we attempt to leverage troves of data to define best practices, we must resist seeing patients as data points rather than individuals. As digital health advocates from different backgrounds and countries, we must keep the patient perspective and health at the center of everything we do.

I GLOBAL HEALTH LANDSCAPE

We begin this book by painting the global health landscape. This is a crucial step before we can dive into the technical component of health information systems. Innovations in health informatics will only reinforce old failed processes unless accompanied by carefully engineered organizational changes that require a deep understanding of the complexities of the issues in global health.

In chapter 1, Stone and company present the evolving global burden of disease resulting from people living longer with chronic diseases and disabilities. Trends differ greatly across countries and regions, reflecting growing health disparities. Mwangi and colleagues zoom in on Kenya as a case study in chapter 2 and describe the infrastructural challenges to health care delivery. In chapter 3, Bradley and Taylor go over the design, implementation, and evaluation of a health system—the organization of the people, the institutions, and the resources that deliver care to a population. Meyers and associates introduce the concept of quality improvement in chapter 4. This pertains to how every member of the system, health care provider or not, is empowered and committed to improving processes and continuous learning. The value of health informatics—or any innovation, for that matter—-is maximized when there is commitment among those in the system to constantly measure and improve the way care is delivered. Evaluation of a health intervention, discussed by Fox and Rothman in chapter 5, is a crucial component of quality improvement. Finally, Peters and Castillo Farias caution readers about potential unintended consequences of technology and introduce social theory as a tool in implementing global health interventions in chapter 6.

The section is but an abbreviated overview of the global health context, and barely scratches the complexity of the problems we are trying to solve with health informatics. We urge our readers to work closely with front-line providers in identifying and understanding the challenges that plague care delivery in resource-constrained settings. The hope that the problems we've had and we continue to have in global health will have technological solutions is very seductive. Disappointments (and failures) are inevitable. The biggest obstacle facing global health is an incomplete understanding of the systems-level issues. We cannot impose a technological solution on what is a problem of weak health care infrastructure.

1 The Global Burden of Disease

Geren S. Stone, Julian Mitton, Jessica Kenney, and Kristian R. Olson

It may be now asked, to what purpose tends all this laborious buzzling, and grouping? To know... what proportion die of each general and particular Casualties? What years are fruitfull, and mortal, and in what space and intervals, they follow each other? [1]

—*John Graunt 1662*

"To ensure a health system is adequately aligned to a population's true health challenges, policymakers must be able to compare the effects of different diseases that kill people prematurely and cause ill health." [2]

—*Global Burden of Disease Report 2012*

Take-Home Messages

- People are living longer than ever before, and they are living more years with chronic disease and disabilities.
- The leading causes of death and disability having shifted from infectious diseases in childhood to noncommunicable diseases in adults.
- These global trends differ greatly across regions, communities, and populations, with marked variation reflecting the growing realities of health disparities.

Introduction

Over 2,000 years ago, Hippocrates first attempted to describe disease from a rational perspective by observing geographical and temporal patterns. From these earliest foundations, epidemiology traces its history through the work and lives of figures including John Graunt, Thomas Sydenham, Ignaz Semmelweiss, John Snow, Louis Pasteur, Robert Koch, and Florence Nightingale [3]. Modern epidemiology—defined as the "study of the distribution and determinants of health-related states or events (including disease) and the application of this to the control of diseases and other health problems"—is an essential component of public health today [4]. Epidemiology helps us to understand the root causes and contexts of disease, and thereby informs health care planning and delivery. The Global Burden of Disease is a concept first published in 1996 that provides summary epidemiology data in order to quantify levels of disease and disability, utilizing metrics such as the disability-adjusted life year (DALY). Whether one is a district health officer in rural Uganda or the director-general of the World Health Organization, it is critical to utilize data and evidence to identify, understand, and address the health issues faced by communities and populations.

The world's population has surpassed 7 billion, with Earth presently supporting "more people than have lived in all of human history" [5,6]. Improvements in agricultural production and sanitation have led to unprecedented population growth [5]. Transitioning into a sustainable development framework, the world is very different than it was when the United Nations General Assembly unanimously adopted the Millennium Declaration and its Millennium Development Goals [7]. Moreover, the rate of change is accelerating with advances in science, technology, communications, and trade. People are more mobile and living longer than ever before. Furthermore, as populations age, people are living longer with chronic diseases and disability. The leading causes of death and disability have shifted from infectious diseases in childhood to noncommunicable diseases in adults [2,6,8,9]. Risk factors for diseases and disability are transitioning. For example, people are now more likely to "suffer from eating too much food rather than too little" [10]. Yet these global trends differ greatly across regions, communities, and populations, with marked variation and divergence highlighting the growing realities of health inequities despite social and scientific advancements.

This chapter addresses and summarizes efforts for measuring the global burden of disease. It begins with a background summary that defines the various means of measuring the global burden of disease and comparing the burdens of different disease and disability states across geography and time. Noting the inherent difficulties and limitations in such research, the chapter then summarizes the most recent data and findings before concluding with a focus on what current trends may predict for the future.

Background

Building on earlier research focused on global mortality patterns, the World Bank and World Health Organization commissioned the initial Global Burden of Disease (GBD) study in 1992 as a comprehensive study of the burden of disease worldwide [11–19]. Under the leadership of physician and health economist Christopher Murray and medical demographer Alan Lopez, the team utilized the best available data to assess the burden of 107 of the most prevalent diseases and injuries along with a study of 10 selected risk factors. The team sought to measure the causes of premature mortality as well as quantify years of healthy life lost as a result of disability. They developed the disability adjusted life year or DALY as a summary measure that combined years of life lost due to premature death and years of healthy life lost weighted by severity of disability [16,20,21]. Thereby, the team sought to quantify the global burden of diseases and injuries—including conditions such as neuropsychiatric and musculoskeletal conditions that lead to ill health but not directly to death. Moreover, as improvements in health care have led to the transition of many formerly fatal conditions to chronic diseases today, the DALY highlighted quantitatively the long-term social and economic burden of disease and injury.

Since that time, there have been numerous assessments of selected diseases, injuries, and risk factors, and the GBD study has undergone various revisions, as the comprehensive review of the state of health in the world [22,23]. In 2012, the Global Burden of Diseases, Injuries, and Risk Factors Study 2010 (GBD 2010) was published. As a major revision to previous efforts, this study, led by the Institute of Health Metrics and Evaluation, involved 488 researchers from 303 institutions and 50 countries. Compared to previous reports, the GBD 2010 employed new and strengthened statistical methods to produce estimates of premature death and disability for 187 countries [2,24]. The most recent update, GBD 2013—now involving over 1,000 researchers from over 100 countries—was published in early 2015. Building on the methods of GBD 2010, the 2013 report utilizes updated statistics, including new subnational and regional data, to focus on 306 causes of death or disability [25]. As such a comprehensive international review and collaborative effort, the GBD study represents a powerful tool to inform global health care delivery.

The GBD study seeks to utilize extensive records as primary sources: surveys, censuses, vital registrations, disease registries, hospital records, surveillance systems, mortuary records, police records, and literature reviews [8,26]. Still, there remain limitations in data from many countries. Due to poor systems of vital registration, studies suggest that nearly 50 million newborn children annually are not registered in health surveillance systems, resulting in one-third of babies globally without a birth certificate before their first birthday. It is estimated that almost 5.5 million stillbirths or neonatal deaths go unrecorded annually, and it is still likely that most people in Africa and Asia are born and die without any legal record [27–31]. The current GBD estimates rely on sophisticated statistical modeling to address areas of limited and inconsistent data, with all outcomes reporting a 95% uncertainty interval, ultimately communicating the strength of the evidence available [8,32–35]. Differences in data sources and statistical modeling have been cited as leading to estimate discrepancies between the GBD and similar World Health Organization (WHO) and United Nations Programme on HIV/AIDS reports, specifically with respect to HIV/AIDS, tuberculosis, and malaria. These discrepancies have led to calls for improved data collection, collaboration, and transparency from those such as WHO Director-General Margaret Chan, especially as estimates have an impact on the distribution of funding and political commitments to global health agendas [27,36,37].

Metrics for Measuring the Global Burden of Disease

Various metrics can be utilized to highlight and compare different aspects of population health. These include life expectancy as well as the leading causes of death and years of life lost caused by specific conditions. Years lived with disability is another measurement that seeks to estimate the short- and long-term loss of health due to a condition, highlighting the social and economic effects of ill health [38]. For the GBD 2010, disability weights for 220 unique health states were derived from pair-comparison surveys of the general population in five countries, along with an open Internet survey. Building on past work on disability weights and acknowledging the limitations of these survey methods, researchers found a surprisingly high degree of consistency across cultural settings. For conditions ranging from mild anemia and secondary infertility to acute schizophrenia and severe multiple sclerosis, the GBD team collected data to derive a scale from ideal health (0.0) to a state of health equivalent to death (1.0) for each condition [39]. Years lived with disability was then calculated as the prevalence of the condition in a population multiplied by the disability weight. As mentioned previously, the DALY is a summary metric of years of life lost, or YLL, due to premature death plus years lived with disability, or YLD, based on disability weight (DALY = YLL + YLD). Another measure of population health is health-adjusted life expectancy (HALE), often referred to as healthy life expectancy. HALE is the number of years a person at a given age can expect to live in good health accounting for age-specific causes of death, illness, and disability [40]. In addition to these measurements, others, such as incidence and prevalence of certain diseases and conditions, along with health indicators in specific populations such as maternal mortality or under-5 mortality rates, serve as important tools and measurements of population health and the burden of disease.

The State of Global Health

The global burden of disease does appear different depending on the measurement tool used to quantify health outcomes. These differences will be highlighted in this section, as we move from more aggregate traditional outcomes (life expectancy and mortality) to more nuanced measurements (such as YLD, HALE, and DALY) that seek to quantify the social and economic impact of ill health and disability. Despite these differences, some trends are constant, such as epidemiologic shifts toward non-communicable diseases, increasing inequities in health outcomes between regions of the world, and a growing burden of chronic disability. Each of these trends will require the global health community to adapt delivery systems to meet the needs of a larger, sicker, and more unequal world.

People are living longer than ever before. The global life expectancy for both sexes has increased from 65.3 years in 1990 to 71.5 in 2013 [25]. Meanwhile, the mean age of death has increased from 46.7 years to 59.3 over this same time period [25,41]. These increases were mainly caused by decreases in mortality from lower respiratory tract infections and diarrheal diseases (contributing 2.2 years of the increased life expectancy); cardiovascular and circulatory diseases (contributing 1.1 years); neonatal conditions (contributing 0.7 years); cancers (contributing 0.4 years); chronic respiratory diseases (contributing 0.5 years); and unintentional injuries (contributing 0.3 year) [25]. For women, reductions in maternal mortality accounted for approximately 0.2 years of increased life expectancy [25]. While these striking advancements in health outcomes are encouraging, they fail to highlight the increasing reality of global health inequity. Figure 1.1 demonstrates changes in the average age of death by region from 1970 to 2010, and while there have been increases in all regions, marked disparity is evident across multiple regions, with those of sub-Saharan Africa demonstrating the lowest mean age at death. Furthermore, in high-income regions, YLL due to premature death account for approximately half of the total disease burden, while in sub-Saharan Africa they staggeringly account for over 80% [2,10,42]. In other words, health is improving in aggregate numbers but not for all, with communities traditionally burdened by poor health outcomes disproportionately marginalized from global health advances in the last four decades.

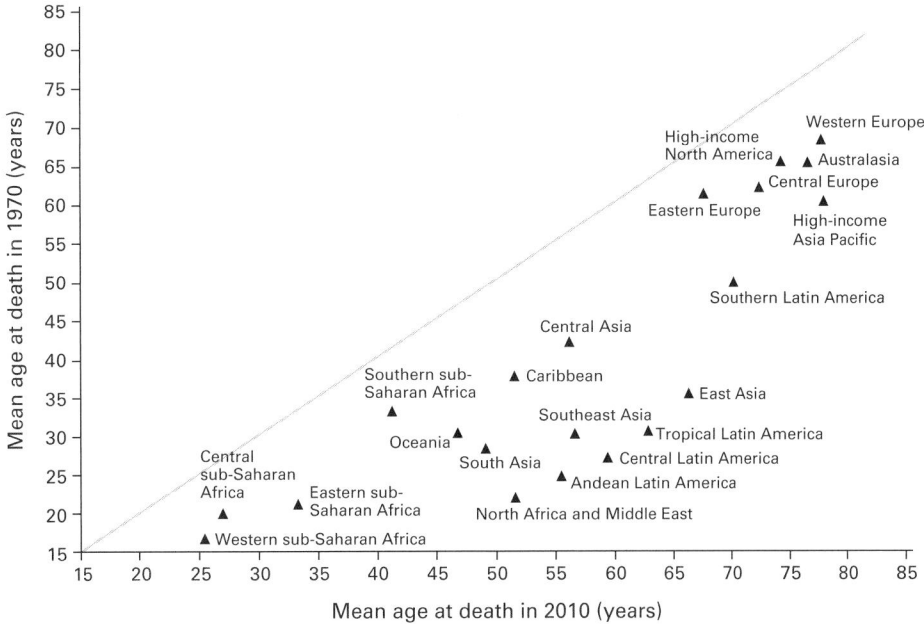

Figure 1.1
Average age of death, 1970, compared with 2010. Reprinted with permission from Institute for Health Metrics and Evaluation, The Global Burden of Disease: Generating Evidence, Guiding Policy. Seattle, WA: IHME; 2013.

Moreover, an increasing proportion of worldwide deaths are occurring at age 70 or older. Death rates have declined in all groups from 1970 to 2010, with the most dramatic decrease in children younger than 5 years, in whom mortality rates declined by nearly 60% (figure 1.2). Yet data suggest that over 6 million children still die annually before 5 years old, with communicable, neonatal, and nutritional conditions accounting for three-quarters of those deaths [25].

While ischemic heart disease remains the leading cause of death, infectious, maternal, neonatal, and nutritional causes combined to lead to 24.9% of deaths worldwide, compared to 34.1% in 1990. Deaths from non-communicable diseases now account for two of every three deaths. Ischemic heart disease alone accounts for one in four deaths worldwide, compared to one in five in 1990. There have also been marked increases in the overall number of deaths attributed to HIV/AIDS, road traffic accidents, diabetes, and various malignancies, including lung, liver, and stomach (figure 1.3) [32]. Despite the increase in the total number of deaths due to cardiovascular disease, the age-standardized death rate—adjusted to reflect the world's demography and changing age structure—for cardiovascular and circulatory diseases decreased from 1990 to 2013 by approximately 22% [25]. Age-standardized death rates, however, did increase over this period for

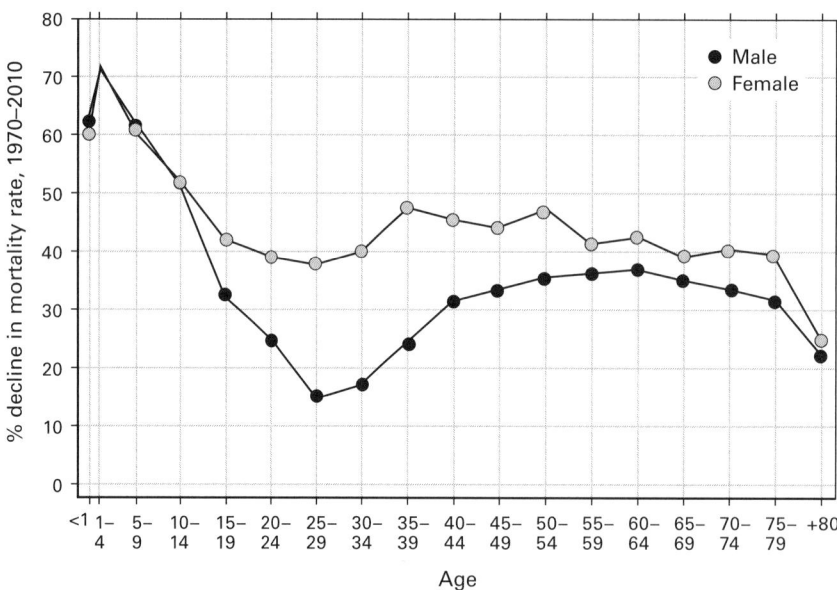

Figure 1.2
Global decline in age-specific mortality rate, 1970–2010. Reprinted with permission from Institute for Health Metrics and Evaluation, The Global Burden of Disease: Generating Evidence, Guiding Policy. Seattle, WA: IHME; 2013.

1990			2010		
Mean rank (95% UI)	**Disorder**		**Disorder**	**Mean rank (95% UI)**	**% change (95% UI)**
1·0 (1 to 2)	1 Ischaemic heart disease		1 Ischaemic heart disease	1·0 (1 to 1)	35 (29 to 39)
2·0 (1 to 2)	2 Stroke		2 Stroke	2·0 (2 to 2)	26 (14 to 32)
3·0 (3 to 4)	3 Lower respiratory infections		3 COPD	3·4 (3 to 4)	−7 (−12 to 0)
4·0 (3 to 4)	4 COPD		4 Lower respiratory infections	3·6 (3 to 4)	−18 (−24 to −11)
5·0 (5 to 5)	5 Diarrhoea		5 Lung cancer	5·8 (5 to 10)	48 (24 to 61)
6·1 (6 to 7)	6 Tuberculosis		6 HIV/AIDS	6·4 (5 to 8)	396 (323 to 465)
7·3 (7 to 9)	7 Preterm birth complications		7 Diarrhoea	6·7 (5 to 9)	−42 (−49 to −35)
8·6 (7 to 12)	8 Lung cancer		8 Road injury	8·4 (5 to 11)	47 (18 to 86)
9·4 (7 to 13)	9 Malaria		9 Diabetes	9·0 (7 to 11)	93 (68 to 102)
10·4 (8 to 14)	10 Road injury		10 Tuberculosis	10·1 (8 to 13)	−18 (−35 to −3)
10·8 (8 to 14)	11 Protein–energy malnutrition		11 Malaria	10·3 (6 to 13)	21 (−9 to 56)
12·8 (11 to 16)	12 Cirrhosis		12 Cirrhosis	11·8 (10 to 14)	33 (25 to 41)
13·2 (9 to 18)	13 Stomach cancer		13 Self-harm	14·1 (11 to 20)	32 (8 to 49)
15·6 (12 to 20)	14 Self-harm		14 Hypertensive heart disease	14·2 (12 to 18)	48 (39 to 56)
15·8 (13 to 19)	15 Diabetes		15 Preterm birth complications	14·4 (12 to 18)	−28 (−39 to −17)
16·1 (12 to 20)	16 Congenital anomalies		16 Liver cancer	16·9 (14 to 20)	63 (49 to 78)
16·9 (13 to 20)	17 Neonatal encephalopathy*		17 Stomach cancer	17·0 (13 to 22)	−2 (−10 to 5)
18·3 (14 to 22)	18 Hypertensive heart disease		18 Chronic kidney disease	17·4 (15 to 21)	82 (65 to 95)
21·1 (6 to 44)	19 Measles		19 Colorectal cancer	18·5 (15 to 21)	46 (36 to 63)
21·1 (12 to 36)	20 Neonatal sepsis		20 Other cardiovascular and circulatory	19·7 (18 to 21)	46 (40 to 55)
21·3 (19 to 26)	21 Colorectal cancer		21 Protein–energy malnutrition	21·5 (19 to 25)	−32 (−42 to −21)
21·6 (18 to 26)	22 Meningitis		22 Falls	23·3 (21 to 29)	56 (20 to 84)
23·2 (21 to 26)	23 Other cardiovascular and circulatory		23 Congenital anomalies	24·4 (21 to 29)	−22 (−40 to −3)
23·7 (20 to 28)	24 Liver cancer		24 Neonatal encephalopathy*	24·4 (21 to 30)	−20 (−33 to −2)
23·8 (20 to 27)	25 Rheumatic heart disease		25 Neonatal sepsis	25·1 (15 to 35)	−3 (−25 to 27)
	27 Chronic kidney disease		29 Meningitis		
	30 Falls		33 Rheumatic heart disease		
	35 HIV/AIDS		62 Measles		

▨ Communicable, maternal, neonatal, and nutritional disorders
☐ Non-communicable diseases
☐ Injuries

—— Ascending order in rank
- - - - Descending order in rank

Figure 1.3
Top 25 causes of mortality in 1990 and 2010, and the percentage change between 1990 and 2010. UI, uncertainty interval. *Includes birth asphyxia/trauma. Reprinted from The Lancet, Vol 380 (2095), Lozano et al., Global and regional mortality from 235 causes of death for 20 age groups in 1990 and 2010: a systematic analysis for the Global Burden of Disease Study 2010, 2095–128, copyright (2012), with permission from Elsevier.

conditions such as HIV/AIDS, diabetes, chronic kidney disease, liver cancer, pancreatic cancer, atrial fibrillation and flutter, drug use disorders, and sickle-cell anemia [25]. According to the GBD 2013, the five main causes of reduced life expectancy worldwide include HIV/AIDS, mental health disorders, intentional injuries, cirrhosis, and diabetes combined with chronic kidney disease and other endocrine disorders [25]. This data highlights the striking shift in global disease burden toward chronic and morbid conditions, reflecting changing demographic trends in income advancement, diet, nutritional insecurities, and lifestyle behaviors (such as smoking and alcohol consumption).

By 2010, ischemic heart disease surpassed lower respiratory infections, diarrheal disease, and preterm birth complications as the worldwide leading cause of YLL (figure 1.4). Moreover, since 1990, there was over a threefold increase in years of life lost to HIV/AIDS, reflecting the global epidemic that reached its climax in the early 2000s but continues to burden much of sub-Saharan Africa and marginalized communities in the developed world [32]. The other conditions with the largest percentage increases from 1990 to 2013 include atrial fibrillation and flutter, peripheral vascular disease, and drug use disorders [25].

Regional variations in disease burden are quite striking. Infectious, maternal, neonatal, and nutritional causes still accounted for 76% of premature mortality in sub-Saharan Africa in 2010 [32]. However, there have been marked reductions in mortality in eastern and southern sub-Saharan Africa since 2004, largely attributable to the simultaneous expansion of antiretroviral treatment for HIV/AIDS and malaria programs' emphasis on insecticide-treated bed nets and artemesinin-combination therapies [43]. Despite these advancements in health care, the regional variations in outcome highlight critical inequities in care delivery and access.

Yet, in the words of the GBD 2010 study, "simply living longer does not mean that people are healthier," and life expectancy and measures of mortality do not account for health and quality of life [2]. Over the past 20 years, there has been an epidemiologic shift in middle- and high-income countries from premature death (mortality) to living longer with ill health (morbidity). Disability as a result of ill health limits economic and social advancements, placing significant stresses on social structures and health care systems managing chronic conditions. While the leading causes of worldwide YLD have been largely constant from 1990 to 2010—with low back pain and major depressive disorder leading the rankings—there were marked increases in overall prevalence for each of the 25 most common conditions, except for iron-deficiency anemia and diarrheal disease (figure 1.5) [33]. Disability aggregates also highlight how more than a quarter of all years lived with disability are due to psychiatric and neurologic conditions, such as major depression and epilepsy [33].

As mentioned previously, healthy life expectancy, or HALE, is another summary measure of population health, since it represents "the number of years that a person at a given age can expect to live in good health" [40]. In 2010, the global male and female

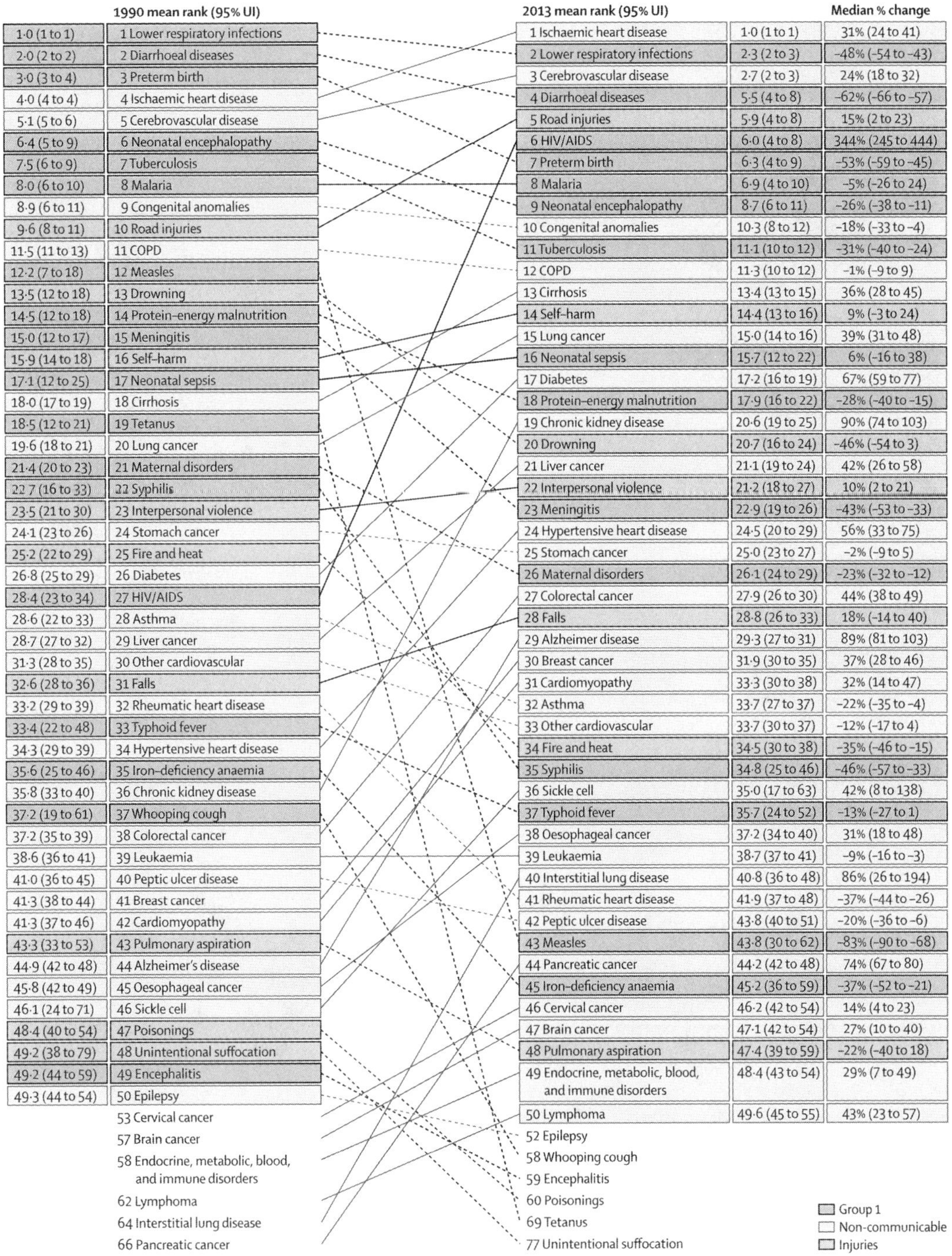

1990 mean rank (95% UI)

Rank (95% UI)	Cause
1·0 (1 to 1)	1 Lower respiratory infections
2·0 (2 to 2)	2 Diarrhoeal diseases
3·0 (3 to 4)	3 Preterm birth
4·0 (4 to 4)	4 Ischaemic heart disease
5·1 (5 to 6)	5 Cerebrovascular disease
6·4 (5 to 9)	6 Neonatal encephalopathy
7·5 (6 to 9)	7 Tuberculosis
8·0 (6 to 10)	8 Malaria
8·9 (6 to 11)	9 Congenital anomalies
9·6 (8 to 11)	10 Road injuries
11·5 (11 to 13)	11 COPD
12·2 (7 to 18)	12 Measles
13·5 (12 to 18)	13 Drowning
14·5 (12 to 18)	14 Protein-energy malnutrition
15·0 (12 to 17)	15 Meningitis
15·9 (14 to 18)	16 Self-harm
17·1 (12 to 25)	17 Neonatal sepsis
18·0 (17 to 19)	18 Cirrhosis
18·5 (12 to 21)	19 Tetanus
19·6 (18 to 21)	20 Lung cancer
21·4 (20 to 23)	21 Maternal disorders
22·7 (16 to 33)	22 Syphilis
23·5 (21 to 30)	23 Interpersonal violence
24·1 (23 to 26)	24 Stomach cancer
25·2 (22 to 29)	25 Fire and heat
26·8 (25 to 29)	26 Diabetes
28·4 (23 to 34)	27 HIV/AIDS
28·6 (22 to 33)	28 Asthma
28·7 (27 to 32)	29 Liver cancer
31·3 (28 to 35)	30 Other cardiovascular
32·6 (28 to 36)	31 Falls
33·2 (29 to 39)	32 Rheumatic heart disease
33·4 (22 to 48)	33 Typhoid fever
34·3 (29 to 39)	34 Hypertensive heart disease
35·6 (25 to 46)	35 Iron-deficiency anaemia
35·8 (33 to 40)	36 Chronic kidney disease
37·2 (19 to 61)	37 Whooping cough
37·2 (35 to 39)	38 Colorectal cancer
38·6 (36 to 41)	39 Leukaemia
41·0 (36 to 45)	40 Peptic ulcer disease
41·3 (38 to 44)	41 Breast cancer
41·3 (37 to 46)	42 Cardiomyopathy
43·3 (33 to 53)	43 Pulmonary aspiration
44·9 (42 to 48)	44 Alzheimer's disease
45·8 (42 to 49)	45 Oesophageal cancer
46·1 (24 to 71)	46 Sickle cell
48·4 (40 to 54)	47 Poisonings
49·2 (38 to 79)	48 Unintentional suffocation
49·2 (44 to 59)	49 Encephalitis
49·3 (44 to 54)	50 Epilepsy

53 Cervical cancer
57 Brain cancer
58 Endocrine, metabolic, blood, and immune disorders
62 Lymphoma
64 Interstitial lung disease
66 Pancreatic cancer

2013 mean rank (95% UI) — **Median % change**

Cause	Rank (95% UI)	Median % change
1 Ischaemic heart disease	1·0 (1 to 1)	31% (24 to 41)
2 Lower respiratory infections	2·3 (2 to 3)	-48% (-54 to -43)
3 Cerebrovascular disease	2·7 (2 to 3)	24% (18 to 32)
4 Diarrhoeal diseases	5·5 (4 to 8)	-62% (-66 to -57)
5 Road injuries	5·9 (4 to 8)	15% (2 to 23)
6 HIV/AIDS	6·0 (4 to 8)	344% (245 to 444)
7 Preterm birth	6·3 (4 to 9)	-53% (-59 to -45)
8 Malaria	6·9 (4 to 10)	-5% (-26 to 24)
9 Neonatal encephalopathy	8·7 (6 to 11)	-26% (-38 to -11)
10 Congenital anomalies	10·3 (8 to 12)	-18% (-33 to -4)
11 Tuberculosis	11·1 (10 to 12)	-31% (-40 to -24)
12 COPD	11·3 (10 to 12)	-1% (-9 to 9)
13 Cirrhosis	13·4 (13 to 15)	36% (28 to 45)
14 Self-harm	14·4 (13 to 16)	9% (-3 to 24)
15 Lung cancer	15·0 (14 to 16)	39% (31 to 48)
16 Neonatal sepsis	15·7 (12 to 22)	6% (-16 to 38)
17 Diabetes	17·2 (16 to 19)	67% (59 to 77)
18 Protein-energy malnutrition	17·9 (16 to 22)	-28% (-40 to -15)
19 Chronic kidney disease	20·6 (19 to 25)	90% (74 to 103)
20 Drowning	20·7 (16 to 24)	-46% (-54 to 3)
21 Liver cancer	21·1 (19 to 24)	42% (26 to 58)
22 Interpersonal violence	21·2 (18 to 27)	10% (2 to 21)
23 Meningitis	22·9 (19 to 26)	-43% (-53 to -33)
24 Hypertensive heart disease	24·5 (20 to 29)	56% (33 to 75)
25 Stomach cancer	25·0 (23 to 27)	-2% (-9 to 5)
26 Maternal disorders	26·1 (24 to 29)	-23% (-32 to -12)
27 Colorectal cancer	27·9 (26 to 30)	44% (38 to 49)
28 Falls	28·8 (26 to 33)	18% (-14 to 40)
29 Alzheimer disease	29·3 (27 to 31)	89% (81 to 103)
30 Breast cancer	31·9 (30 to 35)	37% (28 to 46)
31 Cardiomyopathy	33·3 (30 to 38)	32% (14 to 47)
32 Asthma	33·7 (27 to 37)	-22% (-35 to -4)
33 Other cardiovascular	33·7 (30 to 37)	-12% (-17 to 4)
34 Fire and heat	34·5 (30 to 38)	-35% (-46 to -15)
35 Syphilis	34·8 (25 to 46)	-46% (-57 to -33)
36 Sickle cell	35·0 (17 to 63)	42% (8 to 138)
37 Typhoid fever	35·7 (24 to 52)	-13% (-27 to 1)
38 Oesophageal cancer	37·2 (34 to 40)	31% (18 to 48)
39 Leukaemia	38·7 (37 to 41)	-9% (-16 to -3)
40 Interstitial lung disease	40·8 (36 to 48)	86% (26 to 194)
41 Rheumatic heart disease	41·9 (37 to 48)	-37% (-44 to -26)
42 Peptic ulcer disease	43·8 (40 to 51)	-20% (-36 to -6)
43 Measles	43·8 (30 to 62)	-83% (-90 to -68)
44 Pancreatic cancer	44·2 (42 to 48)	74% (67 to 80)
45 Iron-deficiency anaemia	45·2 (36 to 59)	-37% (-52 to -21)
46 Cervical cancer	46·2 (42 to 54)	14% (4 to 23)
47 Brain cancer	47·1 (42 to 54)	27% (10 to 40)
48 Pulmonary aspiration	47·4 (39 to 59)	-22% (-40 to 18)
49 Endocrine, metabolic, blood, and immune disorders	48·4 (43 to 54)	29% (7 to 49)
50 Lymphoma	49·6 (45 to 55)	43% (23 to 57)

52 Epilepsy
58 Whooping cough
59 Encephalitis
60 Poisonings
69 Tetanus
77 Unintentional suffocation

Legend:
☐ Group 1
☐ Non-communicable
☐ Injuries

Figure 1.4

Top 50 causes of global years of life lost in 1990 and 2010, and the percentage change between 1990 and 2013. UI, uncertainty interval. *Includes birth asphyxia/trauma. Reprinted from The Lancet, Vol 385 (9963), GBD 2013 Mortality and Causes of Death Collaborators, Global, regional, and national age-specific mortality for 240 causes of death, 1990–2013: A systematic analysis for the Global Burden of Disease Study 2013, 117–71, copyright (2015), with permission from Elsevier.

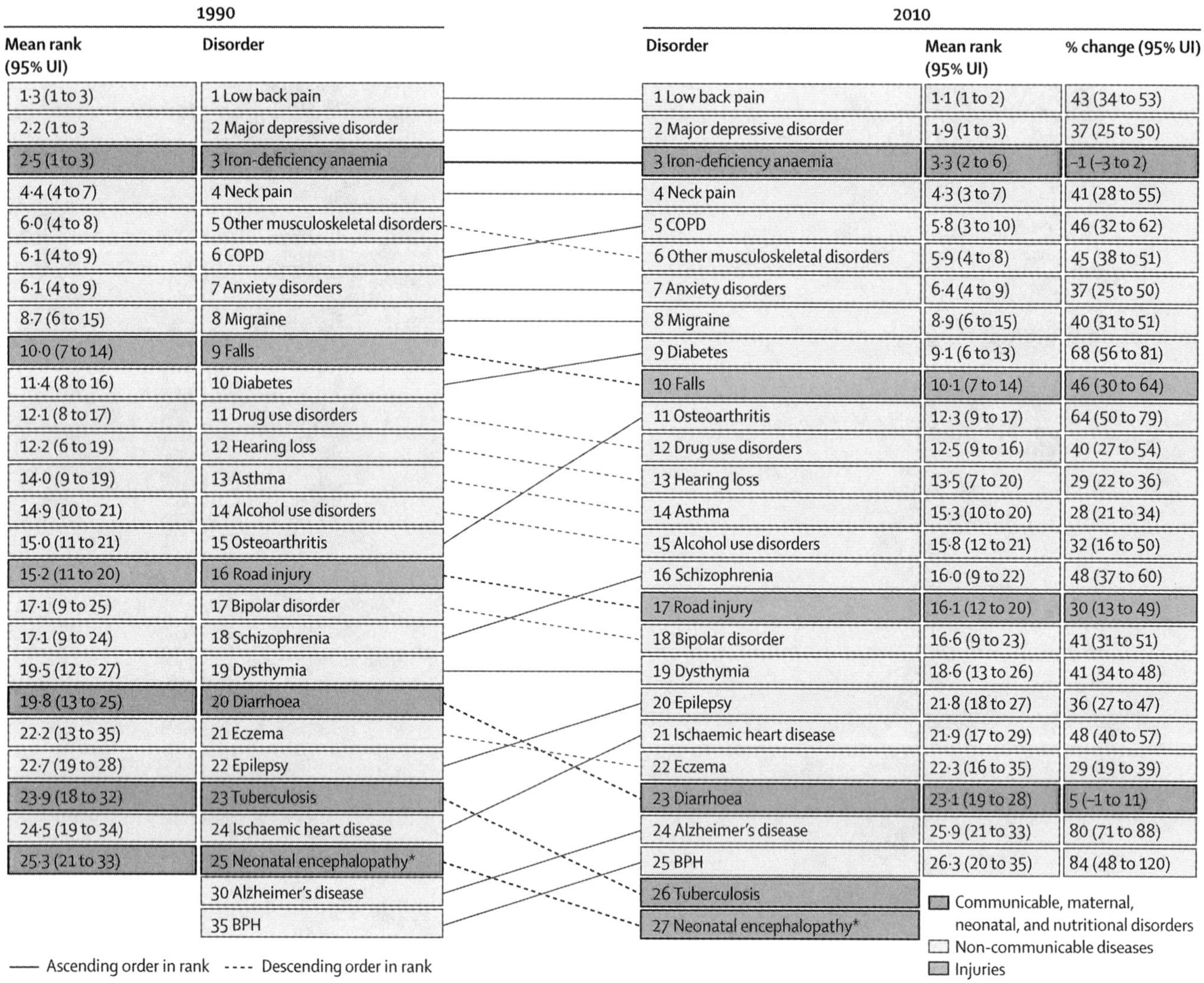

1990

Mean rank (95% UI)	Disorder
1·3 (1 to 3)	1 Low back pain
2·2 (1 to 3)	2 Major depressive disorder
2·5 (1 to 3)	3 Iron-deficiency anaemia
4·4 (4 to 7)	4 Neck pain
6·0 (4 to 8)	5 Other musculoskeletal disorders
6·1 (4 to 9)	6 COPD
6·1 (4 to 9)	7 Anxiety disorders
8·7 (6 to 15)	8 Migraine
10·0 (7 to 14)	9 Falls
11·4 (8 to 16)	10 Diabetes
12·1 (8 to 17)	11 Drug use disorders
12·2 (6 to 19)	12 Hearing loss
14·0 (9 to 19)	13 Asthma
14·9 (10 to 21)	14 Alcohol use disorders
15·0 (11 to 21)	15 Osteoarthritis
15·2 (11 to 20)	16 Road injury
17·1 (9 to 25)	17 Bipolar disorder
17·1 (9 to 24)	18 Schizophrenia
19·5 (12 to 27)	19 Dysthymia
19·8 (13 to 25)	20 Diarrhoea
22·2 (13 to 35)	21 Eczema
22·7 (19 to 28)	22 Epilepsy
23·9 (18 to 32)	23 Tuberculosis
24·5 (19 to 34)	24 Ischaemic heart disease
25·3 (21 to 33)	25 Neonatal encephalopathy*
	30 Alzheimer's disease
	35 BPH

2010

Disorder	Mean rank (95% UI)	% change (95% UI)
1 Low back pain	1·1 (1 to 2)	43 (34 to 53)
2 Major depressive disorder	1·9 (1 to 3)	37 (25 to 50)
3 Iron-deficiency anaemia	3·3 (2 to 6)	–1 (–3 to 2)
4 Neck pain	4·3 (3 to 7)	41 (28 to 55)
5 COPD	5·8 (3 to 10)	46 (32 to 62)
6 Other musculoskeletal disorders	5·9 (4 to 8)	45 (38 to 51)
7 Anxiety disorders	6·4 (4 to 9)	37 (25 to 50)
8 Migraine	8·9 (6 to 15)	40 (31 to 51)
9 Diabetes	9·1 (6 to 13)	68 (56 to 81)
10 Falls	10·1 (7 to 14)	46 (30 to 64)
11 Osteoarthritis	12·3 (9 to 17)	64 (50 to 79)
12 Drug use disorders	12·5 (9 to 16)	40 (27 to 54)
13 Hearing loss	13·5 (7 to 20)	29 (22 to 36)
14 Asthma	15·3 (10 to 20)	28 (21 to 34)
15 Alcohol use disorders	15·8 (12 to 21)	32 (16 to 50)
16 Schizophrenia	16·0 (9 to 22)	48 (37 to 60)
17 Road injury	16·1 (12 to 20)	30 (13 to 49)
18 Bipolar disorder	16·6 (9 to 23)	41 (31 to 51)
19 Dysthymia	18·6 (13 to 26)	41 (34 to 48)
20 Epilepsy	21·8 (18 to 27)	36 (27 to 47)
21 Ischaemic heart disease	21·9 (17 to 29)	48 (40 to 57)
22 Eczema	22·3 (16 to 35)	29 (19 to 39)
23 Diarrhoea	23·1 (19 to 28)	5 (–1 to 11)
24 Alzheimer's disease	25·9 (21 to 33)	80 (71 to 88)
25 BPH	26·3 (20 to 35)	84 (48 to 120)
26 Tuberculosis		
27 Neonatal encephalopathy*		

—— Ascending order in rank   ---- Descending order in rank

■ Communicable, maternal, neonatal, and nutritional disorders
☐ Non-communicable diseases
▨ Injuries

Figure 1.5

Top 25 most common causes of global years lived with disability (YLD) in 1990 and 2010, and percentage change between 1990 and 2010. UI, uncertainty interval. *Includes birth asphyxia/trauma. Reprinted from The Lancet, Vol 380 (9859), Vos et al., Years lived with disability (YLDs) for 1160 sequelae of 289 diseases and injuries 1990–2010: A systematic analysis for the Global Burden of Disease Study 2010, 2163–96, copyright (2012), with permission from Elsevier.

HALE at birth were 59.0 years and 63.2 years, respectively. Reflecting the increase in prevalence of chronic disability, HALE increased at a slower rate than the overall life expectancy at birth since 1990. Strikingly, each year increase in life expectancy at birth was associated with only a 10-month increase in HALE. In other words, the growing epidemiologic trend is toward people living longer, but with those extra years more burdened by disability. Overall, driven by reductions in mortality from 1990 to 2010, HALE rose in nearly every region in the world, with the exception of southern sub-Saharan Africa (the epicenter of the HIV/AIDS epidemic) and the Caribbean (where the 2010 earthquake in Haiti caused extraordinarily high mortality). Once again, though, there is marked variation between countries, with Haiti having the lowest HALE, at 27.8 and 37.1 years for men and women, respectively, and Japan the highest, at 70.6 years and 75.5 years, respectively [40].

Despite population growth, aggregate global DALY remained relatively stable from 1990 to 2010. But, when adjusting for population (per 1,000 people), an overall 23% decrease in outcomes is reassuringly positive, and parallels the decreases in mortality rates over the same period [42]. These aggregate numbers do not, however, show the shifting trends in global disease burdens or the increasing inequity in outcomes. There are some striking success stories, such as the decline in deaths and disability among children under 5 years from 41% to 25% of global DALY from 1990 to 2010. Additionally, the burden of communicable or infectious maternal, neonatal, and nutritional disorders fell from 47% of global DALY to 35% over the same time period. Yet, though there has been a shift away from death in children under 5 years of age, a quarter of the global disease burden remains attributable to preventable disease and injury in the young population. Additionally, the burden of non-communicable diseases rose from 43% to 54% of global DALY from 1990 to 2010 [42]. Over that same period, ischemic heart disease surpassed lower respiratory infections and diarrheal diseases as the leading cause of global DALY, though there was a marked increase in HIV/AIDS-associated DALY over the same period as the epidemic spread across the globe (figure 1.6) [2,8,42]. Despite these notable changing shifts in aggregate epidemiology in both the developing and developed world, preventable communicable diseases remain the leading causes of DALY in the developing world, with striking heterogeneity in regions such as sub-Saharan Africa, where there is marked variation in the burden of disease between rural and urban settings as well as between neighboring countries.

There are a variety of indirect reasons behind the aforementioned epidemiologic shifts in the global burden of disease: advancements in medicine, successful health interventions, economic development, increasing wealth disparities, environmental changes, and demographic shifts of populations. However, many direct reasons can be attributed to changing environmental exposures and behaviors—or risk factors. When examining the factors underlying the global burden of disease in 2010, high blood pressure, tobacco smoking (including secondhand smoke), and household air pollution are the three leading risk

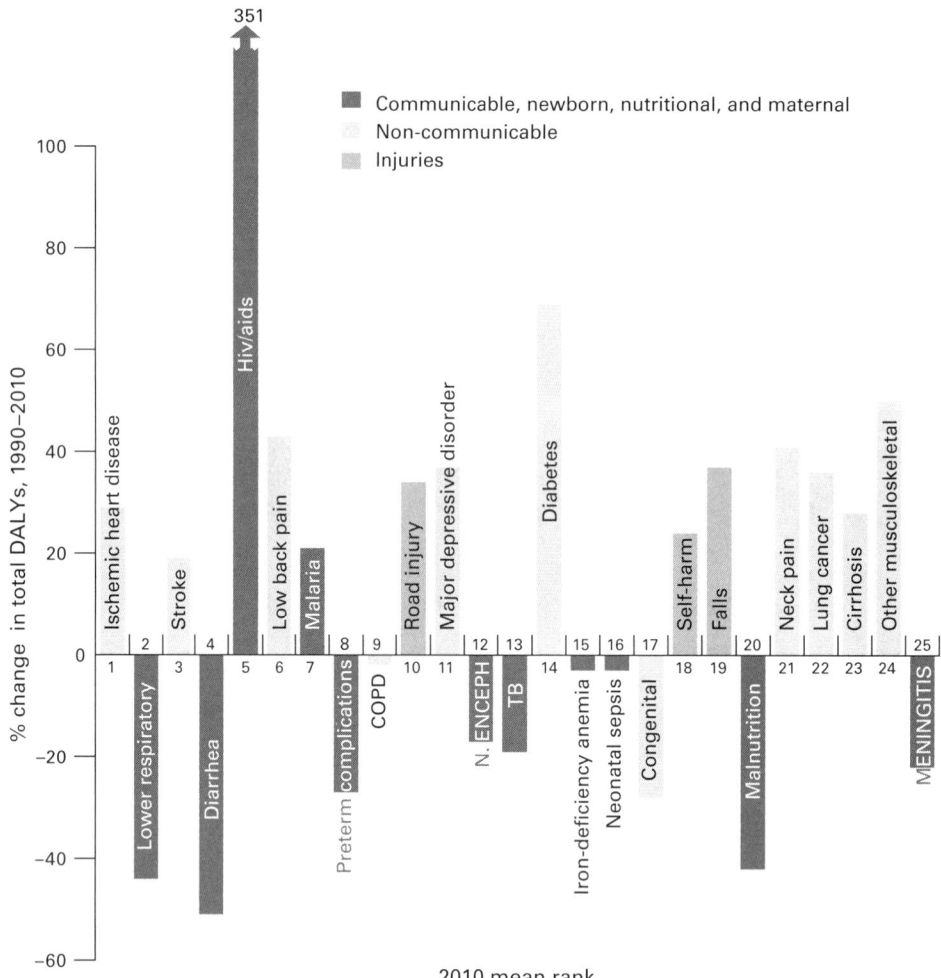

Figure 1.6
Global shifts in leading causes of DALY, 1990–2010. Reprinted with permission from Institute for Health Metrics and Evaluation, The Global Burden of Disease: Generating Evidence, Guiding Policy. Seattle, WA: IHME; 2013.

factors (figure 1.7) [44,45]. In 1990, the leading risk factor was childhood malnourishment (underweight at birth), but in 2010 the proportion of overall disease burden attributed to childhood malnourishment had decreased by more than 50%. Furthermore, malnutrition has been surpassed by multiple other risk factors, including high body mass index. Dietary risks and physical activity altogether accounted for 10% of DALY in 2010 [44]. While there has been a global shift from risk factors that cause communicable illnesses in children to risk factors for non-communicable diseases in adults, there still remains striking regional variation. In most of sub-Saharan Africa, the major risk factors remain those associated with impoverishment: childhood malnourishment, household air pollution, and nonexclusive (or discontinued) breastfeeding. Alternatively, the leading risk factor in 2010 in Eastern Europe, Andean Latin America, and southern sub-Saharan Africa was alcohol use [44,45]. High body mass index has increased, with more than one-third of adults worldwide overweight or obese, and the prevalence continues to increase substantially in children and adolescents in both developed and developing countries [46]. Currently, it is estimated that excess weight accounts for approximately 3.4 million deaths annually and 3.8% of global DALY due to its direct association to conditions with long periods of disability, such as cardiovascular disease and diabetes [44,45].

With the attention brought to HIV, tuberculosis, and malaria through Millennium Development Goal 6, these three diseases have received high priority status in the global community, along with significant resource allocation by programs such as the US President's Emergency Plan for Aids Relief (PEPFAR) and the Global Fund. Substantial progress has been made worldwide, and incidence rates for HIV, tuberculosis, and malaria have all decreased since 2000 [47]. Tuberculosis deaths have been decreasing since 1990, with incidence and prevalence of disease continuing to decrease after 2000, despite increased morbidity from co-infection with HIV. Malaria incidence and mortality began to decline in 2004, with significant progress noted in sub-Saharan Africa since 2008. Incidence peaked in the global epidemic of HIV in 1997, and mortality rates have been declining since 2005. Yet, while the global incidence of HIV is decreasing, it is estimated that more than 100 countries still have increasing HIV incidence rates, while prevalence remains at a staggering 35 million worldwide. Despite progress, these three diseases remain major global health burdens, with mean age of deaths of 15.3 years for malaria, 38.6 years for HIV, and 52.9 for tuberculosis in HIV-negative individuals [47].

Transitions in the Global Burden of Disease

The United Nations General Assembly has held only two meetings to date on health. The first, in 2001, focused on HIV/AIDS. The second, in 2011, focused on non-communicable diseases. The 2011 meeting signified a growing realization of the epidemiologic shifts in the global burden of disease facing all countries and regions around the globe, acknowledging that more than two-thirds of the global DALY now arise from conditions not targeted in the Millennium Development Goals of 2000 [42].

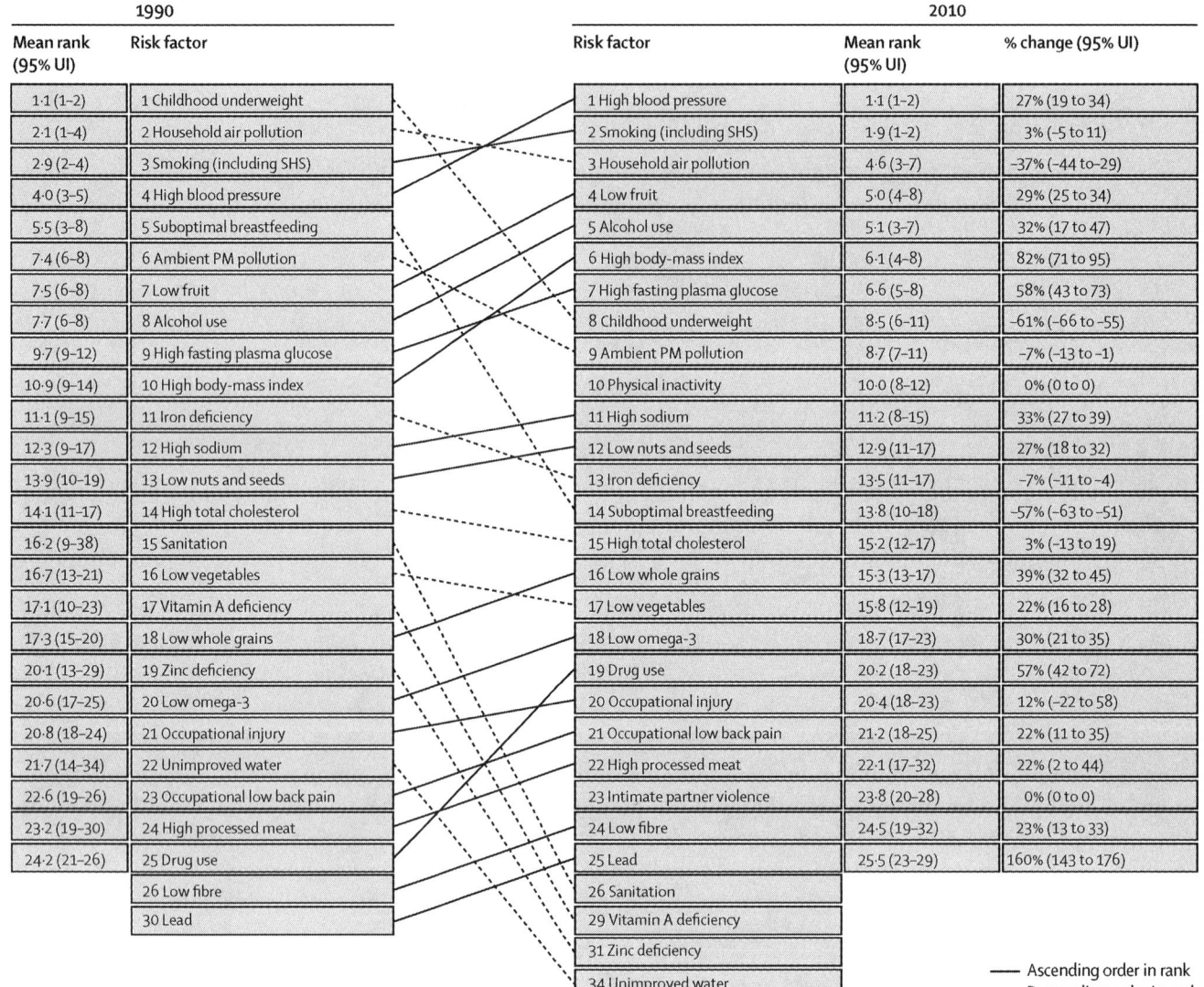

Figure 1.7
Top 25 global risk factors for DALY for all ages and sexes combined in 1990 and 2010, and percentage change between 1990 and 2010. UI, uncertainty interval. *Includes birth asphyxia/trauma. Reprinted from The Lancet, Vol 380(9859), Lim et al., A comparative risk assessment of burden of disease and injury attributable to 67 risk factors and risk factor clusters in 21 regions, 1990–2010: A systematic analysis for the Global Burden of Disease Study 2010, 2224–60, copyright (2012), with permission from Elsevier.

Conclusions and Recommendations

The global burden of disease has significantly shifted in the two decades since the first GBD report. Child mortality has markedly decreased, and people are living longer. There has been a global shift toward non-communicable and chronic diseases, with disability now accounting for a greater overall burden of disease. Moreover, the transition from infectious etiologies to non-communicable diseases highlights changing social behaviors and environmental risk factors such as high blood pressure, obesity, poor nutrition, alcohol consumption, and smoking. Yet there remains marked, staggering inequity and heterogeneity across regions, countries, and communities. The leading causes of DALY in sub-Saharan Africa have changed little over the last three decades, with infectious, maternal, neonatal, and nutritional diseases remaining the primary causes of premature death and disability, even while the prevalence of non-communicable diseases markedly increased. Health disparities are noted worldwide among developed and developing nations, with great disparities among communities even within the same cities or regions. Moreover, while great progress has been made in addressing HIV, tuberculosis, and malaria, these three diseases remain major health burdens worldwide.

Based on demographic and epidemiologic predictions, these trends are likely to persist, with a continued shift toward non-communicable and chronic diseases in aging populations worldwide. Furthermore, without deliberate and intentional efforts, health disparities across regions, counties, and communities will likely continue to grow.

Efforts to examine and describe the global burden of disease have expanded as methods have been refined and the available data has continued to grow. These efforts are vital to governments, policy makers, advocates and health system leaders as they inform discussions, set priorities (including crucial resource allocations), and assess progress. As the Millennium Development Goals came to an end in 2015, continued efforts at strengthening delivery systems and improving data collection are necessary at all levels of the global health community, from the village to international organizations.

These are not new challenges. John Graunt realized the need for robust information systems in 1662 when he presented his summary of observations from the Bills of Mortality in London. He stated that such efforts were "necessary in order to good, certain, and easie Government, and even to balance Parties, and factions" [1]. Those words are no less true today as policy makers, governments, and practitioners try to promote the health of populations they serve around the globe through documenting and responding to these profound health transitions.

Questions for Discussion

- In reviewing the leading causes of disability-adjusted life years worldwide, what surprises or unexpected findings are there?

- What do you believe are the main causes for the epidemiologic transition in the global burden of disease over the last several decades?
- What do you believe will occur over the next 20–30 years?

References

1. Graunt J. Natural and political observations made upon the bills of mortality. 1662.

2. Institute for Health Metrics and Evaluation. *The Global Burden of Disease: Generating Evidence, Guiding Policy.* Seattle, WA: Institute for Health Metrics and Evaluation; 2013.

3. Merrill RM. Introduction to epidemiology. In *Historic Developments in Epidemiology.* Sudbury, MA: Jones and Bartlett Publishers; 2010.

4. World Health Organization. Epidemiology. http://www.who.int/topics/epidemiology/en/.

5. 7 billion of us [editorial]. 2011. Lancet Infect Dis 11(11): 801.

6. Das Gupta M, Engelman R, Levy J, Luchsinger G, Merrick T, Rosen JE. *State of World Population 2014.* United Nations Population Fund; 2014.

7. United Nations General Assembly. 2000. United Nations Millennium Declaration, a/Res/55/2. United Nations General Assembly, fifty-fifth session, agenda item 60(b), September 18.

8. Murray CJ, Lopez AD. 2013. Measuring the global burden of disease. *N Engl J Med* 369(5): 448–457.

9. Hunter DJ, Reddy KS. 2013. Noncommunicable diseases. *N Engl J Med* 369(14): 1336–1343.

10. Murray CJ, Lim S, Lozano R, Naghavi M, Ezzati M, Lopez A. Global burden of disease: Massive shifts reshape the health landscape worldwide [press release]. December 13, 2012. http://www.healthdata.org/news-release/global-burden-disease-massive-shifts-reshape-health-landscape-worldwide.

11. Hakulinen T, Hansluwka H, Lopez AD, Nakada T. 1986. Global and regional mortality patterns by cause of death in 1980. *Int J Epidemiol* 15(2): 226–233.

12. Lopez AD. Causes of death in the industrialized and developing countries: Estimates for 1985–1990. In Jamison D, Mosely WH, Measham AR, and Bobadilla JL, eds. *Disease Control Priorities in Developing Countries.* New York: Oxford University Press; 1993: 15–30.

13. Lopez AD, Murray CJ. 1998. The global burden of disease, 1990–2020. *Nat Med* 4(11): 1241–1243.

14. Murray CJ, Lopez AD. 1996. Evidence-based health policy: Lessons from the global burden of disease study. *Science* 274(5288): 740–743.

15. Murray CJ, Lopez AD, Jamison DT. 1994. The global burden of disease in 1990: Summary results, sensitivity analyses, and future directions. *Bull World Health Organ* 72(3): 495–508.

16. Lopez AD, Mathers CD, Ezzati M, Jamison DT, Murray CJL. Measuring the global burden of disease and risk factors. In Lopez AD, Mathers CD, Ezzati M, Jamison DT, Murray CJL, eds. *Global Burden of Disease and Risk Factors*. Washington, DC: World Bank; 2006: Chapter 1.

17. Murray CJ, Lopez AD. 1997. Mortality by cause for eight regions of the world: Global Burden of Disease study. *Lancet* 349(9061): 1269–1276.

18. Murray CJ, Lopez AD. 1997. Regional patterns of disability-free life expectancy and disability-adjusted life expectancy: Global Burden of Disease study. *Lancet* 349: 1347–1352.

19. Murray CJ, Lopez AD. 1997. Global mortality, disability, and the contribution of risk factors: Global Burden of Disease study. *Lancet* 349: 1498–1504.

20. Murray CJ, Salomon JA, Mathers CD, Lopez AD. *Summary Measures of Population Health: Concepts, Ethics, Measurement, and Applications*. Geneva: World Health Organization; 2002.

21. Murray CJ. Rethinking DALYs. In Murray CJ, Lopez AD, eds. *The Global Burden of Disease*. Cambridge, MA: Harvard University Press; 1996: 1–89.

22. World Health Organization. *The Global Burden of Disease 2004 Update*. Switzerland: World Health Organization; 2008.

23. World Health Organization. *Global Health Risks: Mortality and Burden of Disease Attributable to Selected Major Risks*. France: World Health Organization; 2009.

24. Murray CJL, Ezzati M, Flaxman AD, Lim S, Lozano R, Michaud C, et al. 2012. GBD 2010: Design, definitions, and metrics. *Lancet* 380(9859): 2063–2066.

25. GBD 2013 Mortality and Causes of Death Collaborators. 2015. Global, regional, and national age-sex specific all-cause and cause-specific mortality for 240 causes of death, 1990–2013: A systematic analysis for the Global Burden of Disease study 2013. Lancet 385(9963): 117–171.

26. Speyer P. *Global Burden of Disease: Analyzing and Visualizing Big Data in Global Health*. Washington, DC: Institute for Health Metrics and Evaluation; 2013.

27. Atun R. 2014. Time for a revolution in reporting of global health data. *Lancet* 384(9947): 937–938.

28. Lawn JE, Blencowe H, Oza S, You D, Lee ACC, Waiswa P, et al. 2014. Every newborn: Progress, priorities, and potential beyond survival. *Lancet* 384(9938): 189–205.

29. Setel PW, Macfarlane SB, Szreter S, Mikkelsen L, Jha P, Stout S, AbouZahr C. 2007. A scandal of invisibility: Making everyone count by counting everyone. *Lancet* 370(9598): 1569–1577.

30. UNICEF. *The "Rights" Start to Life. a Statistical Analysis of Birth Registration.* New York: United Nations Children Fund, 2005.

31. Mathers CD, Ma Fat D, Inoue M, Rao C, Lopez AD. 2005. Counting the dead and what they died of: An assessment of the global status of cause of death data. *Bull World Health Organ* 83: 171–177.

32. Lozano R, Naghavi M, Foreman K, Lim S, Shibuya K, Aboyans V, et al. 2012. Global and regional mortality from 235 causes of death for 20 age groups in 1990 and 2010: A systematic analysis for the Global Burden of Disease study 2010. *Lancet* 380(9859): 2095–2128.

33. Vos T, Flaxman AD, Naghavi M, Lozano R, Michaud C, Ezzati M, et al. 2012. Years lived with disability (YLDs) for 1160 sequelae of 289 diseases and injuries 1990–2010: A systematic analysis for the Global Burden of Disease study 2010. *Lancet* 380(9859): 2163–2196.

34. Foreman K, Lozano R, Lopez A, Murray C. 2012. Modeling causes of death: An integrated approach using CODEm. *Popul Health Metr* 10(1): 1.

35. Naghavi M, Makela S, Foreman K, O'Brien J, Pourmalek F, Lozano R. 2010. Algorithms for enhancing public health utility of national causes-of-death data. *Popul Health Metr* 8(1): 9.

36. Chan M. 2012. From new estimates to better data. *Lancet* 380(9859): 2054.

37. Rudan I, Chan KL. 2015. Global health metrics needs collaboration and competition. *Lancet* 385(9963): 92–94.

38. Salomon JA, Mathers CD, Chatterji S, Sadana R, Ustun TB, Murray CJ. Quantifying individual levels of health: Definitions, concepts and measurement issues. In Murray CJ, Evans DB, eds. *Health Systems Performance Assessment: Debates, Methods and Empiricism.* Geneva: World Health Organization; 2003: 301–318.

39. Salomon JA, Vos T, Hogan DR, Gagnon M, Naghavi M, Mokdad A, et al. 2012. Common values in assessing health outcomes from disease and injury: Disability weights measurement study for the Global Burden of Disease study 2010. *Lancet* 380(9859): 2129–2143.

40. Salomon JA, Wang H, Freeman MK, Vos T, Flaxman AD, Lopez AD, Murray CJL. 2012. Healthy life expectancy for 187 countries, 1990–2010: A systematic analysis for the Global Burden of Disease study 2010. *Lancet* 380(9859): 2144–2162.

41. United Nations, Department of Economic and Social Affairs, Population Division. *World Population Ageing 2013.* New York: United Nations; 2013.

42. Murray CJ, Vos T, Lozano R, Naghavi M, Flaxman AD, Michaud C, et al. 2012. Disability-adjusted life years (DALYs) for 291 diseases and injuries in 21 regions, 1990–2010: A systematic analysis for the Global Burden of Disease study 2010. *Lancet* 380(9859): 2197–2223.

43. Wang H, Dwyer-Lindgren L, Lofgren KT, Rajaratnam JK, Marcus JR, Levin-Rector A, Levitz CE, Lopez AD, Murray CJL. 2012. Age-specific and sex-specific mortality in 187 countries, 1970–2010: A systematic analysis for the Global Burden of Disease study 2010. *Lancet* 380(9859): 2071–2094.

44. Lim SS, Vos T, Flaxman AD, Danaei G, Shibuya K, Adair-Rohani H, et al. 2012. A comparative risk assessment of burden of disease and injury attributable to 67 risk factors and risk factor clusters in 21 regions, 1990–2010: A systematic analysis for the Global Burden of Disease study 2010. *Lancet* 380(9859): 2224–2260.

45. Ezzati M, Riboli E. 2013. Behavioral and dietary risk factors for noncommunicable diseases. *N Engl J Med* 369(10): 954–964.

46. Ng M, Fleming T, Robinson M, Thomson B, Graetz N, Margono C, et al. 2014. Global, regional, and national prevalence of overweight and obesity in children and adults during 1980–2013: A systematic analysis for the Global Burden of Disease study 2013. *Lancet* 384(9945): 766–781.

47. Murray CJ, Ortblad KF, Guinovart C, Lim SS, Wolock TM, Roberts DA, et al. 2014. Global, regional, and national incidence and mortality for HIV, tuberculosis, and malaria during 1990–2013: A systematic analysis for the Global Burden of Disease study 2013. *Lancet* 384(9947): 1005–1070.

2 Case Study: Challenges in Providing Universal Health Coverage in Kenya

Jonathan M. Mwangi, Linus Ndegwa, Connie Cheren, and Tony Somers

Take-Home Messages

- Health care requires a multisectoral approach, which includes properly trained and well-compensated personnel, political goodwill, infrastructure, sound policies, and appreciation for different cultural perspectives.
- Policy implementation has been one of the key failures in the health delivery system in developing countries.
- Poor distribution of facilities, poor public transport, weak referral systems, insufficient community health services, and weak collaborations with other service providers have perpetuated poor geographical access to health services.

Introduction

In an ideal world, every human being should enjoy the right to quality and affordable health care, otherwise known as universal health coverage. However, in many countries in the developing world, this remains only an aspiration due to various challenges, including inadequate infrastructure, few trained personnel, inadequate funding, and other factors. This chapter focuses on infrastructural challenges in the delivery of health care, including implementation of health management information systems. While this chapter highlights the situation in Kenya, these challenges are likely to be similar in all low- and middle-income countries. At the end of the chapter, we propose low-cost solutions that have the potential to change the prevalence of some common ailments in Kenya and other developing countries.

In the developing countries, there seems to be a lack of recognition that health is a critical factor to economic development. Therefore, when it comes to budgetary allocations, health does not get the same share as education, transportation, and communication infrastructure. There is also a lack of recognition that health care requires a multisectoral approach, which includes properly trained and well-compensated personnel, political goodwill, infrastructure, sound policies, and appreciation for different cultural perspectives. The government, academia, and industry also need to develop innovative but practical solutions that are geared more toward preventive health.

Background

Since independence in 1963, governance in Kenya has been heavily centralized, with power concentrated in the capital, from which all resources are allocated. As a result, the country has seen marked geographical disparities in resource allocation, including in health care [1].

The country's population is about 43 million, with a total health expenditure of US$1.9 billion (2012), made up of government spending through the Ministry of Health, patients' fees, and grants from multilateral partners and private organizations [2]. This total expenditure works out to about US$27 per capita. According to the World Health Organization (WHO), the government of Kenya covers about 38.7% of overall expenditures on health, while private expenditures account for 61.3% of overall spending. Of note, the government's health budget is only 4.6% of Kenya's GDP, which is far below the 15% that was agreed in the Abuja declaration by African governments [3]. While these figures will certainly change with the recent devolution of health care to counties, it is still very early to determine how the decentralization will impact on the delivery of health care services [1].

Kenya, like other developing countries, is seeing the emergence of a "double burden of disease" because of changing lifestyles and the aging of the population. While communicable diseases remain common, there is also a growing incidence of noncommunicable diseases—such as heart disease, diabetes, cancer, and mental illness—and medical conditions resulting from trauma and accidents. This has put a strain on an already overstretched health care service.

The health sector in Kenya comprises the public system, with major players including the Ministry of Health and parastatal organizations, and the private sector, which includes private for-profit facilities, nongovernmental organizations, and faith-based organizations. Health services are provided through a network of over 9,920 health facilities countrywide, with the public sector system accounting for about 51% of these facilities.

Kenya developed its Health Policy 2012–2030 [4], which gives directions to ensure significant improvement in overall health status in Kenya in line with the country's longterm development agenda, Vision 2030, the Constitution of Kenya 2010, and global commitments. To operationalize the policy, the country developed the Kenya Health Sector Strategic and Investment Plan (KHSSP July 2012–June 2017) after a review of the previous National Health Sector Strategic Plan II (NHSSP II) for 2005–2010 [5]. The plan's mission is "To deliberately build progressive, responsive and sustainable technologically-driven, evidence-based and client-centered health system for accelerated attainment of the highest standard of health to all Kenyans" [6]. The KHSSP has incorporated a revised Kenya Essential Package for Health (KEPH) that defines health services and interventions to be provided for each policy objective by level of care and cohort (where applicable) [6].

The tiers in the KEPH are the levels of care as defined in the Kenya Health Policy (figure 2.1).

1. *Community level.* The foundation of the service delivery system, with both demand creation (health promotion services), and specified supply services that are most effectively delivered at the community level. In the essential package, all nonfacility-based health and related services are classified as community services—not only the interventions provided through the Community Health Strategy as defined in NHSSP II [5].

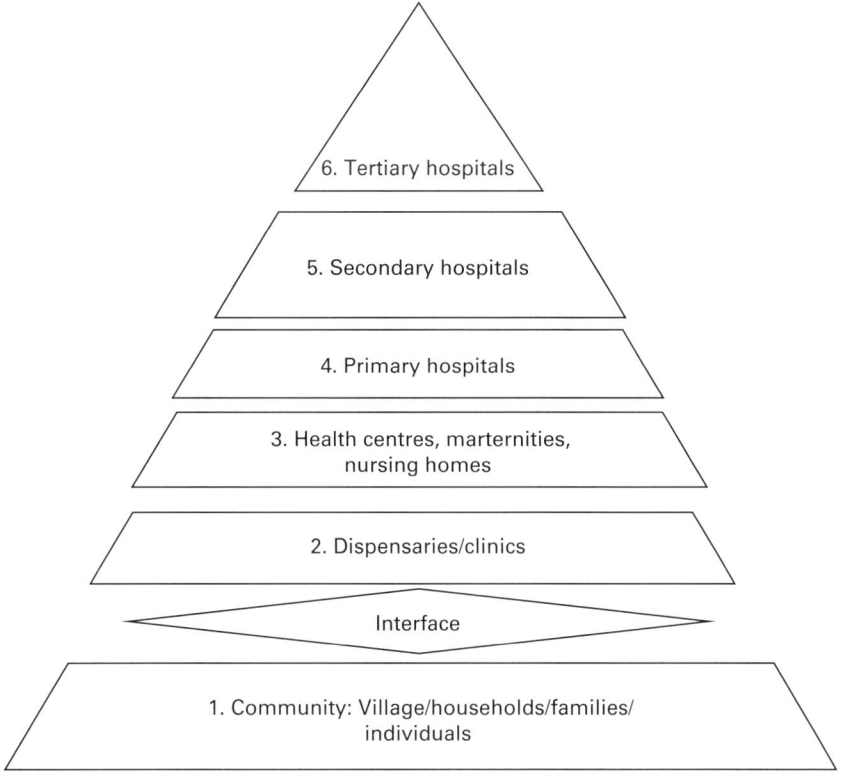

Figure 2.1
Organization of health care service delivery system in Kenya.

2. *Primary care level.* The first physical level of the health system, comprising all dispensaries, health centers, and maternity and nursing homes in the country. This is the first care level, where most clients' health needs should be addressed.

3. *County level.* First-level hospitals, whose services complement the primary care level to allow for a more comprehensive package of close-to-client services.

4. *National level.* Tertiary-level hospitals, whose services are highly specialized and complete the set of care available to persons in Kenya.

The plan KEPH envisions defines health services and interventions to be provided for each of the various policy objectives by level of care (community, primary care, county, and national) and cohort (pregnancy/newborn, childhood, children/youth, adults, elderly) where applicable. Specific interventions to attain have been defined in each policy objective, and services around which the interventions are clustered guide the implementation level and communities regarding what needs to be provided. The existing vertical programs would come together to provide services to the various age groups. Increasingly, they would cooperate and eventually merge into a common set of interventions, each set directed at the various age cohorts at the level of care that they provide. The idea is that once all programs jointly focus on a phase in human development, their combined outputs should be better than each one could have achieved individually.

All services included in the KEPH function through a single delivery point. However, there are several programs that run vertically to the primary health programming (TB, malaria, and HIV/AIDS), other than prevention of mother-to-child transmission, which are planned for and implemented outside of the primary health structures. The referral system among these levels depends on where the skills that are required to address a client's problems are available. The government health service is supplemented by privately owned and operated hospitals and clinics and faith-based hospitals and clinics, which together provide between 30–40% of the hospital beds in Kenya [5].

Various challenges have affected the delivery of health care in Kenya, and consequently hindered the attainment of the Millennium Development Goals and ultimately universal health care coverage for Kenyans. For instance, neonatal and maternal mortality have remained stagnant since 1993 [7]. This chapter discusses some of the challenges affecting health care in Kenya.

Policy Implementation and Monitoring

One of the key failures in the health delivery system in Kenya has been in policy implementation. For instance, in NHSSP II, the essential health services targeted by the sector were defined in the KEPH. This was focused on integration of all health programs into a single package that focused its interventions on the improvement of health at different phases of the human development cycle, at the different levels of the health care delivery system. However, during review of NHSSP II, it was discovered that the KEPH had serious design and operational issues [6] due to the following:

1. difficulty in aligning and planning for crosscutting health services within specific cohorts

2. absence of specific services for some cohorts, such as elderly persons

3. paucity of information to plan and monitor services in some cohorts, such as adolescents

4. disjoint between planning guided by cohorts, operations guided by programs, and budgeting and financing guided by budget areas

5. limitation of a basic package description that doesn't fit with the reality of actual provision of comprehensive services, irrespective of the limited services defined in the KEPH

6. integration of interventions was not appropriately guided by the KEPH, and it didn't define the service areas around which KEPH interventions would be provided (and integration practiced).

By the end of NHSSP II, Kenya's health sector was beginning to see improvements in some health impact targets, in particular adult mortality, infant mortality, and child mortality. However, there were no improvements in neonatal and maternal mortality, while geographic and gender differences in age-specific cohorts persisted all through the policy period [6] (figure 2.2).

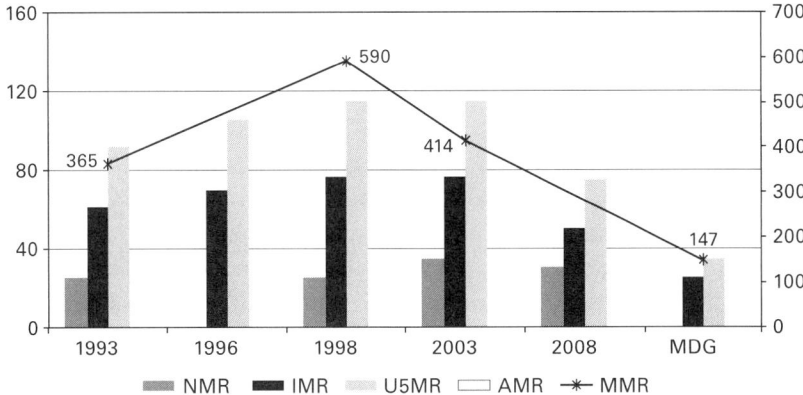

Figure 2.2
Trends in health impact indicators during the period 1993–2013. Key: NMR, neonatal mortality ratio; IMR, infant mortality ratio; U5MR, under-5 mortality ratio; AMR, adult mortality ratio; MMR, maternal mortality ratio; MDG, millennium development goals. Source: Ministry of Health (2013).

While expenditure figures as a proportion of the government's budget remains stagnant, it is also true that inequalities are high, with most resources going to curative hospital care rather than prevention or rural or hard-to-reach areas. The government has also not developed a recent health financing strategy to mobilize resources.

For monitoring and evaluation, the Kenyan health service lacks a strategy to guide the process, and while the public sector has a routine reporting system, there exists no unified comprehensive information system that includes all service providers.

Physical Infrastructure

While good health services can be provided even in minimal service delivery settings, both clients and providers are most likely to be satisfied with a facility if basic amenities and infrastructure components are available. These include a constant supply of clean water, a comfortable waiting area, and a clean latrine for clients, among others. These components also help staff to provide better services.

Geographical Spread and Access

Access is a measure of the ability of a person or community to receive available services. It is a prerequisite to utilization of health services, since it brings services closer to the people. Poor distribution of facilities, poor public transport, weak referral systems, insufficient community health services, and weak collaborations with other service providers have perpetuated poor geographical access to health services. The Kenyan health delivery system is characterized by imbalances in geographical distribution of health facilities in terms of the numbers and types of facilities available. Some areas have disproportionately more facilities than others. Consequently, while the average distance covered to reach the nearest health facility is reasonable (within 5 km for medical services and 2.5 km for public health services, as recommended by WHO), there are underserved areas in the country, particularly in the northern counties of Isiolo, Turkana, Mandera, West Pokot, Marsabit, Samburu, Wajir, and Garissa. Approximately four in every five Kenyans live in rural areas, yet a disproportionate share of health care facilities are located in urban areas [8]. Those in rural areas often have to travel long distances, often on foot, to seek care. According to the World Bank, the index of access to health services (measuring the share of newborns delivered at a health facility) in Kenya, speaks volumes to this disparity. For example, more than eight in 10 children born in Kirinyaga County, which is located in the central part of the country, are delivered in a health facility. In Wajir, which is located in one of the most remote and marginalized regions of the country, one child in 20 is born in a health facility [8] (figure 2.3).

Maternal and child mortality seem to mirror the geographical spread of health care facilities. Complications during pregnancy are a major source of both child and maternal

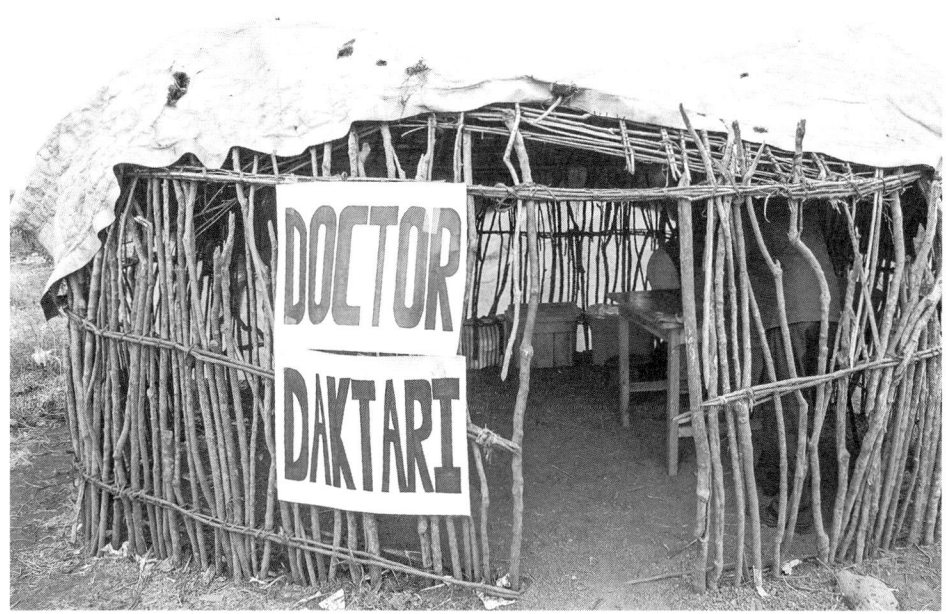

Figure 2.3
A rural medical facility in Marsabit County.

morbidity and mortality. Pregnant women should therefore routinely receive information on the signs of complications (especially anemia and infections) and get tested for them during antenatal visits. In Kenya, however, antenatal care reveals wide disparities across counties, with women from underserved areas having less antenatal care visits compared to their better-served counterparts. For instance, 28.9% of pregnant women from North Eastern province did not receive any antenatal care at all, compared to the national average of 5% [9].

Proper medical care and hygienic environments during delivery also reduce the risk of morbidity and mortality for both the mother and child, which makes it important for mothers to deliver in health facilities. However, in Kenya, only 43% of births take place in health facilities, while 56% occur at home. Disparities in hospital deliveries mirror access to health care facilities, with 81% of all deliveries in North Eastern province taking place at home, compared to about 10% in Nairobi. For the women who delivered at home in North Eastern province, 46.4% cited distance and lack of transport to the facility, while 17.3% cited poor medical services as barriers to deliver in a hospital [9].

Postnatal care is another crucial health care component to reduce infant and child mortality. Access to postnatal care in Kenya also mirrors the spread and access to other health services, with wide provincial differences in the proportion of mothers who do not receive postnatal care. For example, 79% of those in the North Eastern region do not receive postnatal care, compared with 18% of those in the Nairobi region. This disparity continues into early childhood and manifests in geographical variation in child mortality. Universal immunization of children against the six vaccine-preventable diseases (namely, tuberculosis, diphtheria, whooping cough/pertussis, tetanus, polio, and measles) is crucial to reducing infant and child mortality. In the North Eastern region, only 48% are immunized, compared to 86% in the Central region and a national average of 77%. About one in seven children in Nyanza dies before attaining his or her fifth birthday (149 deaths per 1,000), compared with one in 20 children in the Central region (51 deaths per 1,000), which has the lowest rate. Thus, the risk of dying before age five is almost three times higher in Nyanza than in Central province. Infant mortality is also highest in the Nyanza region (95 deaths per 1,000) and lowest in the Eastern region (39 deaths per 1,000) [9]. A major focus of eHealth and mHealth projects in low- and middle-income countries, particularly in East Africa, is increasing access to and use of antenatal services, facility-based childbirth, and immunization [10].

Rural–Urban Migration

Africa's major cities and towns are characterized by some parts of the population with abject poverty that live in informal settlements known as slums [11,12]. These informal settlements are characterized by poor housing conditions, poor social services, poor basic amenities, poor health outcomes, insecurity, and unstable incomes and livelihoods.

In Nairobi, Kenya's capital city and regional economic powerhouse, slum dwellers account for between 60 and 70% of the estimated 4 million residents [12]. The slum settlements usually have no power or water supply, no access to roads, and generally no infrastructure (figure 2.4). Affordable health care in the slums remains a big challenge, and the populations rely on nongovernmental organizations, faith-based organizations, and to a large part on unscrupulous traditional healers. In most slum areas, medical emergencies result in high mortality and disability, because there are no 24-hour health facilities [13,14,15].

Medical Supplies and Equipment

Even in regions where health care infrastructure is available, facilities in Kenya face challenges of stock-outs of medical supplies. A study conducted in 2013 [16] found that non-availability of medicines was the most important barrier to quality cited by health care consumers, and a key factor in the underuse of public health facilities. The 2012 Health Sector Customer Satisfaction, Employee Satisfaction and Work Environment Survey reported that less than half (47%) of clients were able to obtain all prescribed medicines, with the most common explanations being medicines "not available" (77%) and cost

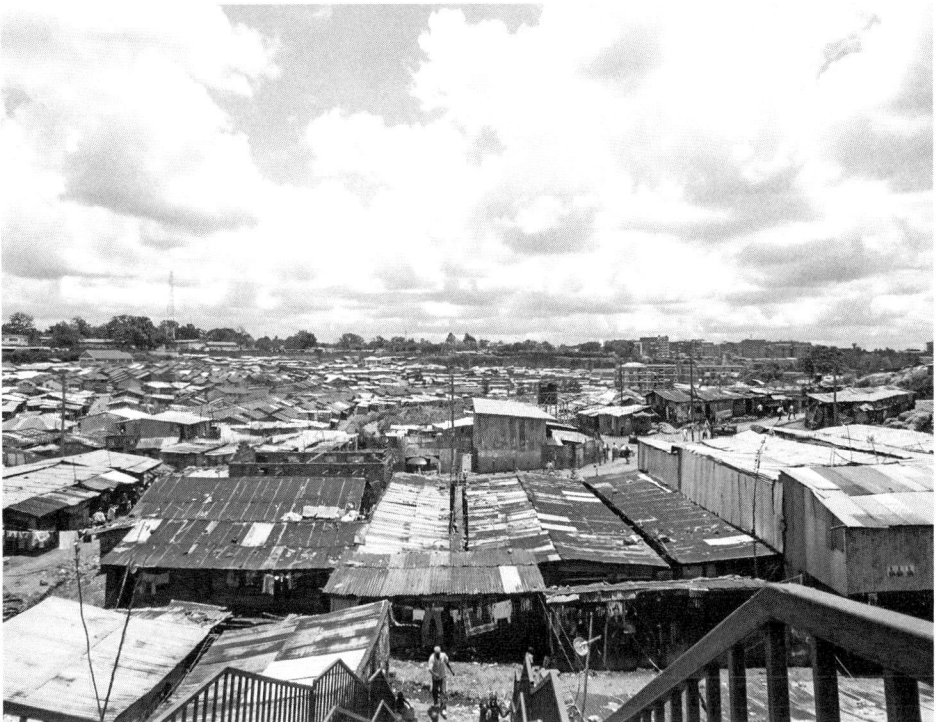

Figure 2.4
A slum settlement in Nairobi, Kenya.

(22%) [17]. A study by Kagema et al. [18] discovered that just over half of facilities (58%) had all of the items needed for infection control, while 63% had medicines for serious obstetric complications, 51% had medicines for common obstetric complications, and 57% had all essential supplies for delivery. Few facilities (20%) had all of the elements needed to support quality during complicated deliveries, such as partographs, guidelines, and delivery providers on staff 24 hours per day.

The 2013 study [16] found that 67% of facilities have the basic equipment required to provide KEPH services. However, there were large discrepancies between public and private health facilities: private nonprofit health facilities had more medical equipment availability (95%) than public facilities (69%) (figure 2.5).

Roads, Water, and Electrical Power Supply

The quality of roads as well as a poor communication network have been cited as reasons for the lack of prompt interventions in health care delivery in many developing countries

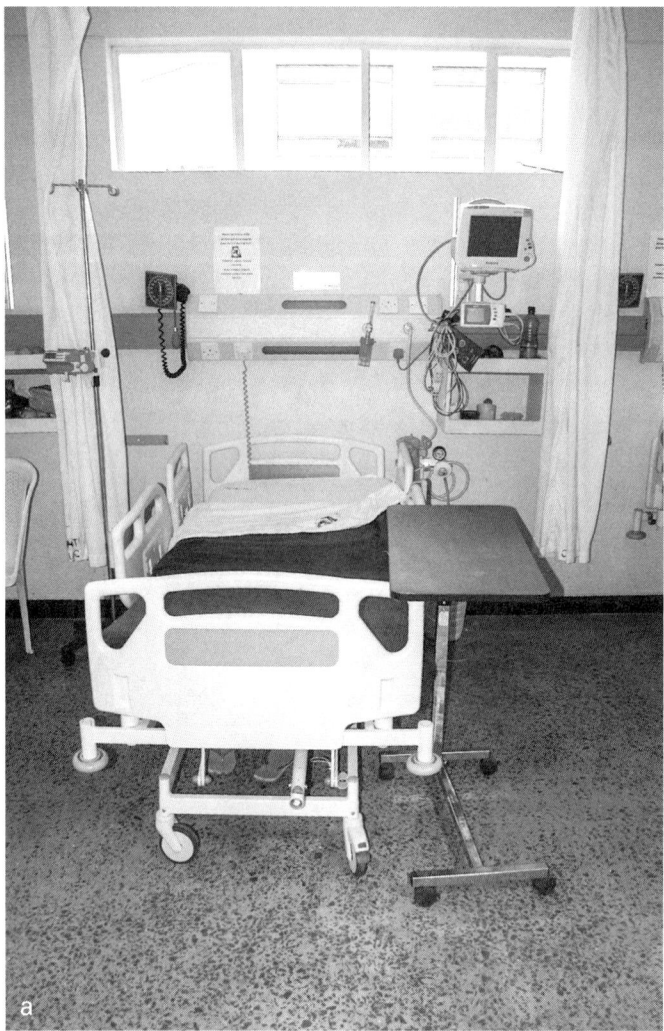

Figure 2.5
A private health facility ward (a) and a public health facility ward (b) showing the disparity of hospital resources.

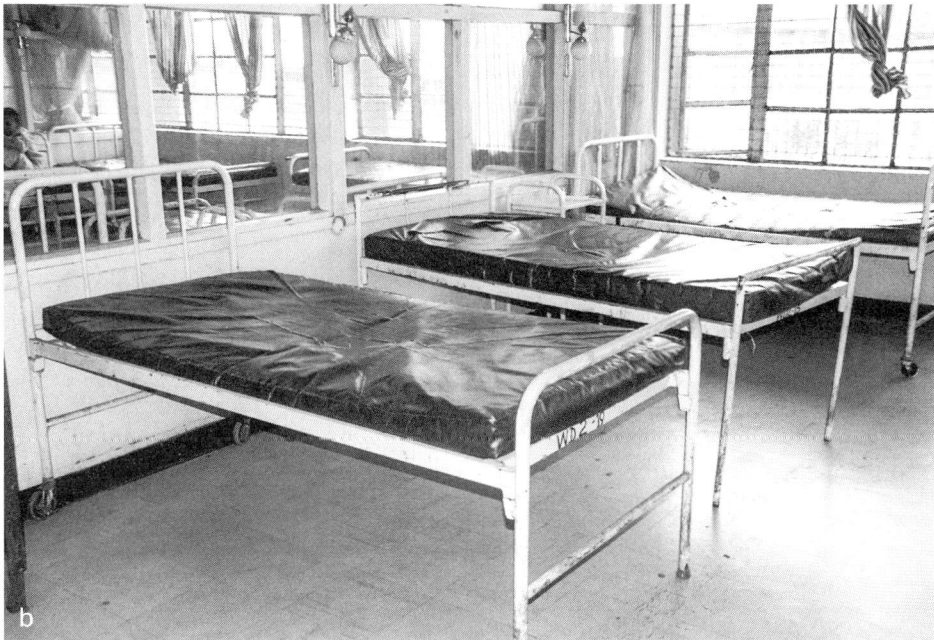

Figure 2.5 (continued)

[19]. It is in this regard that one of the policy objectives of the Kenya Health Policy 2012–2030 [4] is to "strengthen collaboration with other sectors that have an impact on health," which include infrastructure, planning, and transport focusing on improving access among hard-to-reach populations, with a view to facilitate movements of people, goods and services. In some regions of Kenya, it is an arduous task for patients to access hospital facilities due to poor road infrastructure. Roads poorly serve the Northern, Eastern, and Southern parts of the country (figure 2.6). The Northern region, which covers approximately 30% of the country's landmass, has less than 1% of its roads network paved [19]. This status of roads is a significant hindrance to the goal of universal health care coverage in Kenya, and it is not unheard of for patients to die on their way to the hospital.

According to the Kenya Service Provision Assessment report [9], regular water supply (i.e., year-round water supplied by a tap in the facility from a protected or unknown source, or water supplied from a protected well or pump, and water outlet available within 500 meters of the facility), is available in a little under half (46%) of all medical facilities. Only 25% of all facilities have regular, uninterrupted electricity (i.e., the facility is connected to a central power grid, or has solar power, or both, and power is routinely available during regular service hours), or has a functioning generator with fuel.

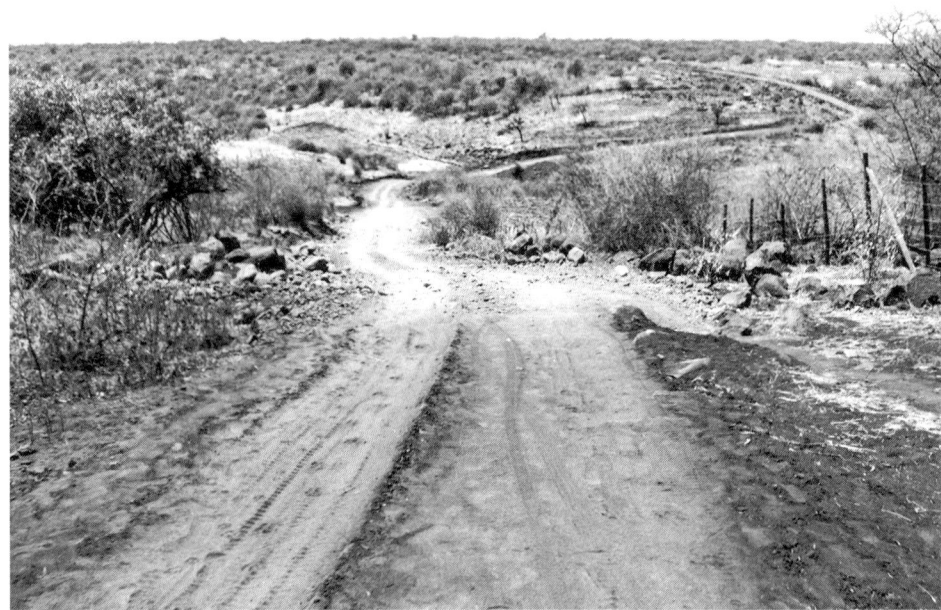

Figure 2.6
A rural road in northeastern Kenya.

According to the same survey, only 13% of the facilities have both of these utilities in regular supply [9].

In those facilities that have installed power from the grid, the supply is sometimes erratic, resulting in equipment failure during critical medical procedures.

Cost and Health Care Facility Utilization

Cost of health care remains a huge barrier to universal health coverage in Kenya, affected by low household income, low prioritization of health at the household level, and low allocation of resources by the state to the health sector [4]. While availability of health care facilities does not guarantee utilization, utilization is an important indicator of health status, health-seeking behavior, and cost and quality of services. The availability of a basic package of health services, the frequency with which these services are offered, the presence of qualified staff for their delivery, and the overall ease of access to the health care system all contribute to client utilization of services in a health facility. The 2007 Kenya

Household Health Expenditure and Utilization Survey shows that overall utilization of health services by people reporting being ill was 77.2%, meaning that 22.8% did not seek health care [20].

Results of the most recent demographic health survey indicate that few Kenyans have health insurance. Only 7% of women and 11% of men age 15–49 are covered by medical insurance, with the largest category of insurance being employer-based policies [9].

Utilization of health care facilities varies greatly across counties. In addition, urban populations access health care services more because they travel shorter distances and have greater financial resources. Those who reported being ill but never sought treatment cited health care costs (44%) and distance to health facility (18%) as the main barriers to utilization [20].

Kenyans who are employed and whose income exceeds a set threshold participate in the National Health Insurance Fund. According to the WHO, the government of Kenya covers about 38.7% the overall expenditures on health, while private expenditures account for 61.3% of overall spending. In 2006, 80% of private expenditures were out-of-pocket payments for health services [21].

Human Capacity

The health workforce is defined as the stock of people engaged in operations whose primary intent is to enhance health. The availability of appropriate and equitably distributed health workers, attraction and retention of required health workers, improvement of institutional and health worker performance, and capacity building and development of the health workforce are essential to meeting this basic need of health.

Geographic Spread and Adequacy

According to data from the Ministry of Health, Kenya has a total of 4,500 specialists and medical officers, only about 1,000 of whom work in the public sector, which serves the majority of Kenyans [6]. Of these doctors, 530 work at the 12 national referral hospitals— Kenyatta National Hospital, Moi Teaching and Referral Hospital, Spinal Injury Hospital, Pumwani Hospital, Mathari Hospital, and the seven Provincial General Hospitals. About 37000 nurses supplement physician care, as do traditional midwives, clinical officers, pharmacists, and community health workers. The total number of health workers is just over 17 per 10,000 people. Medical staff (medical and clinical officers) in Kenya represent just over 1 per 10,000 people; in comparison, the United States counts on 26 physicians per 10,000 people. Their distribution, however, is not equitable, with many areas of the county having significant health workforce gaps. More than 50% of Kenyan physicians practice in Nairobi, which, with an estimated 4 million people, represents a small fraction of the country's population. As a result, in Kenya, any complicated medical case is always referred to Nairobi because this is where almost all experienced consultants can be found.

The main reasons for this skewed distribution of health workers are low budgetary support, high levels of attrition, unfavorable terms and conditions of work, lack of incentives for hard-to-reach areas, lack of equity in remuneration, low employee satisfaction, and stagnation due to unfavorable career trajectories. In a study done in Marsabit County (a northern frontier area in Kenya) on employee satisfaction, it was notable that 68% and 63% of health workers cited conditions of work (hospital supplies) and lack of career progression, respectively, as the biggest contributors to low employee satisfaction (Mwangi, Cheren & Partners for Care, manuscript in preparation).

Training and Continuous Education

Apart from inadequate numbers of health workers, the Kenyan health care system is also hampered by a lack of skills inventory to guide deployment of workers to ensure equitable distribution of existing skills, but also inform areas where more training is required. Even where training needs have been identified, there exist challenges in budgetary support, lack of mechanisms to link training institutions with service needs, lack of a training policy for the health sector, and inadequate facilities for training.

Brain Drain

Human resource is critical in strengthening health systems. It takes a lot of time and capital for a country and individual to train health workers. An estimated $500 million is spent annually on medical education of workers from Africa who will eventually emigrate [22]. In Kenya alone, US$65,997 is spent educating a single medical doctor from primary school to university, and for every doctor who emigrates, US$517,931 returns in investment are lost [23]. Each country requires their skilled health workforce to meet their health needs [21]. The migration of trained health workers from the public sector to higher-paying positions in the private sector, or away from Kenya altogether, has made retaining qualified health personnel a persistent challenge. Kenya has one of the highest net emigration rates for doctors in the world, with 51% leaving the country to work elsewhere, according to a 2000 study. The presence of so few health personnel in Kenya can make it difficult for the government to carry out adequate disease surveillance, maintain accurate statistics regarding disease outbreaks, and report relevant findings to neighboring countries and international organizations.

The Way Forward

Improving geographical access. For the Kenyan government to roll out a universal health coverage program, it will need to improve physical access to health care facilities for at least 90% of the population. The KHSSP aims to achieve this through upgrading 40% of dispensaries to full primary care units, operationalizing 100% of health centers to fully functional primary care facilities, and putting in place a fully functional referral system in at least 80% of counties. Current infrastructure improvement efforts, especially on roads, is also expected to improve access to health care. However, there is still a long way to go with regard to access to some facilities; for example, only the Kenyatta national referral hospital in Nairobi is able to offer radiotherapy treatment.

Quality of care. It is recognized that quality of care is influenced by the capacity to use available inputs to deliver desired outcomes. Apart from physical facilities, quality of care is also affected by the "soft inputs" needed to deliver care, which include health workers' attitudes, motivation, equipment management, and leadership skills, among others. The government has identified priority actions to improve quality of care during the KHSSP term, which include:

- improving services' relevance and acceptability by use of regular service charters by all service delivery points, conducting regular client satisfaction surveys to continually ensure clients expectations are informing intervention provisions, and ensuring patient safety in provision of services.

- improving continuity of care through strengthening referral services and improving patient experiences in utilization of services.

- integration of services by linking provision of similar interventions together through the KEPH defined service groupings.

- ensuring a comprehensive approach to services is applied and used, not one focusing solely on programs. The sector has also committed itself to developing quality monitoring and evaluation indicators, which will be incorporated into a facilitative supervision system.

- application of an accreditation framework for health services and training institutions, and legislating compliance to the Kenya Quality Model for Health as the framework for quality improvement.

Sociocultural barriers. Strongly held traditional beliefs and, in some instances, low literacy levels, religious beliefs, and gender bias hinder access to health services, especially for women, children, adolescents, the disabled, and other vulnerable groups. Recognizing this problem, the government has to make the provision of health services more humane, compassionate, and dignified. Targeted measures include ensuring privacy in the course of service delivery, especially for women.

Information gathering and access. To improve its information gathering and better track its progress in meeting the health-related Millennium Development Goals, Kenya has developed a health management information system and is currently working with international partners to improve its capacity to provide timely and relevant data regarding the country's health situation to policy makers and other stakeholders.

Questions for Discussion

- What are the biggest challenges that face the health sector in developing countries? How can these challenges be addressed?
- What is the role of the international academic partnerships in improving access to health care in poor countries?
- How can developing countries make use of available health data to inform prioritization of resources considering their budgetary constraints?
- How can health systems in developing countries be designed to empower the health workforce to deliver effective care?
- What is the role, if any, of informal health care providers in universal health care access?
- Developed countries have innovative therapies for improving the health of their populations. Should these be rolled out in developing countries?
- How can developing countries improve the impact evaluation of the different health care solutions that are implemented to improve access?

References

1. World Bank Fiscal Decentralization Knowledge Programme Team. 2012. *Devolution Without Disruption: Pathways to a Successful New Kenya*. World Bank.

2. World Health Organization. 2012. *World Health Statistics Report 2012*. Geneva, Switzerland: World Health Organization.

3. African Union. 2001. Abuja Declaration on HIV/AIDS, Tuberculosis and Other Related Infectious Diseases. African Summit on HIV/AIDS, Tuberculosis and Other Related Infectious Diseases. Abuja, Nigeria, April 24–27, 2001. http://www.un.org/ga/aids/pdf/abuja_declaration.pdf. Accessed December 1, 2015.

4. Government of Kenya. 2013. Kenya. Health Policy 2012–2030. Nairobi, Kenya: Government of Kenya.

5. Ministry of Health. 2005. Reversing the trends: The second national health sector strategic plan of Kenya (NHSSP II), 2005–2010. Nairobi, Kenya: Government of Kenya.

6. Ministry of Health. 2013. Accelerating attainment of health goals: The Kenya health sector strategic and investment plan (KHSSP), July 2012–June 2017. Nairobi, Kenya: Government of Kenya.

7. Government of Kenya. 2010. Review of the Kenya Health Policy Framework, 1994–2010. Nairobi, Kenya: Government of Kenya.

8. World Bank. 2013. *Global Monitoring Report 2013: Rural-Urban Disparities and Dynamics and the Millennium Development Goals.* Washington, DC: World Bank.

9. Kenya National Bureau of Statistics and ICF Macro. 2010. *Kenya Demographic and Health Survey 2008–09.* Calverton, MD: Kenya National Bureau of Statistics and ICF Macro.

10. Mushamiri I, Luo C, Iiams-Hauser C, Ben Amor Y. 2015. Evaluation of the impact of a mobile health system on adherence to antenatal and postnatal care and prevention of mother-to-child transmission of HIV programs in Kenya. *BMC Public Health* 15: 102. doi:10.1186/s12889-015-1358-5.

11. UN-Habitat. 2008. *The State of African Cities 2008: A Framework for Addressing Urban Challenges in Africa.* Nairobi, Kenya: UN-Habitat.

12. UN-Habitat. 2010. *State of African cities 2010: Governance, Inequalities and Urban Land Markets.* Nairobi, Kenya: UN-Habitat.

13. Fotso JC, Ezeh A, Madise N, Ziraba A, Ogollah R. 2009. What does access to maternal care mean among the urban poor? Factors associated with use of appropriate maternal health services in the slum settlements of Nairobi, Kenya. *Matern Child Health J* 13(1): 130–137.

14. Ziraba AK, Mills S, Madise N, Saliku T, Fotso JC. 2009. The state of emergency obstetric care services in Nairobi informal settlements and environs: Results from a maternity health facility survey. *BMC Health Serv Res* 9: 46.

15. Taffa N, Chepngeno G, Amuyunzu-Nyamongo M. 2009. Child morbidity and health-care utilization in the slums of Nairobi, Kenya. *J Trop Pediatr* 51(5): 279–284.

16. Ministry of Health. 2014. Kenya service availability and readiness assessment mapping. Nairobi, Kenya: Government of Kenya.

17. Ministry of Medical Services and Ministry of Public Health and Sanitation. 2012. Health sector customer satisfaction, employee satisfaction and work environment survey. Nairobi, Kenya: Government of Kenya.

18. Kagema F, Ricca J, Rawlins B, Rosen H, Mukhwana W, Lynam P, et al. 2010. *Quality of Care for Prevention and Management of Common Maternal and Newborn Complications: Findings from a National Health Facility Survey in Kenya.* Nairobi: USAID and MCHIP.

19. Noor A, Amin A, Gething P, Atkinson P, Hay S, Snow R. 2006. Modelling distances travelled to government health services in Kenya. *Trop Med Int Health* 11: 188–196.

20. Ministry of Transport. 2009. Integrated national transport policy: Moving a working nation. Nairobi, Kenya: Government of Kenya.

21. Ministry of Health. 2009. Kenya household health expenditure and utilization survey 2007. Nairobi, Kenya: Government of Kenya.

22. Willis-Shattuck M, Bidwell P, Thomas S, Wyness L, Blaauw D, Ditlopo P. 2008. Motivation and retention of health workers in developing countries: A systematic review. *BMC Health Serv Res* 8: 247.

23. Oyelere UR. 2007. Brain drain, waste or gain? What we know about the Kenyan case. *J Global Initiatives* 2: 113–129.

3 Health Systems in Low- and Middle-Income Countries

Elizabeth H. Bradley and Lauren A. Taylor

Take-Home Messages

- There is no one perfect health system design. A number of short-, mid-, and long-range health goals may be equally worthy to pursue on behalf of a population. Each low- or middle-income country makes trade-offs to design a system that suits its health goals and operates within relevant constraints.
- Effective management of low- or middle-income countries health systems often requires coordinated efforts between the Ministry of Health, Ministry of Finance, other government offices, nongovernmental organizations, and faith-based organizations. This coordination can be challenging, but also allows a health system to more directly address the social determinants of health in addition to providing health care services.
- Many health system performance schemes aim to assess the health system on the basis of accessibility, quality, and cost of health care services. Measuring impact of health systems on the health of the population is important but can pose challenges.

Health systems comprise a vast scope of inputs, including providers of health and health care around the globe (figure 3.1). The World Health Organization describes a health system as all organizations, institutions, resources, and people whose primary purpose is to improve human health [1,2]. The design of health systems draws on the expertise of multiple disciplines; for instance, economists and political scientists examine the impact of financial incentives or regulatory efforts, while anthropologists, sociologists, and organizational psychologists study the effect of differences in community and organizational constraints on health services. Still further, computer scientists, biologists, and engineers develop novel technologies to improve clinical, management, or communication challenges within health systems.

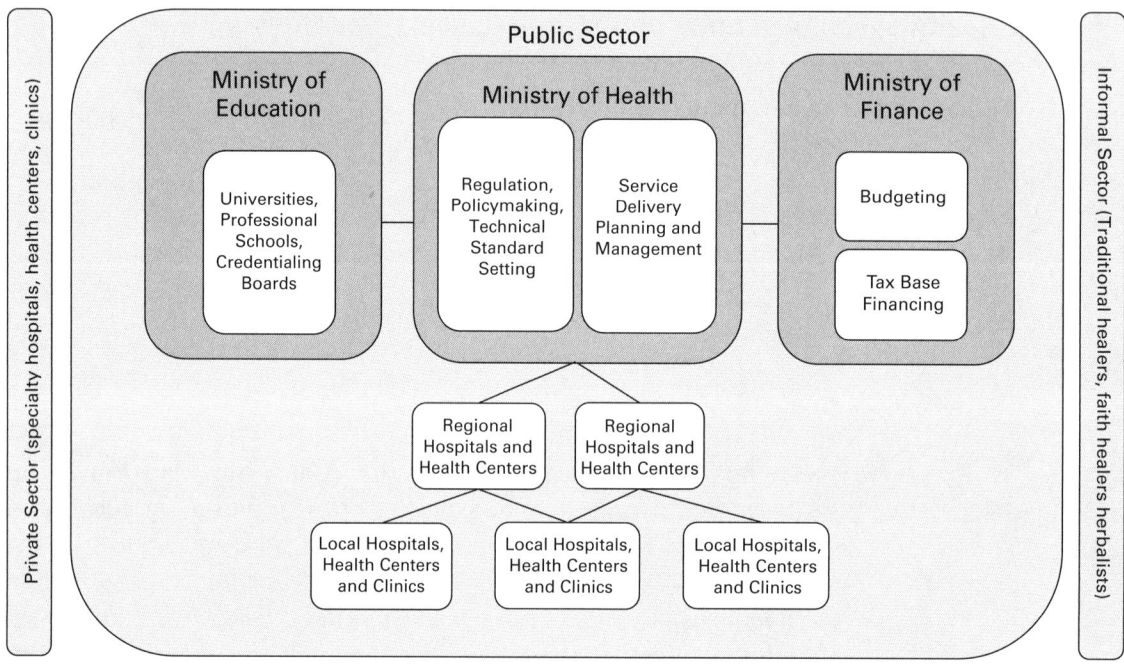

Figure 3.1
Components of the health system.

Several framing questions can provide a useful starting place in the examination of health systems. Evaluation of health systems in low- and middle-income countries begins with fundamental issues with regard to their purpose, diversity in their design and financing, and their performance. In seeking to understand these parameters, several broad questions may be useful to ask: what is the goal of the health system? How is the health system financed and managed? How do we measure performance of the health system? The answers to these questions vary considerably across countries and over time within countries, based on economic development and shifts in political security and philosophy.

What Is the Goal?

Goals can be shorter-term, medium-term, or longer-term, and may pertain to the primary care system (that is, the part of the health care system—often health posts or clinics, or community health workers—for preventive or chronic care or less serious acute care) or to curative care (that is, the part of the system—often hospitals—that is used to treat illness and require secondary or tertiary levels of care). Shorter-term goals in low- and middle-income health systems might be to expand access to at least basic services (e.g., antenatal care, skilled birth attendance, and vaccination services) for the population. Medium-term goals might be to enhance not only access to but also the quality of services delivered (e.g., prompt emergency care, proper medication regimens, and effective chronic care). Longer-term goals might be to promote and sustain the health of individuals and communities as well as promote health equity across communities. A critical distinction in health system goals is between the provision of medical care and the promotion of health. Provision of medical care focuses primarily on people who are already ill or at risk for illness in so much as they require medical care, whereas promotion of health focuses more broadly on social determinants of health (e.g., housing, income support, education, nutrition) and the degree to which health systems may support and sustain the population's health. Many health systems aim to accomplish both of these goals, but inevitably prioritize one end over the other in their strategies.

Most health systems have historically emphasized the management of physicians, hospitals, nursing homes, and other health care providers. However, researchers have increasingly demonstrated that the contribution of medical care (e.g., physicians, clinics, hospitals) is relatively modest compared with the influence of diet, exercise, environment, occupation, and income on the population's health. As a result, many health systems are finally recognizing that the target of their action—health—should include services such as assistance with employment, education, and housing. As a result, these services are being incorporated into the responsibilities of the health system to varying degrees. Paradoxically, as low- and middle-income countries (LMIC) experience economic development, an emerging middle class often demands increasingly medicalized approaches to health, inflating health care costs disproportionate to improvement in health outcomes [3]. Although increased spending in health care from less than 5% of GDP to 6–10% of GDP has been associated with substantial improvements in life expectancy [4], over-investment in health technology can also limit health improvements if it diverts funding from more basic health and social services [3].

How Are Health Systems Financed and Managed?

A second question that can be helpful in assessing how a system is organized is to investigate how it is financed and managed. LMIC vary in the percentage of GDP allocated to health systems. In countries with very low income, less than 5% of GDP is spent on health care and is largely financed by global development aid [5,6]. The remainder of health care expenditures is borne by individuals through private, out-of-pocket, and informal payments. In these countries, the government is often ill-equipped to direct significant resources toward health and health care, and without a strong economy, employer-based or community-based insurance or payment schemes are not feasible. Middle-income countries typically spend between 5% and 10% of their GDP on health and health care [6], and such economies are often able to support a social health insurance scheme funded by general tax revenues or other sources. Such a scheme may be accompanied by efforts to establish community-based health insurance funded by contributions from the community to finance primary care [7,8]. Nevertheless, for 1.3 billion people living in LMIC, financial concerns limit individuals' access to health care, leaving significant treatment gaps in critically important areas such as HIV and mental health care [9,10].

The management of health systems in LMIC is generally the shared responsibility of the Ministry of Health (for policy, regulation, and financing of health delivery) and Ministry of Education (for medical, nursing, and other health provider educational institutions, which ultimately develop the human resources needed to provide health care). Coordination of efforts between the ministries can be complex, but has been quite successful in Rwanda's Human Resources for Health project [11] and in Ethiopia's scale-up of medical schools [12], to name two examples. Within the Ministry of Health, a distinction is often made between a policy-making and financing entity and a service-delivery entity. Most hospitals are managed by the government, although nongovernmental organizations, faith-based organizations, and private and traditional sector providers also oversee some hospitals and health centers. Although some countries are moving toward monitoring quality in hospitals and health centers using health management information systems, this capability can be hampered by limited automation and connectivity, limited staff training in information technology and data analysis, and poor accountability throughout the health system. Many LMIC have also sought to decentralize the management of health systems through the establishment of local governing boards and management capacity building [13,14,15], but much of the human resources administration, operating budget allocations, and capital investment decisions, including those that involve information technology, are made at the regional or federal levels.

How Do We Measure Health System Performance?

Indicators of health system performance typically pertain to accessibility, quality, and cost of health care services [16]. Accessibility refers not only to physical and economic access to services, but also to adequate information about service availability, delivered in a nondiscriminatory and culturally appropriate manner [17]. Quality refers to both technical and experiential domains, and is often assessed by self-reported patient experience and health service provider adherence to clinical and management guidelines [18]. Cost includes the overall cost to society of delivering health services, often measured as a percent of GDP, with particular attention to the portion of the financial burden born by individuals and families. In LMIC, health systems have historically been focused on combating infectious disease (typically responsible for a large portion of deaths) and promoting reproductive health, including maternal, newborn, and child health (e.g., family planning, antenatal and postnatal care, vaccination). Although noncommunicable disease burdens are increasing in LMIC, health systems there have limited experience and capacity to manage chronic diseases. If performance metrics are not revisited frequently by a wide range of stakeholders, a performance evaluation effort can give way to a myopic focus on metrics tied to one disease or intervention type. Additionally, although quality of care is acknowledged to be an important consideration [18], achieving widespread access to basic health services such as antenatal care, family planning, and vaccinations is generally the more dominant metric by which health systems are evaluated in LMIC.

Because capital and transportation infrastructure can be limited and the shortage of health care providers can be extreme [19], a common model of health care delivery in LMIC is to leverage community health workers [20]. These workers are typically high school graduates with up to a year of training in health education and primary care who may or may not be paid for their services. Measuring community health worker output and impact has proved difficult for various reasons: their integration into the Ministry of Health may be challenged at the local level, their training is often variable, and their supervision and oversight are inadequate. Use of mobile technology is increasing and holds promise for supporting, managing, and monitoring community health workers in LMIC [21]. However, ensuring adequate compensation for these front-line staff remain of utmost importance for sustaining health system performance.

Conclusion

The *goals* of health systems in LMIC are diverse and change over time. Increasing attention is being paid not only to access, but also to quality of health care services. Furthermore, the development of effective health systems requires models that equally address both the medical and the social determinants of health. The *financing and management* of health systems varies substantially across LMIC, although integrating country-specific resources, external funding, and service providers is invariably a challenge across countries. *Performance* of health systems is often measured by access, cost, and quality of care, and various indicators of health. These are typically tailored to the priorities of the country, although global actors such as the World Bank and World Health Organization also influence select performance measures. In addition, eHealth can be particularly useful for health system performance evaluation—capturing data on clinical care, management, supply chains, financing, and staff employment and training.

Questions for Discussion

- How might short-, medium-, and long-term goals for a health system be in conflict with one another?
- What kinds of challenges might a Ministry of Health face in building cross-sector partnerships with other ministries, nongovernmental organizations, or faith-based organizations? What might the benefits be?

References

1. World Health Organization. 2000. World Health Report. Geneva, Switzerland: World Health Organization. http://www.who.int/whr/2000/en/whr00_en.pdf.

2. World Health Organization. 2007. Strengthening Health Systems to Improve Health Outcomes: WHO's Framework for Action. http://www.who.int/healthsystems/strategy/everybodys_business.pdf.

3. Bradley EH, Taylor LA. 2013. *Paradox and Promise in American Health Care: Why Spending More is Getting Us Less.* New York, NY: Public Affairs Press.

4. OECD. 2013. *Health at a Glance 2013: OECD Indicators.* Paris, France: OECD Publishing. doi:10.1787/Health_Glance-2013-En.

5. Lu C, Schneider MT, Gubbins P, Leach-Kemon K, Jamison D, Murray CJ. 2010. Public financing of health in developing countries: A cross-national systematic analysis. *Lancet* 375(9723): 1375–1387. doi:10.1016/S0140-6736(10)60233-4.

6. World Bank Group. 2015. Health expenditure, total. World Health Organization Global Health Expenditure database. http://data.worldbank.org/indicator/SH.XPD.TOTL.ZS.

7. Ekman B. 2004. Community-based health insurance in low-income countries: A systematic review of the evidence. *Health Policy Plan* 19(5): 249–270.

8. Lagarde M, Palmer N. 2006. The impact of health financing strategies on access to health services in low and middle income countries (protocol). *Cochrane Database Syst Rev* 3, CD006092. doi:10.1002/14651858.CD006092.

9. Preker A, Carrin G, Dror D, Jakab M, Hsiao W, Arhin D. Rich-poor differences in health care financing. In Preker AS, Carrin G, eds. *Health Financing for Poor People: Resource Mobilisation and Risk-Sharing.* Washington, DC: World Bank; 2004: 3–51.

10. Xu K, Evans DB, Kawabata K, Zeramdini R, Klavus J, Murray CJ. 2003. Household catastrophic health expenditure: A multicountry analysis. *Lancet* 362(9378): 111–117. doi:10.1016/S0140-6736(03)13861-5.

11. Binagwaho A, Kyamanywa P, Farmer PE, Nuthulaganti T, Umubyeyi B, Nyemazi JP, et al. 2013. The human resources for health program in Rwanda—a new partnership. *N Engl J Med* 369(21): 2054–2059. doi:10.1056/NEJMsr1302176.

12. Derbew M, Animut N, Talib ZM, Mehtsun S, Hamburger EK. 2014. Ethiopian medical schools' rapid scale-up to support the government's goal of universal coverage. *Acad Med* 89(8 Suppl): S40–S44. doi:10.1097/ACM.0000000000000326.

13. Bossert TJ, Beauvais JC. 2002. Decentralization of health systems in Ghana, Zambia, Uganda and the Philippines: A comparative analysis of decision space. *Health Policy Plan* 17(1): 14–31.

14. Bossert TJ, Larranaga O, Giedion U, Arbelaez JJ, Bowser DM. 2003. Decentralization and equity of resource allocation: Evidence from Colombia and Chile. *Bull World Health Organ* 81(2): 95–100.

15. McNatt Z, Thompson JW, Endeshaw A, Tatek D, Linnander E, Ageze L, et al. 2014. Implementation of hospital governing boards: Views from the field. *BMC Health Serv Res* 14: 78. doi:10.1186/1472-6963-14-178.

16. Mills A. 2012. Health policy and systems research: Defining the terrain; identifying the methods. *Health Policy Plan* 27: 1–7.

17. Committee on Economic Social and Cultural Rights. 2000. General comment 14: The right to the highest attainable standard of health (twenty-second session). http://www1.umn.edu/humanrts/gencomm/escgencom14.htm.

18. Kruk ME, Freedman LP. 2008. Assessing health system performance in developing countries: A review of the literature. *Health Policy* 85(3): 263–276.

19. Chen L, Evans T, Anand S, Boufford JI, Brown H, Chowdhury M, et al. 2004. Human resources for health: Overcoming the crisis. *Lancet* 364(9449): 1984–1990. doi:10.1016/S0140-6736(04)17482-5.

20. Pallas SW, Minhas D, Pérez-Escamilla R, Taylor L, Curry L, Bradley EH. 2013. Community health workers in low-and middle-income countries: What do we know about scaling up and sustainability? *Am J Public Health* 103: E74–e82. doi:10.2105/AJPH.2012.301102.

21. Derenzi B, Borriello G, Jackson J, Kumar VS, Parikh TS, Virk P, 2011. Mobile phone tools for field-based health care workers in low-income countries. *Mt Sinai J Med* 78(3): 406–418. doi:10.1002/msj.20256.

4 Culture of Quality and Safety: A Prerequisite for Any Informatics Intervention

David J. Meyers, Tiara M. Forsyth, and Adrian Velasquez

Take-Home Messages

- Health informatics interventions should be considered quality improvement interventions.
- It is vital to have a culture of quality and safety for health informatics interventions to succeed.
- To build and sustain a culture of quality and safety, both top-down and bottom-up methods are necessary, and should leverage the power of both stories and data. Positive deviance is an example of a useful framework.

Introduction

With over 6.8 billion cell phones on the planet [1], mobile communication plays an increasingly fundamental role in daily life. Many groups have tried to leverage this phenomenon to improve health care delivery through cell phone applications that educate and increase medication compliance among patients or to empower community health workers to carry out tasks that would otherwise require intensive training. Through these applications, implementers aim to reach patients who would not otherwise seek health care because of access difficulty, and to expand capacity in communities facing health care provider shortages.

Digital health has seen some success in low- and middle-income countries (LMIC) to date: electronic medical record systems (EMRs) have improved quality of care through increased efficiency and better patient tracking [2–5]. In some instances, mobile phone applications for health interventions—known as mHealth—have been found to improve outcomes when compared with traditional methods [6–13]. However, numerous mHealth interventions do not advance past the pilot stage [14], and very few large-scale studies have been performed to evaluate their effectiveness. In a 2012 WHO survey, 83% of countries surveyed had one or more ongoing mHealth programs, yet over 50% faced barriers making mHealth a national area of priority. 47% reported that lack of knowledge about mHealth posed a significant barrier in scaling up interventions, and 44% cited a lack of policy regarding mHealth as a crucial factor [15]. While governments and NGOs are excited about mHealth, its potential as a tool to improve clinical outcomes requires deliberate and thoughtful planning. In this chapter, we argue that one of the major issues contributing to this phenomenon—dubbed "pilot-it is," in which mHealth projects fail to go beyond a feasibility phase, is the lack of an adequate culture of quality and safety within health delivery organizations.

What is the purpose of global health informatics? Is it to test a new piece of technology? To implement a new system or workflow? Or to improve the effectiveness and efficiency of care with the goal of improving patient outcomes and quality of life? If one subscribes to this last purpose, then it is important to acknowledge that an intervention in health informatics is an intervention in quality improvement (QI), a growing movement in health care worldwide over the past thirty years [16].

Health care quality improvement can be defined as "the combined and unceasing efforts of everyone—healthcare professionals, patients and their families, researchers, payers, planners and educators—to make the changes that will lead to better patient outcomes (health), better system performance (care) and better professional development" [16]. QI initiatives in the United States have been responsible for substantial improvements in patient health outcomes [17–19], and QI methodologies have been effectively implemented in resource-limited settings around the world [20–24].

In order for a QI intervention to be successful, there must first be a culture of quality and patient safety in place [25–28]; if people within an organization are not committed to continuous improvement in the services they provide, innovations in health care delivery, including those in information systems, are unlikely to sustain or scale. This chapter will describe what comprises this culture of quality and patient safety and methods for fostering one.

Defining a Culture of Quality and Safety

The Advisory Committee on the Safety of Nuclear Installations defines a culture of quality and safety as follows:

The safety culture of an organization is the product of individual and group values, attitudes, perceptions, competencies, and patterns of behavior that determine the commitment to, and the style and proficiency of, an organization's health and safety management. Organizations with a positive safety culture are characterized by communications founded on mutual trust, by shared perceptions of the importance of safety, and by confidence in the efficacy of preventive measures. [29]

We believe three important aspects of any culture of quality and safety include (1) an environment where everyone feels empowered to contribute; (2) a focus on continuous learning; and (3) frequent evaluation through concrete measures.

Several studies highlight the importance of building an ecosystem where everyone can contribute to improving quality of care [30,31]. This environment allows interventions to be crafted in a manner that is both realistic and culturally sensitive in order to encourage buy-in among organization members. For example, if a mobile phone intervention in a community health worker program is implemented before consulting with health workers to elicit their ideas and suggestions, the chance of success is diminished [30]. When team members feel that they played an important role in the program design, they perceive ownership of the project, leading to a greater accountability and program success [32]. A recent study in Uzbekistan found that several hospital staff were not interested in embracing evidence-based treatments, contributing to the failure of a quality improvement intervention [33]. If, from the outset, adequate buy-in from the staff had been solicited, perhaps the failure of the program could have been avoided. In another example, a US hospital had quality issues due to a lack of engagement of the hospital's board [34]. A case study found that many of the board members had backgrounds in finance but lacked an appreciation of the value of continuous quality improvement. It was not until the board began attending sessions on developing a culture of quality and safety that the hospital was able to improve health outcomes. This is a widespread issue: one study found only about 20% of hospital leaders believe it is the job of the board to promote quality [35]. Studies reveal that buy-in from hospital boards is linked to quality improvement outcomes [36,37].

A second important component of this culture of quality and patient safety is a focus on continuous learning. QI is often misrepresented as a one-time "fix" for an organization's problems. In reality, it must be a round-the-clock process built into the organization. Continuous quality improvement methods such as plan-do-study-act (PDSA) cycles have been found effective in reducing costs and improving quality of care [38–40]. In the health informatics context, while staff might be initially enthusiastic about a new tool as it is implemented, a commitment to continuous learning and improvement within the organization is vital for sustainability and scalability once the novelty wears off.

To track whether quality is maintained or improved, an organization needs a system to measure changes in quality [41]. This brings us to the third important aspect of quality and patient safety culture: monitoring and evaluation through concrete measures. Performance measurement plays an important role. But in order for relevant measurements to take place, the organization must be dedicated to collecting and analyzing data [42,43].

While these three aspects do not comprise a culture of quality and patient safety in its entirety, they are key components for such a culture to thrive in an organization. There are a number of approaches that can be used to help engender this culture in order to lay the groundwork for future interventions, including those in health informatics.

Past Successes and Potential Solutions

Creating a culture of quality and safety to implement and sustain technological innovations has challenges that are not insurmountable. Recent reviews have described several effective interventions for promoting such a culture [44]. In this section, we outline strategies and describe success stories in a variety of international low-resource settings.

Two recent reviews found that the characteristics of this culture fall within seven domains: leadership, teamwork, evidence-based intervention, communication, learning, justice, and a patient-centered focus [45,46]. Leadership interventions focus on strong management built around supporting improvements in quality and safety. Teamwork interventions center on building a spirit of collaboration among care providers and other stakeholders, which include informatics personnel. Communication interventions aim to improve dialogue between management, providers, and patients. Evidence interventions focus on substantiating and demonstrating the effectiveness of quality improvement initiatives as well as current practice. Learning interventions feature educational programs for all staff, including the managers. Finally, interventions that have a social justice drive and patient-centered focus are more likely to flourish. While the evidence for successful change in each of these domains is limited, individual interventions targeting each of these domains have been successful in the past [45]. Leadership and team-based interventions have demonstrated the most notable success in the literature to date.

Interventions for improving quality and patient safety culture can be initiated at different levels of an organization. Top-down approaches involve leadership and the larger policies of an institution to encourage change, while bottom-up methods engage front-line staff to lay the groundwork. In the Philippines, the national insurance provider PhilHealth implemented national benchmarks that all health centers must meet for reimbursements, which is an example of a top-down strategy that has had some success in other countries around the world [47,48]. A problem that arises with top-down strategies is that they may not lead to real culture change and only impose significant strain on already overburdened health care workers.

Possible, an international NGO that provides access to free health care in rural Nepal, successfully employs a bottom-up intervention for staff engagement. Possible operates a district health care system in rural Achham, Nepal, through a public-private partnership with the Nepali Ministry of Health. Bayalpata Hospital is the district-level hospital and hub of this system, and is surrounded by 13 village clinics and over 150 community health workers. Like many hospitals in LMICs, Bayalpata Hospital faces challenges with maternal mortality and post-hospitalization complications. To address these concerns, Possible implements a program in which clinical staff and administrators engage in daily continuing medical education sessions at the start of the workday and weekly morbidity and mortality conferences. At the morbidity and mortality conferences, a hospital staff member presents a case study of a patient the hospital might have failed to serve at the highest level of quality. Members of the hospital team provide data detailing the context. The combination of stories and data analysis from these meetings demonstrates and justifies the need for continuous quality improvement among the participants. The assembly of doctors, nurses, and administrators help foster the culture at all levels of the organization. This approach has proven successful across resource-limited settings [49,50].

One topic under much debate is the role of resource constraints and financial incentives in forging a culture of quality and patient safety. It is well known that staffing deficits contribute to burnout and fatigue [51]. Physician trainees who work 24-hour shifts make 36% more serious medical errors and up to five times more diagnostic errors than their colleagues who work shorter shifts [52]. Given these staffing deficits, it is often difficult for resource-constrained settings to engage workers in adopting innovations, including new technologies [53]. While the solution that first comes to mind is to increase the level of staffing or the funding of departments, recent studies have found that quality improvement is not driven by resources alone. Increased resources and financial incentives might lead to temporary improvements, but might not result in long-term, sustainable change [54,55]. While an adequate level of resources, including staffing, is crucial, budget-neutral approaches to improving quality have been successful. One such approach is positive deviance.

Positive deviance, a method that can be employed top-down or bottom-up, has been particularly successful in LMIC [56]. Positive deviance approaches were first designed for use in nutrition interventions in Vietnam [57] and are rooted in the idea that every community, even in the presence of resource constraints, has individuals who are already doing things well from whom others can learn. These "positive deviants" are first identified and then observed to see how they achieve success, and are then presented to other members of the community as models [56]. Researchers have documented the effectiveness of positive deviance in improving the quality of care and demonstrated its potential as a tool, especially in resource-limited settings [58–60]. Most health systems have some facilities that perform exceptionally well; through identifying these facilities and what makes them "tick," other health facilities may learn how to improve their care delivery. As these facilities are working with similar resources, it can often be relatively budget-neutral for a facility to modify their practices and replicate that of the identified "deviants."

Conclusions

A culture of quality and patient safety does not develop overnight. It takes time to instill the values of measurement, continuous learning, and engagement at all levels of an organization. Without such a culture, time and resources will be wasted in implementing a program that has little chance of being sustained or scaled. While launching a positive-deviance initiative to address problems in organizational culture may be a lofty initial goal to start, there are several simple first steps. Engaging staff in discussions about quality or conducting one of many available surveys of quality and patient safety culture are great ways to start [61].

The goal of health informatics interventions is to improve quality of care through the services provided by a health system. This makes health informatics a tool of quality improvement. A robust culture of quality and safety is necessary for the success of these interventions.

Questions for Discussion

- What barriers exist that hinder the development of a culture of quality and safety?
- What other approaches might be useful in building a culture of quality and safety in a rural health care setting?
- Are there situations in which a technological intervention can be successfully scaled without a culture of quality or safety?

References

1. International Telecommunication Union. *The World in 2013: ICT Facts and Figures.* Geneva, Switzerland: International Telecommunication Union; 2013.

2. Vilella A, Bayas J-M, Diaz M-T, Guinovart C, Diez C, Simó D, et al. 2004. The role of mobile phones in improving vaccination rates in travelers. *Prev Med* 38: 503–509. doi:10.1016/j.ypmed.2003.12.005.

3. Fraser HS, Biondich P, Moodley D, Choi S, Mamlin BW, Szolovits P. 2005. Implementing electronic medical record systems in developing countries. *Inform Prim Care* 13: 83–96.

4. Mamlin BW, Biondich PG, Wolfe BA, Fraser H, Jazayeri D, Allen C, et al. 2006. Cooking up an open source EMR for developing countries: OpenMRS—A recipe for successful collaboration. *AMIA Annu Symp Proc* 529–533.

5. Samal L, Wright A, Healey MJ, Linder JA, Bates DW. 2014. Meaningful use and quality of care. *JAMA Intern Med* 174: 997–998. doi:10.1001/jamainternmed.2014.662.

6. Littman-Quinn R, Chandra A, Schwartz A, Fadlelmola FM, Ghose S, Luberti AA, et al. 2011. mHealth applications for telemedicine and public health intervention in Botswana. IST-Africa Conference Proceedings: 1–11.

7. Free C, Phillips G, Felix L, Galli L, Patel V, Edwards P. 2010. The effectiveness of mHealth technologies for improving health and health services: A systematic review protocol. *BMC Res Notes* 3: 250. doi:10.1186/1756-0500-3-250.

8. Blaya JA, Fraser HSF, Holt B. 2010. E-health technologies show promise in developing countries. *Health Aff (Millwood)* 29: 244–251. doi:10.1377/hlthaff.2009.0894.

9. Blaya J, Cohen T, Rodriquez P, Kim J, Fraser H. 2009. Personal digital assistants to collect tuberculosis bacteriology data in Peru reduce delays, errors, and workload, and are acceptable to users: Cluster randomized controlled trial. *Int J Infect Dis* 410–418.

10. Lindquist AM, Johansson PE, Petersson GI, Saveman B-I, Nilsson GC. 2008. The use of the Personal Digital Assistant (PDA) among personnel and students in health care: A review. *J Med Internet Res* 10: E31. doi:10.2196/jmir.1038.

11. Cole-Lewis H, Kershaw T. 2010. Text messaging as a tool for behavior change in disease prevention and management. *Epidemiol Rev* 32: 56–69. doi:10.1093/epirev/mxq004.

12. Burton C, Weller D, Sharpe M. 2007. Are electronic diaries useful for symptoms research? A systematic review. *J Psychosom Res* 62: 553–561. doi:10.1016/j.jpsychores.2006.12.022.

13. Dale O, Hagen KB. 2007. Despite technical problems personal digital assistants outperform pen and paper when collecting patient diary data. *J Clin Epidemiol* 60: 8–17. doi:10.1016/j.jclinepi.2006.04.005.

14. Tomlinson M, Rotheram-Borus MJ, Swartz L, Tsai AC. 2013. Scaling up mHealth: Where is the evidence? *PLoS Med* 10: E1001382. doi:10.1371/journal.pmed.1001382.

15. World Health Organization. 2012. Global observatory for eHealth series. Vol. 3. http://www.who.int/goe/publications/ehealth_series_vol3/en/index.html. Accessed April 9, 2013.

16. Batalden PB, Davidoff F. 2007. What is "quality improvement" and how can it transform healthcare? *Qual Saf Health Care* 16: 2–3. doi:10.1136/qshc.2006.022046.

17. Weiner BJ, Shortell SM, Alexander J. 1997. Promoting clinical involvement in hospital quality improvement efforts: The effects of top management, board, and physician leadership. *Health Serv Res* 32: 491–510.

18. Shojania KG, Ranji SR, McDonald KM, Grimshaw JM, Sundaram V, Rushakoff RJ, et al. 2006. Effects of quality improvement strategies for type 2 diabetes on glycemic control: A meta-regression analysis. *JAMA* 296: 427–440. doi:10.1001/jama.296.4.427.

19. Jha AK, Perlin JB, Kizer KW, Dudley RA. 2003. Effect of the transformation of the Veterans Affairs health care system on the quality of care. *N Engl J Med* 348: 2218–2227. doi:10.1056/NEJMsa021899.

20. El-Jardali F, Saleh S, Ataya N, Jamal D. 2011. Design, implementation and scaling up of the balanced scorecard for hospitals in Lebanon: Policy coherence and application lessons for low and middle income countries. *Health Policy* 103: 305–314. doi:10.1016/j.healthpol.2011.05.006.

21. Maru DS, Andrews J, Schwarz D, Schwarz R, Acharya B, Ramaiya A, et al. 2012. Crossing the quality chasm in resource-limited settings. *Global Health* 8: 41. doi:10.1186/1744-8603-8-41.

22. Sifrim ZK, Barker PM, Mate KS. 2012. What gets published: The characteristics of quality improvement research articles from low- and middle-income countries. *BMJ Qual Saf* 21(5): 423–431. doi:10.1136/bmjqs-2011-000445.

23. Stelfox HT, Joshipura M, Chadbunchachai W, Ellawala RN, O'Reilly G, Nguyen TS, et al. 2012. Trauma quality improvement in low and middle income countries of the Asia-Pacific region: A mixed methods study. *World J Surg* 36: 1978–1992. doi:10.1007/s00268-012-1593-1.

24. Wilson RM, Michel P, Olsen S, Gibberd RW, Vincent C, El-Assady R, et al. 2012. Patient safety in developing countries: Retrospective estimation of scale and nature of harm to patients in hospital. *BMJ* 344: e832. doi:10.1136/bmj.e832.

25. Boudreaux AM, Vetter TR. 2013. The creation and impact of a dedicated section on quality and patient safety in a clinical academic department. *Acad Med* 88: 173–178. doi:10.1097/ACM.0b013e31827b53dd.

26. Cohen MM, Eustis MA, Gribbins RE. 2003. Changing the culture of patient safety: Leadership's role in health care quality improvement. *Jt Comm J Qual Patient Saf* 29: 329–335.

27. Mitchell PH. Defining patient safety and quality care. In Hughes RG, ed. *Patient Safety and Quality: An Evidence-Based Handbook for Nurses.* Rockville, MD: Agency for Healthcare Research and Quality; 2008. http://www.ncbi.nlm.nih.gov/books/NBK2681/.

28. Sherwood G, Barnsteiner J. *Quality and Safety in Nursing: A Competency Approach to Improving Outcomes.* John Wiley & Sons; 2012.

29. Advisory Committee on the Safety of Nuclear Installations Study Group on Human Factors. *Third Report—Organising for Safety.* London: HSE Books; 1993.

30. Minvielle E, Sicotte C, Champagne F, Contandriopoulos A-P, Jeantet M, Préaubert N, et al. 2008. Hospital performance: Competing or shared values? *Health Policy* 87: 8–19. doi:10.1016/j.healthpol.2007.09.017.

31. Holleman G, Poot E, Mintjes-de Groot J, van Achterberg T. 2009. The relevance of team characteristics and team directed strategies in the implementation of nursing innovations: A literature review. *Int J Nurs Stud* 46: 1256–1264. doi:10.1016/j.ijnurstu.2009.01.005.

32. Jain M, Miller L, Belt D, King D, Berwick DM. 2006. Decline in ICU adverse events, nosocomial infections and cost through a quality improvement initiative focusing on teamwork and culture change. *Qual Saf Health Care* 15: 235–239. doi:10.1136/qshc.2005.016576.

33. Ahmedov M, Green J, Azimov R, Avezova G, Inakov S, Mamatkulov B. 2013. Addressing the challenges of improving primary care quality in Uzbekistan: A qualita-

tive study of chronic heart failure management. *Health Policy Plan* 28: 458–466. doi:10.1093/heapol/czs091.

34. Slessor SR, Crandall JB, Nielsen GA. 2008. Case study: Getting boards on board at Allen Memorial Hospital, Iowa Health System. *Jt Comm J Qual Patient Saf* 34: 221–227.

35. Jha A, Epstein A. 2010. Hospital governance and the quality of care. *Health Aff* 29: 182–187. doi:10.1377/hlthaff.2009.0297.

36. Joshi MS. 2006. Getting the board on board: Engaging hospital boards in quality and patient safety. *Jt Comm J Qual Patient Saf* 32: 179–187.

37. Curry LA, Spatz E, Cherlin E, Thompson JW, Berg D, Ting HH, et al. 2011. What distinguishes top-performing hospitals in acute myocardial infarction mortality rates? A qualitative study. *Ann Intern Med* 154: 384–390. doi:10.7326/0003-4819-154-6-201103150-00003.

38. Shortell SM, Jones RH, Rademaker AW, Gillies RR, Dranove DS, Hughes EF, et al. 2000. Assessing the impact of total quality management and organizational culture on multiple outcomes of care for coronary artery bypass graft surgery patients. *Med Care* 38: 207–217.

39. McLaughlin C. *Continuous Quality Improvement in Health Care: Theory, Implementation, and Applications.* Jones & Bartlett Learning; 2004.

40. Nadeem E, Olin SS, Hill LC, Hoagwood KE, Horwitz SM, and the Understanding the Components of Quality Improvement Collaborative. 2013. A systematic literature review. *Milbank Q* 91: 354–394. doi:10.1111/milq.12016.

41. Conway PH, Mostashari F, Clancy C. 2013. The future of quality measurement for improvement and accountability. *JAMA* 309: 2215–2216. doi:10.1001/jama.2013.4929.

42. Chassin MR, Loeb JM, Schmaltz SP, Wachter RM. 2010. Accountability measures—using measurement to promote quality improvement. *N Engl J Med* 363: 683–688. doi:10.1056/NEJMsb1002320.

43. Cagnazzo L, Taticchi P, Brun A. 2010. The role of performance measurement systems to support quality improvement initiatives at supply chain level. *Int J Prod Perform Manag* 59: 163–185. doi:10.1108/17410401011014249.

44. Morello RT, Lowthian JA, Barker AL, McGinnes R, Dunt D, Brand C. 2013. Strategies for improving patient safety culture in hospitals: A systematic review. *BMJ Qual Saf* 22: 11–18. doi:10.1136/bmjqs-2011-000582.

45. Sammer CE, Lykens K, Singh KP, Mains DA, Lackan NA. 2010. What is patient safety culture? A review of the literature. *J Nurs Scholarsh* 42: 156–165. doi:10.1111/j.1547-5069.2009.01330.x.

46. Halligan M, Zecevic A. 2011. Safety culture in healthcare: A review of concepts, dimensions, measures and progress. *BMJ Qual Saf* 20: 338–343. doi:10.1136/bmjqs .2010.040964.

47. Quimbo SA, Peabody JW, Shimkhada R, Woo K, Solon O. 2008. Should we have confidence if a physician is accredited? A study of the relative impacts of accreditation and insurance payments on quality of care in the Philippines. *Soc Sci Med* 67: 505–510. doi:10.1016/j.socscimed.2008.04.013.

48. Philippine Health Insurance Corporation. 2004. Benchbook on performance improvement of health services. http://www.philhealth.gov.ph/partners/providers/benchbook/QualityAssuranceProgram_Benchbook.pdf.

49. Pham HH, Coughlan J, O'Malley AS. 2006. The impact of quality-reporting programs on hospital operations. *Health Aff* 25: 1412–1422. doi:10.1377/hlthaff.25.5.1412.

50. Sexton JB, Helmreich RL, Neilands TB, Rowan K, Vella K, Boyden J, et al. 2006. The Safety Attitudes Questionnaire: Psychometric properties, benchmarking data, and emerging research. *BMC Health Serv Res* 6: 44. doi:10.1186/1472-6963-6-44.

51. Galadanci HS. 2013. Protecting patient safety in resource-poor settings. *Best Pract Res Clin Obstet Gynaecol* 27: 497–508. doi:10.1016/j.bpobgyn.2013.03.006.

52. Landrigan CP, Rothschild JM, Cronin JW, Kaushal R, Burdick E, Katz JT, et al. 2004. Effect of reducing interns' work hours on serious medical errors in intensive care units. *N Engl J Med* 351: 1838–1848. doi:10.1056/NEJMoa041406.

53. Were MC, Shen C, Bwana M, Emenyonu N, Musinguzi N, Nkuyahaga F, et al. 2010. Creation and evaluation of EMR-based paper clinical summaries to support HIV-care in Uganda, Africa. *Int J Med Inform* 79: 90–96. doi:10.1016/j.ijmedinf.2009.11.006.

54. Carroll A. 2014. The problem with "pay for performance" in medicine. *New York Times*, July 28.

55. Scott A, Sivey P, Ait Ouakrim D, Willenberg L, Naccarella L, Furler J, et al. 2011. The effect of financial incentives on the quality of health care provided by primary care physicians. *Cochrane Database Syst Rev* 9: CD008451. doi:10.1002/14651858.CD008451 .pub2.

56. Marsh DR, Schroeder DG, Dearden KA, Sternin J, Sternin M. 2004. The power of positive deviance. *BMJ* 329: 1177–1179.

57. Zeitlin MF, Ghassemi H, Mansour M, and the United Nations University. *Positive Deviance in Child Nutrition: With Emphasis on Psychosocial and Behavioural Aspects and Implications for Development.* Tokyo, Japan: United Nations University; 1990.

58. Bradley EH, Curry LA, Ramanadhan S, Rowe L, Nembhard IM, Krumholz HM. 2009. Research in action: Using positive deviance to improve quality of health care. *Implement Sci* 4: 25. doi:10.1186/1748-5908-4-25.

59. Marra AR, Reis Guastelli L, Pereira de Araújo CM, Saraiva dos Santos JL, Filho MAO, Silva CV, et al. 2011. Positive deviance: A program for sustained improvement in hand hygiene compliance. *Am J Infect Control* 39: 1–5. doi:10.1016/j.ajic.2010.05.024.

60. Mustaphi P, Dobe M. 2005. Positive deviance—The West Bengal experience. *Indian J Public Health* 49: 207–213.

61. Agency for Healthcare Research and Quality. 2014. Surveys on patient safety culture. http://www.ahrq.gov/professionals/quality-patient-safety/patientsafetyculture/index.html.

5 Modern Epidemiology and Global Health in the Era of Information Systems and mHealth

Matthew P. Fox and Kenneth J. Rothman

Take-Home Messages

- Public-health interventions may seem as if they would be effective based on logic or intuition, but nonetheless may in reality have no worthwhile effect and, in some cases, even be harmful. Before implementing or advocating for interventions, we need to assess their effectiveness rigorously.
- To be able to evaluate whether an intervention has a causal effect on an outcome, careful data collection and comparisons need to be made. The epidemiologic method can help design valid studies to assess cause and effect.
- Researchers have several major design options available to them to evaluate the effectiveness of an intervention, including cohort, case-control and cross-sectional studies. Each approach has its own strengths and limitations.

As eHealth and mHealth programs and interventions continue to play a bigger role in how we deliver and monitor health care, particularly to underserved and geographically remote populations, it is tempting to take at face value the bromide that bringing more technology to more people will be better for the health of populations, and that investments in these approaches should be made without delay. Unfortunately, the history of health care has shown us that interventions that seem like a good idea may not achieve the expected benefit despite substantial costs. In other cases, approaches that we expect will have a substantial positive effect on health because some epidemiologic studies point toward a benefit may turn out to be harmful. For example, our understanding of what constitutes a healthy diet has vacillated over the past few decades as studies indicate harms or benefits of dietary constituents such as red meat, margarine, butter, eggs, chocolate, alcohol, and refined sugars. This experience should at least give us pause before we rush to implement appealing eHealth and mHealth interventions, despite expectations that these interventions would be beneficial.

Prudence requires that before we conclude that new technology and approaches will achieve worthwhile benefits in terms of survival, quality of life, or other health outcomes, we evaluate the effectiveness of new interventions using rigorous methods. Epidemiology, which is the study of disease occurrence and the application of that knowledge to disease control, provides a toolkit to assess which of these approaches, and in what contexts, are most effective. For a more comprehensive description of epidemiologic methods, the interested reader can consult introductory epidemiology texts [1–4]. Here we focus on epidemiologic methods to help assess the extent to which an intervention causally affects one or more specified health outcomes. For example, if we offered an eHealth intervention to people at a local health clinic and we observe that those who chose to take the intervention experienced better health than those who chose not to do so, how can we infer that the intervention was the cause of better health? It is possible, for example, that those who chose to accept the intervention did so because they are better educated about their own health and engage in more healthful activities such as eating a low-fat diet and engaging in regular exercise. Epidemiologic methods seek to tease out causal connections from associations that reflect the effect of extraneous factors.

The emphasis on methodology in epidemiologic research stems, in large part, from epidemiology's focus on human health. In science that does not involve humans (say, lab experiments on mice or physical experiments) the scientist can exert considerable control over the environment in which she works and can limit many sources of error or bias. For example, we do not let mice choose whether or not to get our test treatment, but instead we choose a population of mice that are genetically similar and randomly assign them to get the intervention or not. This approach allows us to create similar mouse populations, one of which will get the treatment and the other of which will not. Such a design limits the possibility that an imbalance between the populations in one or more extraneous factors (referred to as confounders in the epidemiologic literature), such as genetics and diet, might explain an observed association between the intervention and the outcome.

In studies of humans, there are many instances when it is unethical or impractical to randomize people to the interventions we would like to evaluate. For example, we cannot ethically assign people to be smokers to assess the health effects of smoking. This limitation means that we have to compare populations in which people decide for themselves whether or not to take a given treatment or engage in a particular behavior. Those who opt to be treated may differ considerably from those who opt not to be treated, just as those who become smokers differ in various ways from those who remain nonsmokers. To redress imbalances between the self-selected groups that epidemiologists study, we design studies to limit possible imbalances in extraneous factors, or else adjust for these imbalances as part of the data analysis. Well-designed and conducted nonexperimental studies (studies in which people are not assigned a treatment, but make their own decisions about which treatment they receive) should arrive at the same result obtainable through experiments of similar populations that assign treatments to patients randomly. For example, there is a lower risk of acquiring HIV in males who are circumcised compared with those who are not. This benefit of circumcision was seen in many epidemiologic studies that did not use random assignment of circumcision [5], but later three studies that used randomization found a consistent benefit to circumcision of roughly a 50% reduction in acquisition of HIV [6–8].

Suppose an investigator has decided she wants to assess the utility of an eHealth intervention that electronically monitors pill taking. Specifically, she would like to measure improvement in getting patients to complete three months of therapy for tuberculosis in a clinic in Kenya. The investigator must make critical decisions about how to gather and analyze the information on the study population. Each of these decisions will have implications for how to collect and analyze the resulting data and how well the results will serve as a guide to assessing cause and effect between the pill-monitoring device and tuberculosis. The textbooks cited above provide excellent guidance on each of these aspects, but we will briefly summarize the major issues here.

Study Design

Investigators looking to study the effects of particular eHealth or mHealth interventions typically want to make a straightforward comparison. They wish to compare the proportion of people who get the disease (or other outcome of interest) in those who received the intervention and those who did not receive the intervention. This comparison helps to gauge the extent to which the intervention is associated with a change in the risk of the outcome. To achieve this end, investigators have several study designs available to them to evaluate the effectiveness of an intervention like the pill-monitoring device. These designs include ecologic studies, case series, cohort studies, case-control studies, and cross-sectional studies. We will focus on the last three mentioned, which are those most commonly used for evaluating causal effects.

In a cohort study, investigators typically start with two populations, one exposed to the intervention and one not exposed, and follow these populations forward in time to compare their health outcomes. When doing so, we can improve the study validity by making the intervention and comparison cohorts as similar as possible with respect to other factors that cause the outcome. Such factors are called confounding factors. This balance of possible confounding factors can be achieved through the study design, using restriction, matching, or where possible random assignment. It is not necessary, however, to achieve balance for possible confounders in the study design, because any imbalances for variables that are measured well can be rectified through data analysis, using either stratification or regression modeling. As an example, suppose we wanted to evaluate the effect of electronic step-counters on blood pressure six months later. In a cohort design to evaluate the effectiveness of these devices, we would find and enroll a group of people who chose to use the step-counters and another group who chose not to use them. We could then follow them for six months, measuring the difference in the average blood pressure of each group at the end of the follow-up period. This design is conceptually straightforward and makes it clear that the intervention occurs before the health outcome, an essential requirement for the intervention to cause the outcome. One disadvantage is that if the outcome is unusual, it may require that large populations be enrolled, at considerable expense. A special case of the cohort design is the experimental study, in which people are assigned, usually at random, to receive one of two or more possible interventions. The strength of this design is that the random assignment will lead to approximate balance for all potential confounding variables, even those that are not measured, if enough people are randomized. As noted above, however, it is often ethically difficult or impractical to assign interventions.

Another approach would be a case-control study. With this approach, instead of classifying everyone in a population with respect to their intervention status, the investigator takes a sample of the population and uses that sample, which is called the "control" group, to estimate the proportion of the population that receives the intervention. Consider as an example a study of SMS pill reminders among HIV-positive patients taking antiretroviral therapy to reduce the need to switch to second-line treatment. Suppose we had a way to identify all those within a population of patients starting treatment for HIV who switched from first-line to second-line treatment. Let us consider switching to second-line treatment to be the outcome of interest. We could conduct a case-control study by enrolling all patients who switched to second-line treatment, and a sample of the study population who started HIV treatment. We can then see what proportion of the cases got SMS reminders and compare that with the proportion of the study population who got SMS reminders to assess how much the reminders reduced the need to switch. This design has the advantage of obtaining most of the information about the relation of SMS messages to treatment-switching with fewer people than the corresponding cohort study would require. It is a more efficient and less expensive approach. Some have criticized case-control studies for looking backward from disease to exposure rather than forward from exposure to disease, and consequently being less reliable than cohort studies. These concerns are misplaced. Case-control studies, when properly designed and executed, are valid and efficient [9]. One can consider them to be cohort studies with a sampling of the population to improve study efficiency. For a more complete description of cohort versus case-control studies, the reader should consult one of the previously cited introductory epidemiology texts.

Finally, we can also choose to enroll people in a study and find out about their current exposure to the intervention we are interested in and their current status regarding the outcome. This design is called a cross-sectional study. It is efficient because it does not involve following people over time. On the other hand, it may be difficult to determine whether the exposure preceded the outcome or vice versa. For example, in our study of electronic step-counters and blood pressure, we could ask people if they are currently using a step-counter, and we can measure their blood pressure. But finding an association between the two might reflect a health concern of some people with high blood pressure that causes them to use step-counters as a response to their elevated pressure.

Sources of Bias and Study Error

When epidemiologists design their studies, they need to consider the ways in which sources of bias can cause them to get the wrong answer about cause and effect. There are three general categories of bias that epidemiologists focus on: confounding, selection bias, and information bias.

Confounding factors, mentioned earlier, are risk factors for the outcome that are unbalanced between intervention groups. Confounding itself is the bias in study results that occurs when potential confounding factors are imbalanced. Confounding produces a difference in the study outcome that is attributable to one or more of these confounding factors. To illustrate confounding, return to our example of electronic step-counters and blood pressure, and further suppose we conducted a nonrandomized prospective cohort study. In this study, we allow people to decide for themselves whether or not to use the step-counter. Suppose further that those who do choose to use one do so for reasons that are associated with other factors that affect their health. For example, those who choose to use a step-counter may exercise more, refrain from smoking, and have a more healthful diet than those who do not. Each of these factors could have an effect on blood pressure unrelated to the effect of the step-counter. If we ignore these other factors, using a step-counter would appear to have a bigger effect on blood pressure than it actually has.

There are several strategies that epidemiologists use to control confounding. One approach, for example, is matching each patient who uses a step-counter with a similar patient who does not. The matching characteristics would be potential confounding factors such as age, smoking behavior, level of exercise, and so forth. Matching on these factors will prevent any of them from producing a difference in outcome between step-counters and those not using a step-counter. Matching is useful but expensive, and as stated earlier, it is not a necessary design feature. Other approaches may also be used, either in the design of the study or in the data analysis.

The second bias we are typically concerned about is selection bias, which is bias that occurs as a result of the way that people are selected into or out of the study. Selection bias occurs when the results we observe in those who are included in the study are different from the results we would have observed had everyone who was eligible to be in our study been included and completed the study. Suppose, for example, we conducted a study of the effectiveness of a portable oxygen saturation monitor on pneumonia treatment cure rates. If 20% of those who got the monitor and 10% of those who didn't couldn't be located at the end of the study, we wouldn't be able to observe their outcomes. If this is the case, it might be that those who are left in the study are different from those who remain, giving us a biased result.

The third source of bias we are concerned with is information bias, which is bias that occurs when we are not able to get accurate information from people in our study on important variables like their exposure or their outcome status. Suppose, for example, in a study of the effect of a remote pill-counter device on tuberculosis cure, we assess whether or not tuberculosis is present at the end of the study using microscopy. Because microscopy is not perfect, some people who still have tuberculosis at the end of the study may get classified as if they do not have tuberculosis. These errors can affect our results and prevent us from drawing correct inferences about the magnitude of the relation between pill reminders and tuberculosis cure.

Design Issues for eHealth and mHealth

There are several issues relating specifically to studies of eHealth and mHealth interventions that are worth considering before designing studies of these types of interventions. First, because many eHealth and mHealth interventions involve the collection of data from patients, these tools also have a role to play in the evaluation of interventions. For example, the remote pill-monitoring device collects adherence data on patients in the intervention group of the study and is thought to be better than self-report [10,11]. The improved accuracy the device provides has the potential to reduce the cost of research by reducing the amount of data that would otherwise need to be collected. In other cases, such as the pooled HIV treatment databases being funded by the National Institutes of Health [12], the use of already collected electronic medical records may obviate the need for direct patient contact entirely (see chapter 15, on the secondary use of health data, for more). For Internet-based studies such as the Snart-Gravid and Snart Foraeldre studies in Denmark [13], participants can enter much of their data online, reducing the cost to conduct the study. In addition, because data are entered by participants without direct supervision from the researcher, participants may be more inclined to answer questions honestly, which helps to reduce bias. Each of these benefits, however, may also have drawbacks. For example, whereas using existing patient records may be less expensive than collecting data solely for research purposes, the existing information from records may not be as detailed or have the same quality as data collected expressly for a study. Information on key variables might be missing as well. Such trade-offs must be weighed before deciding whether to employ eHealth and mHealth techniques in data collection.

In addition to the design issues related to eHealth interventions, eHealth also has a critical role to play as a tool for measurement in global epidemiologic research. As cell phone and smartphone penetration reach further into resource-limited settings, data can be collected at remote sites directly from participants and uploaded promptly to remote servers, with large cost savings. Even in cases where it is desirable to have a person gather data, programs to collect data that can be run on tablets or cell phones can reduce the cost of data collection and reduce the need for expensive storage of paper records. These devices are capable of capturing images to record medical conditions or verifying medications, scanning fingerprints for identification and signing consent forms, assessing vital signs like heart rate, using voice recognition to turn voice recordings into text, scanning bar codes, and noting and storing GPS coordinates to allow for spatial analysis. These novel approaches to data collection offer great potential to improve the way new health interventions are evaluated. (See chapter 29 for more discussion of these opportunities.) Nonetheless, as we stated at the start of this chapter, before being adopted these approaches should be assessed with healthy skepticism, as many of them have yet to be rigorously evaluated.

Questions for Discussion

- Suppose you wish to study the extent to which wearing an electronic fitness band reduces the risk of a heart attack. If you simply compare the proportion of fitness-band wearers that have a heart attack with the corresponding proportion among those who do not wear a fitness band, describe a variable that might confound the difference in the two proportions. What could you do to address this problem?

- Imagine a study reporting results from users of a heart-rate monitor program on a smartphone. It shows that the average heart rate among users of the monitor is 84 beats per minute. Would you expect this heart rate to be higher or lower than the heart rate of a comparable group that does not use the heart-rate monitor? Why? Would you expect 84 beats per minute to be a good characterization of the average heart rate among those using the phone app? Why or why not?

References

1. Rothman KJ. 2012. *Epidemiology: An Introduction.* 2nd ed. New York, NY: Oxford University Press.

2. Aschengrau A, Seage GP. 2003. *Essentials of Epidemiology for Public Health* 1st ed. Sudbury, MA: Jones & Bartlett Publishers.

3. Friis RH. 2009. *Epidemiology 101: Essential Public Health.* 1st ed. Sudbury, MA: Jones & Bartlett Publishers.

4. Gordis L. 2008. *Epidemiology.* 4th ed. Philadelphia, PA: W. B. Saunders Company.

5. Siegfried N, Muller M, Deeks J, Volmink J, Egger M, Low N, et al. 2005. HIV and male circumcision—a systematic review with assessment of the quality of studies. *Lancet Infect Dis* 5: 165–173. doi:10.1016/S1473-3099(05)01309-5.

6. Auvert B, Taljaard D, Lagarde E, Sobngwi-Tambekou J, Sitta R, Puren A. 2005. Randomized, controlled intervention trial of male circumcision for reduction of HIV infection risk: The ANRS 1265 Trial. *PLoS Med* 2: e298. doi:10.1371/journal.pmed.0020298.

7. Bailey RC, Moses S, Parker CB, Agot K, Maclean I, Krieger JN, et al. 2007. Male circumcision for HIV prevention in young men in Kisumu, Kenya: A randomised controlled trial. *Lancet* 369: 643–656. doi:10.1016/S0140-6736(07)60312-2.

8. Gray RH, Kigozi G, Serwadda D, Makumbi F, Watya S, Nalugoda F, et al. 2007. Male circumcision for HIV prevention in men in Rakai, Uganda: A randomised trial. *Lancet* 369: 657–666. doi:10.1016/S0140-6736(07)60313-4.

9. Rothman KJ. 2014. Six persistent research misconceptions. *J Gen Intern Med* 29: 1060–1064. doi:10.1007/s11606-013-2755-z.

10. Haberer JE, Kahane J, Kigozi I, Emenyonu N, Hunt P, Martin J, et al. 2010. Real-time adherence monitoring for HIV antiretroviral therapy. *AIDS Behav* 14: 1340–1346. doi:10.1007/s10461-010-9799-4.

11. Bachman Desilva M, Gifford AL, Keyi X, Li Z, Feng C, Brooks M, et al. 2013. Feasibility and acceptability of a real-time adherence device among HIV-positive IDU patients in China. *AIDS Res Treat* 2013: 957862. doi:10.1155/2013/957862.

12. Egger M, Ekouevi D, Williams C. 2011. Cohort profile: The international epidemiological databases to evaluate AIDS (IeDEA) in sub-Saharan Africa. *Int J Epidemiol* 41: 1256–1264.

13. Huybrechts KF, Mikkelsen EM, Christensen T, Riis AH, Hatch EE, Wise LA, et al. 2010. A successful implementation of e-epidemiology: The Danish pregnancy planning study "Snart-Gravid." *Eur J Epidemiol* 25: 297–304. doi:10.1007/s10654-010-9431-y.

6 Global Health and Social Theory

Jesse Feierabend-Peters and Kristin Castillo Farias

Take-Home Messages

- Social theory is a useful tool in designing and implementing successful global health interventions.
- Project implementers should strive to understand the local context in which an intervention is employed through interdisciplinary collaboration, by asking detailed questions about the lives and experiences of stakeholders and community members, and through a consideration of the ways that social forces systematically constrain people's choices and access to health services.
- These steps will help to avert unintended consequences and to foster global health endeavors that offer meaningful improvements in the lives of those who need care the most.

Introduction

Whereas the natural sciences generally operate in a closed system in which variables can be controlled and results replicated, the social sciences seek to unravel the seemingly unpredictable nature of human behavior and interactions. Social theory provides useful intellectual frameworks by which to examine human behavior and the impact that actions might have on a community or an individual. When applied to global health, social theory can also be useful in helping to design successful initiatives and to understand the reasons why well-intentioned interventions may not always yield the desired outcomes.

This chapter will illustrate the ways in which two social theories—Robert Merton's theory of unintended consequences and Paul Farmer's notion of structural violence—can be used to critically analyze and improve global health interventions. First, we will define each theory and examine it within the context of global health. Using examples, we will then illustrate the ways in which these social theories provide a framework by which to evaluate pitfalls that plague global health endeavors when they are not keenly attuned to the context in which they are employed. Recognizing that local contexts can change, and will undoubtedly *be* changed, by the introduction of new technologies, we then argue that interdisciplinary collaboration between the natural and social sciences is indispensable to designing global health interventions that are effective and sustainable, and that offer meaningful improvements in the lives of the people whom they are trying to reach.

Robert Merton's Theory of Unanticipated Consequences

Robert Merton's theory of unanticipated consequences can be used to better understand why some global health interventions yield undesired effects. Merton defines "unanticipated consequences" as outcomes that arise as a direct result of an initial action, but deviate from the designated goal. He identifies that a lack of knowledge is often what predisposes toward unanticipated consequences. Human behavior—as well as sociocultural, political, and economic forces—can be so dynamic and nuanced that attempts to predict the outcome of an intervention may be challenging or virtually impossible. However, Merton asserts that most negative unintended consequences can be overcome by avoiding "ignorance," which he defines as a state in which attainable knowledge is missing [1].

Unanticipated consequences can arise when new technologies are introduced into local contexts. Prenatal sex determination in China provides one example of such unanticipated consequences. In the late 1970s and early 1980s, ultrasounds became recognized as a novel technology that could be used to monitor pregnancy, identify potential complications, and provide other useful diagnostic information. It also offered a reliable means of verifying a fetus' sex, whereas prenatal sex determination had previously been imprecise. As ultrasound technology became more widespread throughout China in the late 1980s, the sex ratio at birth in China rose from 106 males per 100 females born to 111.9 males per 100 females by early 1990 [2]. Supported by population trends, as well as sociological surveys and ethnographic data, many researchers began to postulate that the widespread use of prenatal sex determination and sex-selective abortion of female fetuses may be playing a role in these changing population trends. In one survey of 820 women in rural central China, Junhong found that 36% of abortions conducted among surveyed women were acknowledged to be female sex-selective abortions [3]. According to the 2000 Population Census, the sex ratio for the second child while the first child is a girl reached as high as 191.3 males per 100 females, compared to 103.9 when the first child was a boy [2]. In a context in which strong beliefs about son preference became intensified by China's birth-limitation programs, an important piece of medical technology was utilized in unanticipated ways, thereby altering population trends. Despite the government's attempts to ban prenatal sex determination by ultrasonography, this technology ultimately became a means by which gender inequalities were created and maintained on a population-wide scale.

In order to avoid unintended consequences of new technologies or interventions, project implementers must be cognizant of the fact that any global health endeavor or technical solution is enmeshed in the specific local context in which it is employed and that a project has the potential to impact people and places in ways that its implementers do not expect or intend. Thus, prior to implementing a project, there should be an attempt to formulate a deep understanding of local contexts. Practical means of meeting these ends include involving stakeholders and community members in designing project solutions as well as engaging in multidisciplinary collaboration. Such collaboration should mean that knowledge is gathered and generated in a wider variety of ways, an appreciation of local contexts can be furnished, and ignorance can be more easily avoided.

Structural Violence

Paul Farmer uses the concept of "structural violence" to describe the systematic nature with which the social, economic, and political forces organizing our world exert a form of violence on those who suffer from the most severe forms of inequality [4–7]. Evidence of this violence is visible in the extreme disparities in distribution, morbidity, and mortality from preventable diseases such as HIV, tuberculosis, and malaria. Structural violence can also be used to understand the ways in which the choices of certain populations are systematically limited. Suffering and risk for HIV, Farmer argues, are "'structured' by processes and forces that conspire—whether through routine, ritual, or, more commonly, the hard surfaces of economics and politics—to constrain agency" [8].

Farmer's work in Haiti illustrates the connection between poverty, ill health, and structural violence. Farmer discusses the hardships faced by women with AIDS in rural Haiti and explains that, without a consideration of the ways that these women's lives are shaped by structural violence, one could assume they "had contracted [AIDS] ... because—to use the language that casts them as free agents—they chose to be promiscuous" [9]. Instead, Farmer demonstrates how simply by virtue of inhabiting a world marred by poverty and sexism, some women are at greater risk of contracting HIV [7,8]. Specifically, Farmer's ethnographic research highlights the fact that "the main difference between women in rural Haiti who had HIV and those who did not was the occupation of their primary sexual partner" [9].

In a context with scarce earning opportunities for women, it is advantageous to form amorous relationships with drivers or soldiers—men with higher incomes. These men in turn were more likely to have multiple sexual partners or to interact with sex tourists from abroad, and thus rural women who partnered with these upwardly mobile men were more likely to contract HIV than those whose sexual partners were local farmers. In this environment, rural women contracted HIV, not through a choice to be promiscuous, but rather by seizing one of the few opportunities to make ends meet in a context rife with poverty, limitation, and sexism [9]. In this way, the concept of structural violence addresses the manner in which the agency and choices of certain populations are constrained by factors such as "racism, sexism, political violence, and grinding poverty."

In the case of global health interventions, it is readily apparent that without careful consideration of the forms of structural violence at play in a particular context, unintended consequences may ensue. In particular, the poorest inhabitants of a region may have difficulty accessing the intervention, or the intervention itself may promote greater disparities among various subsets of a population. As Fischer illustrates, "history shows the benefits conferred by technology: lowland malaria clearance in Nepal, south of Rome, and in southern Africa. But these successes also had the effect of allowing higher-caste or wealthier populations to displace or subordinate the original inhabitants" [10]. Thus, while an intervention may improve the quality of life for a particular population, it may also serve to marginalize other groups.

Those employing global health interventions should be cognizant of the ways that structural violence touches the lives of people in the region so that those who most desperately need care can access it. Moreover, as the example of malaria illustrates, though an intervention has seemingly succeeded in addressing an identified need, it may simultaneously cause harm or limit the options of certain individuals. As the notion of structural violence makes clear, there may be systematic barriers that make it difficult for certain individuals to access care. Thus implementers should be keenly aware of the ways that the voiceless, the poorest, and the most marginalized subsets of a population navigate the systems in place so that these groups can also reap the benefits of a particular health endeavor [11].

Conclusion

While a single technology has the potential to benefit an array of communities around the globe, the implementation of this technology in a specific location must be informed by knowledge about that particular context and must strive to predict and to prevent adverse effects. Ultimately, an interdisciplinary approach to global endeavors that includes ethnographic data, and asks detailed questions about the lives and experiences of community members, may improve project outcomes and help mitigate undesirable consequences [11]. Global health technologies should not be imposed upon communities from the outside but should arise from within the community, should have local value, should be operated by members of the community when possible, and should be accessible to the poorest and most marginalized subsets of a population. Local contexts can change, and undoubtedly will be changed, by the introduction of new technologies. Therefore, project implementers must continue to monitor for and evaluate unintended conse-quences even after rolling out an intervention. It is in this fashion that global health interventions will promote equity and increase the likelihood that all people in a region—especially the invisible, the voiceless, the poorest, and the most marginalized—receive quality care.

Questions for Discussion

- What is social theory, and how might it be useful in informing global health practice? What are its limitations?
- How might attention to local context and experience be important when designing global health programs? Provide examples.

References

1. Merton RK. 1936. The unanticipated consequences of purposive social action. *Am Sociol Rev* 1(6): 894–904.

2. World Bank. 2006. Gender gaps in China: Facts and figures. October. http://sitere sources.worldbank.org/INTEAPREGTOPGENDER/Resources/Gender-Gaps -Figures&Facts.pdf.

3. Junhong C. 2001. Prenatal sex determination and sex-selective abortion in rural central China. *Popul Dev Rev* 27(2): 259–281.

4. Farmer P. *Pathologies of Power: Health, Human Rights, and the New War on the Poor.* Berkeley, CA: University of California Press; 2005.

5. Saussy H, Farmer P, eds. *In Partner to the Poor: A Paul Farmer Reader.* Berkeley, CA: University of California Press; 2010.

6. Walton DA, Farmer PE, Lambert W, Léandre F, Koenig SP, Mukherjee JS. 2004. Integrated HIV prevention and care strengthens primary health care: Lessons from rural Haiti. *J Public Health Policy* 25(2): 137–158.

7. Farmer PB, Nizeye B, Stulac S, Keshavjee S. 2006. Structural violence and clinical medicine. *PLoS Med* 3(10): E449.

8. Farmer P. 1996. On suffering and structural violence: A view from below. *Daedalus* 125(1): 261–283.

9. Farmer P, Kim JY, Kleinman A, Basilico M. *Reimagining Global Health: An Introduc-tion.* Berkeley, CA: University of California Press; 2013.

10. Biehl J, Petryna A, eds. *When People Come First: Critical Studies in Global Health.* Princeton, NJ: Princeton University Press; 2013.

11. Gupta A, Ferguson J, eds. *Discipline and Practice: "The Field" as Site, Method, and Location in Anthropology.* Berkeley, CA: University of California Press; 1997.

II INTRODUCTION TO HEALTH INFORMATION TECHNOLOGY

Hamish S. F. Fraser

This section describes the key building blocks for creating and deploying a successful health information system (HIS). It includes a mix of policy and technical issues reflecting the sociotechnical nature of the field.

Chapter 7—entitled "What Are Informatics, eHealth and mHealth?"—provides a brief overview of the background and history of HISs, commonly referred to as eHealth and mHealth. It includes definitions of these terms and what their meaning is in this book. Chapter 8, "Understanding Local Policy and the National eHealth Strategy," introduces key concepts in developing strategy and policies for health informatics. This includes aligning plans with government policy and preparing for successful scale-up and longer-term use of an HIS. Chapter 9, "Databases and Registries," introduces key technical components for almost any HIS and key design issues and lessons learned in the context of existing databases, typically SQL bases and newer designs. Registries are in some sense the precursors of the modern HIS, and this functionality continues to be improved as a component of a scaled-up HIS. Chapter 10, "Electronic Health Records," builds on the previous chapter, broadening it to encompass key functions of electronic health records (EHRs) in a wide range of settings. Many of these core functions and components are described in detail in other chapters, but the EHR pulls them together into one integrated system. Chapter 11, "Communication Networks and Global Health," is included because of the key role these play in most modern HISs, including mHealth systems, EHRs, and national reporting systems such as DHIS2. Network infrastructure and availability is improving rapidly worldwide, but limitations and breakdowns can have a profound effect on the success or failure of projects. Chapter 12, "Health Information Standards and Interoperability," focuses on the foundational issue of incorporating open data storage and transmission standards to create scalable, interoperable, and maintainable HISs. While this can seem complex, with potential slowdown in development, it is an example of the importance of building on the experience of other projects worldwide and leapfrogging many older systems. Chapter 13, "Data Security for Mobile Health Care," addresses another key issue that all HISs must solve, especially if they collect and use personally identifiable data. With the globalization of software and the Internet, data breaches that are seen frequently in the United States and Europe will inevitably afflict all countries if precautions are not taken in the design and use of HIS. Chapter 14, "Enterprise Architectures for eHealth," takes the process of scaling up HIS a step further. It describes how to combine the components, standards, and tools for interoperability and security with user requirements and policy and strategy goals. It also describes a number of tools and frameworks to facilitate this process and successful examples of these approaches in use. Chapter 15, "Secondary Data Use," discusses the essential process of extraction and analysis of health data from HISs such as EHR systems, in many ways the "deliverable" from the creation and use of a HIS. The analyses can support clinical care, resource management, and research. Data analysis from HISs is becoming a key priority in high-income countries, and they have great potential in low- and middle-income countries, particularly with the standardization on a small number of open systems in many low-income settings.

7 What Are Health Informatics, eHealth, and mHealth?

Balwant Godara and Vipan Nikore

Take-Home Messages

- Two of the most common information and communication technology (ICT) terms in health care today are health informatics and eHealth.
- Various terms to define eHealth have arisen, such as "the use of ICT for health" by the World Health Organization and "ICT tools and services that can improve prevention, diagnosis, treatment, monitoring and management" by the European Commission.
- Examples of eHealth include personal health applications such as decision support systems for clinicians, telemedicine, and point-of-care diagnostics, as well as public health applications such as supply-chain management, education for health care professionals, and surveillance applications.
- Challenges in developing and scaling ICT solutions for global health include evaluation, interoperability, privacy, appropriate user design, literacy and language barriers, questions around use of data, and physical infrastructure.

Introduction

There are several well-known bottlenecks in the typical health care process, such as delay in acting on symptoms, delayed or wrong diagnosis, noncompliance with treatment regimens, loss of patients to follow-up, and incomplete self-management. Additional bottlenecks are introduced by inefficiencies of the health system itself—supply-chain management, human resources ill-adapted in number and skills to population's health needs, poor information management, and fragmented care with weak links between primary, secondary, and tertiary care. Resource-limited settings suffer the most from these bottlenecks. This leads to poor health outcomes, such as those defined by the

Millennium Development Goals [1]. For example, the Asia-Pacific regional report for 2011–2012 [2] assesses country performance in eight indicators directly related to the health-related Millennium Development Goals. Of these eight indicators, India is "slow" on five, "regressing" on one, "on track" on one, and an "early achiever" on one. This situation is representative of several low- and middle-income countries (LMIC) the world over.

New alternatives thus have to be sought to strengthen health systems and make care processes more efficient. Information and communications technology (ICT) are proving to be a viable new choice for this. The term ICT includes IT, telecommunications, PCs, mobile phones, sensing systems, and so on. First, mobiles are near-ubiquitous and have become "humanity's most pervasive platform" [3]. This spread is accompanied by an increase in the variety of applications, with voice being exceeded by texting, video, and Internet. Finally, cost per feature is being driven down. A consequence of this accessibility to technology and increase in speed of digital data transfer is an increasing variety of uses of ICT, from agriculture and commerce to politics and governance, and of course to health care.

Defining eHealth, Global Health Informatics, and mHealth

We are still learning the full potential of ICT's impact on the health of individuals and health systems. Thus, as the field remains in its infancy and waits for its true identity to reveal itself, its accompanying definitions and terms also remain in flux, with little agreement around terminology.

Various terms to define the field have arisen, progressing from *electronic data processing in health* to terms such as *medical informatics*, *health informatics*, *eHealth*, *mHealth*, and *ICT-for-health*. Some terms have taken distinct definitions, while some, such as electronic data processing in health, are now rarely used. Subcategories and related terms with similar names, such as clinical informatics and biomedical informatics, cloud the nomenclature even more.

Two of the most common ICT terms in health care today are health informatics and eHealth. The difference between them is intensely debated among professionals in the field, particularly around which term is a parent to the other. There is also debate over whether these terms refer to ICT in the field, or whether they are more broad and focused on any use of computers in health care (for more on this debate, see appendix A at the end of chapter).

The term eHealth is a new definition, dating back to the late 1990s. In the nascent years of the term, there will continue to be debate over what is and what is not considered eHealth, as well as the difference between eHealth and health informatics. Our goal in this book is to help readers develop tools that will empower them to impact and improve health, rather than get caught up in this nomenclature debate. For simplicity, we will use the terms eHealth, health informatics, and digital health interchangeably in this book. We will specifically define the following related but key terms.

- *eHealth.* Recent efforts have tried to define eHealth as follows.
  - o "The use, in the health sector, of digital data—transmitted, stored and retrieved electronically—in support of health care, both at the local site and at a distance" [4].
  - o "The cost-effective and secure use of ICT in support of health and health-related fields, including health care services, health surveillance, health literature, and health education, knowledge and research" [5].
  - o The World Health Organization (WHO) defines eHealth as "the use of ICT for health."
  - o The European Commission refers to eHealth as "ICT tools and services that can improve prevention, diagnosis, treatment, monitoring and management" |6|.
  - o Scott and Varghese describe eHealth as a collection of various implementations within two interrelated domains: telehealth and health informatics [7]. Under each domain are examples such as telemedicine, electronic health records, decision-support systems, and so on. This can be best illustrated by figure 7.1.

Because the WHO definition is very broad, we will start from the definition developed by the European Commission, which is still somewhat broad but more descriptive.

- *Global health informatics.*
  - o "The informatics discipline focused on empowering people to use appropriate technology to provide information-based solutions with a global perspective that supports health care for all" [8].
- *mHealth.*

  Similarly to eHealth, the definition of mHealth has undergone an evolution over the past decade (see appendix B at the end of chapter), but we will define it as "the subset of eHealth that includes mobile phones, other mobile devices, and services delivered via telecommunications networks, the software, platforms, devices, and infrastructure that are used by the mobile" [9].

What Is the Current Status of eHealth?

This past decade has seen a very high number of health programs that integrate ICT elements. These "tech-enabled" programs are to be found in both the public and private health sectors. For example, the WHO's Global Observatory on eHealth (GOe) survey in 2009, wherein WHO member countries self-assessed the ICT integration of their health systems, reported that 83% of the 112 responding countries had at least one mHealth program running [10]. The 2013 eHealth survey by the GOe, which surveyed eHealth in

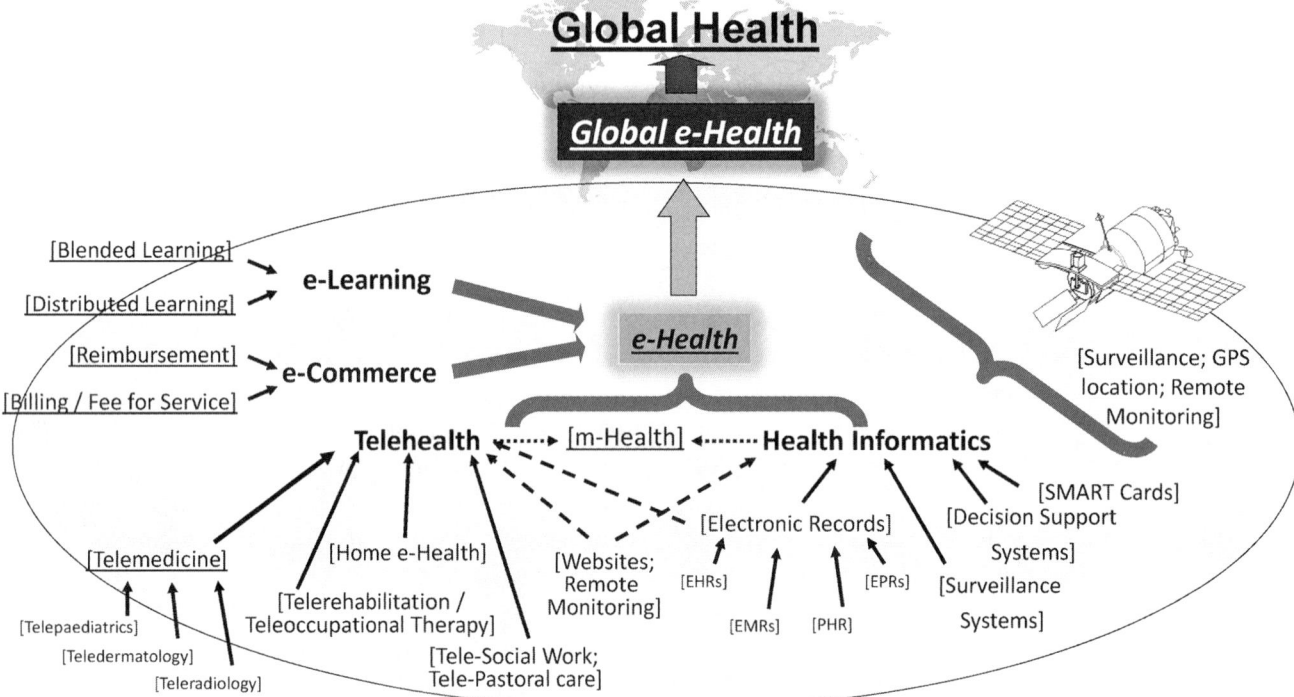

Figure 7.1
Global eHealth. © Dr. Richard E. Scott 2004, 2006, 2009, 2012, 2015; www.ntcehc.ca.

the 75 countries of the Commission on Information and Accountability in maternal and child health, identifies a "quiet revolution" at work in the use of ICT tools to collect data on health indicators, as well as the use of health services by these target populations, and to assess the quality of these services [11]. This picture is completed by a positive sign from the Centre for Health Market Innovations 2012 survey of eHealth in the private sector, which is often stronger than the public health sector in many LMIC: 27% of the 650-plus programs surveyed had "expressly" integrated ICT elements to help achieve their goals [12].

Several recent efforts aim to make sense of this rising corpus of eHealth initiatives by classifying them into different applications [3,4,13–17]. One of the most relevant recent classifications seeks to place mHealth (and, by extension, eHealth) within the context of universal health coverage [18], which is seen as the third global health transition after the demographic and epidemiological. This work is itself built on a 1978 cascading model that illustrates how health systems lose performance because of bottlenecks at successive levels, each dependent on the previous layer. The authors adapt the model to illustrate where eHealth investments can have the greatest impact toward the achievement of universal health coverage. The components of the health system into which eHealth ought to be integrated are grouped into categories of accountability, supply, demand, quality, and cost; suites of eHealth strategies could contribute to efforts in strengthening any given category. This superposition of mHealth strategies on layers of health systems is shown in figure 7.2 below, wherein the different "mHealth strategies" can be considered synonymous with "areas of application of eHealth."

A lack of harmonization of innovations across these different layers of the health system is often responsible for a lack of interest from government entities, and ultimately the failure of many eHealth initiatives.

The following examples illustrate how eHealth is currently impacting global health communities.

- Personal health applications
  o Decision making for diagnosis: decision support systems for clinicians, point-of-care diagnostics, call centers, and teleconsultations.
  o Patient reminders: appointments, adherence, and more.
  o Emergency medical response to persons
  o Self-management devices

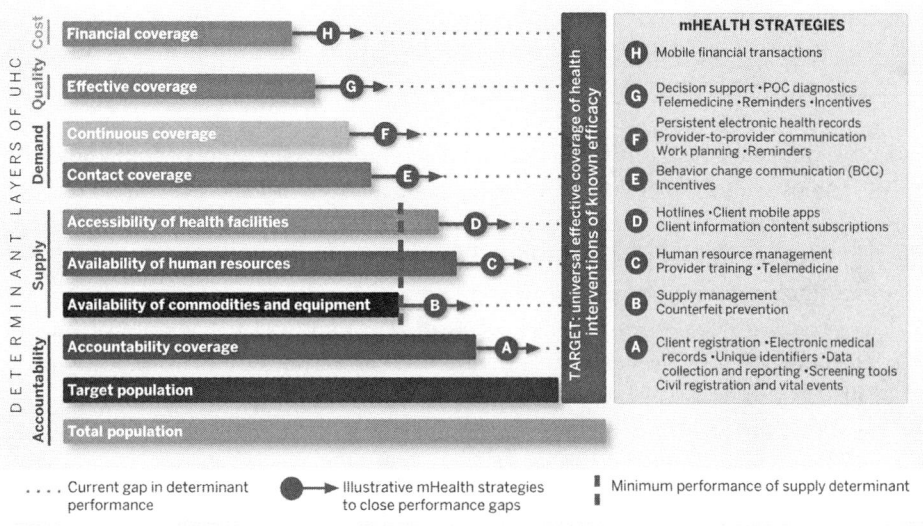

Figure 7.2
mHealth strategies. From Mehl and Labrique, *Science* 345, 1284 (2014). doi:10.1126/science.1258926

- Public health or institutional applications
  - o Data gathering: routine surveillance, disease outbreaks, and so on
  - o Supply-chain management
  - o Financing: payments, insurance, and so on
  - o Training and support to health care professionals
  - o Accountability
- Interaction between individual and public health
  - o Health awareness, information, and promotion to populations
  - o Electronic medical records

The health care area where eHealth is commonly used is disease surveillance, whereas an area that has been slower to adopt eHealth is diagnostic and clinical decision support.

What Challenges Does eHealth Face?

These past two decades have seen an eruption of eHealth initiatives. As a discipline, eHealth is considered to be at a "tipping point" [19,20] between a multitude of small-scale pilots and scaled and long-term integration into health practice. The reality is that most eHealth initiatives fail to reach scale or create desired impacts. Some fear we are being plagued by "pilotitis," with many small initiatives sprouting up without any real coordination or ability to scale. Several challenges prevent most eHealth initiatives from scaling *up* in numbers, scaling *out* across different settings, scaling *in* across different groups in a setting, and scaling *across* different disease areas [21].

One important challenge is interoperability. eHealth has to co-exist and cooperate with offline legacy systems (such as mandatory paper-based reporting and health surveillance). Moreover, technical interoperability is needed within the existing eHealth landscape in a given setting. The example of Kenya is telling: before the government decided to impose interoperability as a precondition to new initiatives, the eHealth landscape had become an "incompatible patchwork of solutions" [3].

A second challenge is a lack of evidence regarding the impact of eHealth on health system performance and on individual health. The lack of formal evaluations of most eHealth initiatives prevents the formation of a solid evidence base, which is essential to gather interest (and investment) from the multiple stakeholders that are invariably needed for any eHealth initiative to scale. The 2009 GOe survey on eHealth found that only 7% of the countries with mHealth initiatives actually evaluated their impact [3]. This evaluation is certainly very difficult, for several reasons. eHealth is often used in conjunction with other health initiatives, and it becomes difficult to ascertain the contribution of the eHealth element alone to any improvements in health care outcomes. Moreover, eHealth initiatives for behavioral change must be evaluated over very long periods of time to discern any palpable impact on the health behavior of individuals or the population. Further, evaluation is a challenge, because technology evolves rapidly and often outpaces the speed of our evaluation methods. For example, it may take months or years to rigorously evaluate a new system that uses a new technology, but by the end of the evaluation period the technology is obsolete. Evaluation is also a challenge because a technology could be successful in one environment, and then in a different environment with different users and workflow it could fail miserably. However, given that there exists a history of failed technology initiatives that have caused serious financial harm to many health systems, it is essential to conduct such evaluations, and indeed to build them into the initial design of the solution itself. Chapter 24 discusses evaluation of health information systems in more detail.

The third major challenge is concern about the privacy and security of data, which are inherent to any system storing and exchanging digital data and exacerbated because of the critically private nature of health data. The confidentiality of data is even more necessary in the case of diseases with stigma attached to them (such as HIV), and in cases where the exchange of information takes place over commercial mobile networks and the storage takes place on off-site cloud platforms (which is increasingly the case).

Other challenges arise from the physical infrastructure available in a particular setting, such as the availability of power supply and connectivity as well as physical devices like servers. User-centric design is also a major challenge, as an oft-overlooked concern is the acceptability of the solution by the destined users. Literacy and language barriers could significantly limit the technology options available for the design, and insufficient user training and perceived "ownership" of the solution by the user could lead to rejection of the solution altogether.

Finally, the most recent, and least understood, challenge is the use of the data. As we see ever-larger stores of data about individuals, populations, and health systems, questions arise about the use of this data to inform decisions related to the health of persons and policies of health systems. Thus, these vast stores of data can and should also be converted into health intelligence. This, unfortunately, is not being done sufficiently.

What Is the Technology Used in eHealth?

Our extensive study of the landscape has allowed us to conclude that, from the technology perspective, most eHealth solutions present a similar architecture, comprised of the following three elements.

- The *front end*, which is the user device and the user interface (website, SMS, or an "app")
- The *back end*, which is the underlying ICT infrastructure (including cloud storage and data analytics)
- The *controller*, which interfaces the front and back ends and decides on the information to be exchanged between the two.

Some examples of these common architectures (front, controller, back) are shown in figure 7.3 below:

In LMIC with minimal resources, for the *front end* it is sometimes better to use mobile devices and connections, which are more accessible and reliable than computers and fixed-line Internet in many settings. Mobile devices can work despite poor fixed-line infrastructure, such as IT material and power supplies. Further, many individuals find them easier to use than computers. These factors make the mobile phone the user device of choice for many eHealth initiatives, depending on the eHealth service provided. The increasing feature per cost and feature per size are likely to further aid the use of mobile devices (be they basic phones, feature phones, smartphones, or tablets) in eHealth.

Remote monitoring allows physiological parameter measurement (and even some microbiology analyses) to be done closest to the patient for a quicker response (such as further referral, start of treatment, epidemic control measures, etc.). This monitoring requires a set of sensors at the point of care, often in the form of a "box" (such as the RxBox deployed in government health centers in the Philippines, or ReMeDi/mDOC used by World Health Partners in India). These devices are often used in conjunction with teleconsultation and electronic medical records.

In terms of *communication*, SMS is considered the best "common-denominator" service for eHealth: it is available in all mobile devices, featured in all generations of mobile standards, used by the largest majority of mobile users, and is the most cost-effective communications means in many settings. The added advantages of asynchronous communication and notification of delivery make SMS a good choice in non-real-time situations. Accordingly, most eHealth solutions today are either designed for SMS or also integrate SMS as one of their data-delivery tools. The disadvantages of SMS are message-size limitations and lack of guaranteed delivery. This is discussed more in chapter 11, "Communication Networks."

The rise of "*apps*," with increasing mobile broadband connectivity and enabling devices, make them an interesting option as future eHealth user interfaces. Most app developers adapt their apps to more than one operating system [3], making them potentially device-agnostic, but each new operating system often increases the cost of the development.

At the back end, there have been several recent efforts to use *cloud computing*, "dynamically scalable and often virtualized resources provided as a service over the Internet" [22]. This relieves the eHealth implementers from heavy infrastructural investments for the back end, besides ensuring data backup in case of problems on site, and the possibility of accessing data from anywhere. The main perceived challenge to cloud computing, especially in the sensitive area of health, is the concern of data security (both for storage and communication). That said, some recent large-scale eHealth programs in resource-limited settings integrate cloud back ends, such as GxAlert for diagnostics and surveillance of tuberculosis in Nigeria. The other major challenge is, of course, the need for 24/7

A Representative implementation: remote monitoring and telemedicine

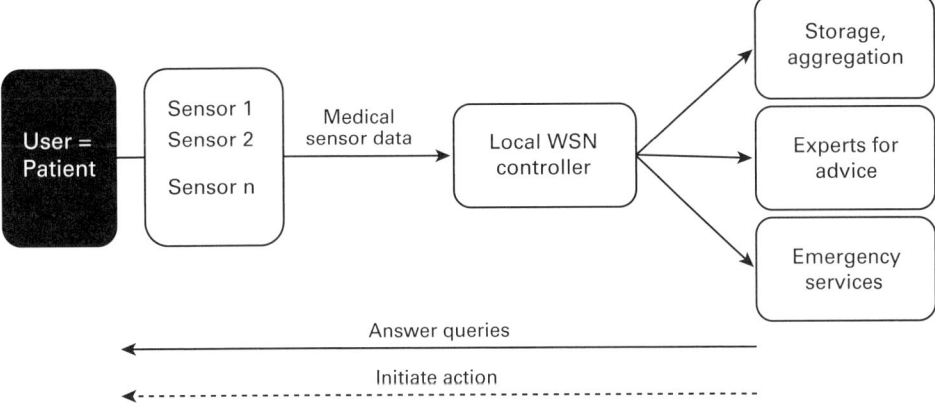

B Representative implementation: treatment compliance

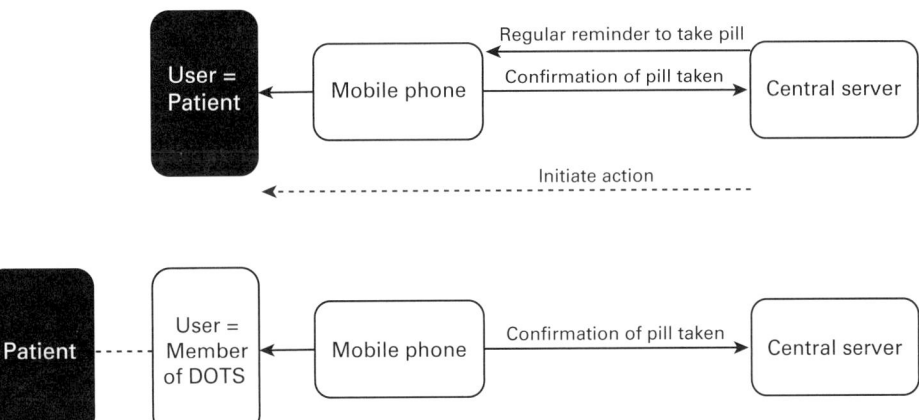

C Representative implementation: disease surveillance

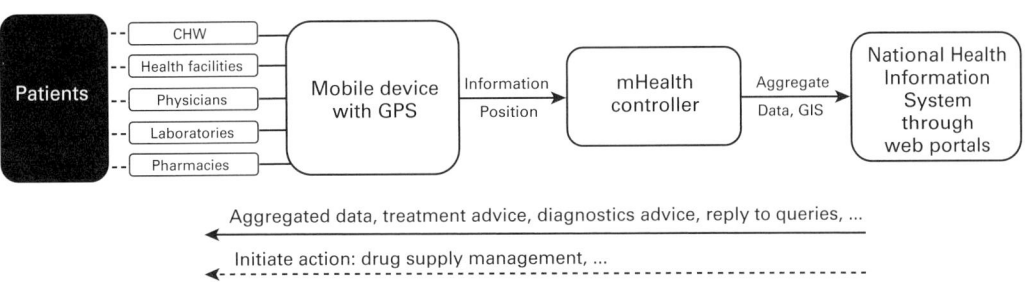

Figure 7.3
(A) Remote monitoring. Critical element: reliable, adapted, and comprehensive sensing technology. (B) Treatment adherence. Critical element: way to ensure direct observation of adherence. (C) Disease surveillance. Critical element: geographical information system.

connectivity (or at least 8/5 for ambulatory care), which is by no means guaranteed in most low-income settings.

Open-source development is also gaining ground for the end-to-end design of eHealth solutions, as evidenced by the enormous spread of platforms like RapidSMS (used in the excellent Project Mwana for diagnosis and follow-up of infant HIV in Zambia [11,23]). Magpi (formerly Episurveyor) and the OpenRosa consortium's CommCare are telling examples of open-source solutions for mobile data collection, aggregation, analysis, and reporting. OpenMRS (Open-Source Medical Record System) was initially developed for HIV and TB, but is also used for cardiac diseases and primary care and in many other clinical areas. Being open source, it can be adapted at several levels, from form creation to addition of software modules and modification of the core code. OpenMRS is reportedly used at large scales in over 25 countries, and many eHealth initiatives (including GxAlert mentioned above) interface with OpenMRS.

Conclusion

The future success of eHealth, both individual initiatives and as a collective discipline, will depend on how well it is able to address the challenges mentioned above. This can be done to a great extent by adopting a systematic approach to designing solutions, choosing the technology best suited to the health care goal being addressed, studying the existing landscape of settings, ensuring interoperability, implementing usability engineering to ensure user acceptance, and building in evaluation mechanisms and models for long-term economic viability. Finally, it is important to stress the "health" part of eHealth rather than emphasize the technology.

Questions for Discussion

- What are five examples of eHealth applications?
- What are seven challenges facing eHealth?

Appendix A

This debate over which is the parent term—eHealth or medical informatics—can be illustrated by a 2005 paper comparing various definitions, which noted that eHealth as a "general theme relates to electronic communication, which is supported by the fact that most definitions specify the use of networked digital information and communications technologies, primarily the Internet. This differentiates eHealth from its parent field of medical informatics, which encompasses fixed technologies, such as X-ray equipment, and pure bioinformatics research" [24]. This definition frames the newer eHealth term as a subset of medical informatics, yet many in the community define eHealth as the umbrella term, one that encompasses the subsets of health and medical informatics.

Appendix B

Similarly to eHealth, the definition of mHealth has undergone an evolution over the past decade.

- In 2010, a definition was advanced to use wireless communications as a means of providing health information [13]: "mHealth is the use of portable electronic devices for mobile voice or data communication over a cellular or other wireless network of base stations to provide health information."

- As the number and variety of projects (and stakeholders) increased, a new definition of mHealth was advanced in 2011 by the WHO's Global Observatory for eHealth [10]: "medical and public health practice supported by mobile devices, such as mobile phones, patient monitoring devices, personal digital assistants (PDAs), and other wireless devices."

- In 2012, another (and broader) definition was proposed [3]: "mHealth encompasses any use of mobile technology to address health care challenges such as access, quality, affordability, matching of resources, and behavioural norms through the exchange of information."

- In 2013, mHealth was described as "the subset of eHealth that includes mobile phones, other mobile devices, and services delivered via telecommunications networks, the software, platforms, devices, and infrastructure that are used by the mobile device" [9].

References

1. United Nations. 2013. The Millennium Development Goals report.

2. UN Economic and Social Commission for Asia and the Pacific. 2012. Accelerating equitable achievement of the MDGs. Closing gaps in health and nutrition outcomes. Asia-Pacific regional Millennium Development Goals report.

3. World Bank. 2012. Information and communications for development: Maximizing mobile. doi:10.1596/978-0-8213-8991-1. http://www.worldbank.org/ict/IC4D2012.

4. Interactive Research and Development. 2012. mHealth to improve TB care. Commissioned by Stop TB partnership. http://www.stoptb.org/assets/documents/resources/publications/acsm/mHealth%20to%20Improve%20TB%20Care.pdf.

5. Blaya JA, Fraser HSF, Holt B. 2010. E-health technologies show promise in developing countries. *Health Aff* 29(2): 244–251. doi:10.1377/hlthaff.2009.0894.

6. European Commission. http://ec.europa.eu/health/ehealth.

7. Varghese S, Scott RE. 2004. Categorizing the telehealth policy response of countries and their implications for complementarity of telehealth policy. *Telemed J E Health* 10(1): 61–69.

8. Richards J, Douglas G, Fraser H. Global public health informatics. In Magnuson JA, Fu PC Jr, eds. *Public Health Informatics and Information Systems*. London: Springer-Verlag; 2013: 623.

9. Payne JD. 2013. The state of standards and interoperability for mHealth among low- and middle-income countries. mHealth Alliance. https://www.k4health.org/toolkits/mhealth-planning-guide/state-standards-and-interoperability-mhealth-among-low-and-middle-income-countries.

10. World Health Organization. 2011. mHealth. New horizons for health through mobile technologies. Global observatory for eHealth series; vol. 3. http://www.who.int/goe/publications/goe_mhealth_web.pdf.

11. World Health Organization. 2013. Global observatory for eHealth. eHealth for women's and children's health. Survey. http://www.who.int/goe/survey/ehealth_survey 2013_en.pdf.

12. Lewis T, Synowiec C, Lagomarsino G, Schweitzer J. 2012. E-health in low- and middle-income countries: Findings from the Center for Health Market Innovations. *Bull World Health Organ* 90: 332–340. doi:10.2471/BLT.11.099820.

13. Kahn JG, Yang JS, Kahn JS. 2010. "Mobile" health needs and opportunities in developing countries. *Health Aff* 29(2): 252–258. doi:10.1377/hlthaff.2009.0965.

14. GSMA and McKinsey & Company. 2010. mHealth: A new vision for healthcare. http://www.gsma.com/connectedliving/wp-content/uploads/2012/03/gsmamckinseym-healthreport.pdf.

15. Piette JD, Lun KC, Moura LA Jr, Fraser HSF, Mechael PN, Powell J, et al. 2012. Impacts of e-health on the outcomes of care in low- and middle-income countries: Where do we go from here? *Bull World Health Organ* 90: 365–372. doi:10.2471/BLT .11.099069.

16. World Economic Forum. 2010. Advancing mHealth solutions: Proceedings of the mHealth Summit at the World Economic Forum, San Diego, California, June 28, 2010.

17. iHeed Institute and Dalberg Global Development Advisors. 2011. mHealth education: Harnessing the mobile revolution to bridge the health education and training gap in developing countries. Report for mHealthEd 2011 at the Mobile Health Summit, June 2011.

18. Mehl G, Labrique A. 2014. Prioritizing integrated mHealth strategies for universal health coverage. *Science* 345: 1284.

19. VitalWave Consulting. 2013. Sustainable financing for mobile health (mHealth): Options and opportunities for mHealth financial models in low and middle-income countries. Commissioned by mHealth Alliance. http://digitalprinciples.org/wp-content/uploads/2015/12/Sustainable-Financing-mHealth.pdf.

20. mHealth Alliance. 2012. Pushing the frontier: The role of mHealth in the fight against tuberculosis. Commissioned by the Stop TB Partnership. http://www.stoptb.org/assets/documents/getinvolved/psc/mHealth%20&%20TB%20by%20mHA%20&%20STBP%202012.pdf.

21. Tolle KM, Curioso WH. 2010. Improving global public health through devices, sensors and mobility. Microsoft Research Faculty Summit, Guaruja, Brazil, May 12–14, 2010.

22. Alamri A. 2012. Cloud-based e-Health multimedia framework for heterogeneous network. 2012 IEEE International Conference on Multimedia and Expo Workshops, pp. 447–452. doi:10.1109/ICMEW.2012.84.

23. Seidenberg P, Nicholson S, Schaefer M, Semrau K, Bweupe M, Masese N, et al. 2012. Early infant diagnosis of HIV infection in Zambia through mobile phone texting of blood test results. *Bull World Health Organ* 90: 348–356. doi:10.2471/BLT.11.100032.

24. Pagliari C, Sloan D, Gregor P, Sullivan F, Detmer D, Kahan JP, et al. 2005. What is eHealth (4): A scoping exercise to map the field. *J Med Internet Res* 7(1): E9.

8 Understanding Local Policy and the National eHealth Strategy

Alvin B. Marcelo

Take-Home Messages

- To successfully implement a national health information system, an eHealth strategy supported by active governance, guided by a clear enterprise architecture, and implemented with effective program management must be established. These elements are foundational and should be made transparent to all stakeholders in order to reap the benefits of eHealth in a country.

Summary

Health information systems are challenging to build because they are complex. They are composed of several components that must work together cohesively for the whole system to be effective.

This chapter describes a programmatic approach to building national-scale health information systems, starting with a thorough understanding of local policies and followed by crafting the national eHealth strategy aligned with those policies. Thereafter, the leadership structure adopts an information technology (IT) governance framework, which activates a series of distinct processes that begin with clarifying what benefits should be achieved within acceptable risks and available resources. These benefits, risks, and resources are then forwarded to a program management team who supervises responsible entities to ensure their timely delivery. The ultimate goal of IT governance is to provide assurance to stakeholders that all activities in a complex, country-wide health information system are aligned toward achieving the objectives of the national health strategy.

Introduction

Various definitions of eHealth exist, ranging from the World Health Organization (WHO) definition of eHealth as "the use of information and communication technologies…for health" [1] to Scott's definition that categorizes eHealth activities related to two domains, telehealth and health informatics [2]. Examples of eHealth include treating patients, conducting research, educating the health workforce, tracking diseases, and monitoring public health. Chapter 7 in this section discusses this topic in depth.

At the macro level, the Global Observatory for eHealth publishes an analysis of the state of eHealth implementation in many countries [3]. In the eHealth Atlas of 2013, a few countries already reported having national eHealth strategies, but many listed have challenges with governance, privacy, and capability [4].

Challenges with Implementing eHealth

Various difficulties in the design, implementation, and maintenance of health information systems have been described [5,6]. These challenges can be categorized along familiar issues such as poor infrastructure, weak organization structures, poor benefits definition, poor analysis of requirements and workflow, poor software design and testing, and lack of rigorous evaluation, to name a few.

In a hospital, for example, hardware, software, network, data, people, and policies must be combined at the right sequence to enable information to flow within the facility. It is widely known and accepted that hospital information systems can be expensive and time-consuming to develop and maintain [7,8].

Such is the seemingly insurmountable challenge that a developing country faces when tasked with crafting its national eHealth strategy. If single installations of hospital information systems are formidable, how much more difficult will it be to do the same for all hospitals in the country? Adding to this complexity is the need to also connect clinics, drug stores, laboratories, and radiology suites, as well as involving key stakeholders of the health care system, such as citizens.

State of eHealth in Asia

While IT has been applied in varying degrees in different parts of the health sector (clinics, hospitals, pharmacies, etc.), country-wide implementations are rare. The Asia eHealth Information Network [9], a network created by WHO to assist countries with their national eHealth programs, has embarked on monitoring country progress as part of its support to its membership. Preliminary results show that while several countries are advancing, their progress is mostly tentative, and all are faced with varying types of challenges.

Why Are National-Scale eHealth Systems Difficult to Implement?

The most common reason given for the scarcity of national-scale eHealth solutions is lack of capacity to design, implement, and support a system [10]. While most of the health IT practitioners in a country tend to focus on facility-based information systems (hospitals, clinics, laboratories, pharmacies), it is rare to find experts who have experience working on projects that directly serve the needs of the whole country. Because a typical health system environment is multicomponent and multistakeholder, designing, developing, implementing, and deploying country-wide health information systems are beyond any single ministry's expertise. Although many ministries of health now accept the important role of IT in health service delivery, most do not have the expertise and language to articulate this desire with enough clarity and eloquence to advocate for and lead the activities required to initiate the necessary reforms.

Local Policy and National Health Objectives

The language needed to support country-wide health IT solutions is ideally expressed in a national eHealth strategy. But the greatest challenge in some countries is primarily the lack of even a national health strategy—one that clarifies the main health issues affecting the population and those that must be addressed in order of priority [11]. If a national health strategy exists, it can serve as the foundation for a national eHealth strategy.

Local policies on health priorities are crucial prerequisites to crafting an effective national eHealth strategy. These priorities define the "business indicators" that are measured to check whether any intervention, eHealth included, is successful or not. Without clearly defined health or business indicators, it will be difficult to justify the high cost of IT as applied to the health sector.

Since decreasing costs of IT has made it accessible to citizens, many stakeholders have started creating their own eHealth solutions to problems they encounter in their environment. Although this enthusiasm and eagerness are welcome, these implementations which proceed without alignment with the national eHealth strategy can further worsen an already fragmented health information system.

It is therefore important that before widespread deployment of eHealth solutions, a national health strategy be formulated, promoted widely, and accepted by civil society. The strategy clarifies what benefits will be targeted in order of priority and simplifies the selection of appropriate eHealth solutions for the country.

In the Philippines, for example, the National Health Objectives 2011–2016 [12] listed the key indicators for each problem domain (e.g., maternal care, child care, tuberculosis, and so on). Moreover, recent policy statements and political strategy constrain which among these indicators get preference. Upon assuming office in 2010, President Benigno Aquino stated achieving the Millennium Development Goals and universal health coverage were his priorities for health [13]. This pronouncement provides a basis for the first domain areas that will become the focus of the Philippine national eHealth strategy.

Challenges with Translating Health Priorities into an eHealth Strategy

Despite the clarity of national health priorities, they do not easily translate into an eHealth strategy. For one, there is a dearth of eHealth strategy frameworks to guide countries. For another, the capacity to write such a strategy would be limited in many developing countries. Scott and Mars [14] published their principles and framework only recently in 2013.

In 2012, the WHO and the International Telecommunications Union (ITU) jointly published the National eHealth Strategy Toolkit. The three-part toolkit describes processes by which a country may be able to define a vision, craft an action plan, implement, and monitor its national eHealth strategy. It is "an expert, practical guide that provides governments, their ministries and stakeholders with a solid foundation and method for the development and implementation of a national eHealth vision, action plan and monitoring framework" [15].

The toolkit specified seven major areas in a national eHealth strategy and provided a methodology for transitioning from vision to an action plan to monitoring (see figure 8.1).

Information Technology Governance

As prescribed by the toolkit, an eHealth vision is an important first step to the national eHealth strategy, but many countries have remained uncertain of what to do next after crafting their action plan. Often, this is due to the unfamiliarity with the role of governance bodies in national-scale eHealth implementation. In reality, technical matters pertaining to the national eHealth strategy are often left to a strategy team. But because

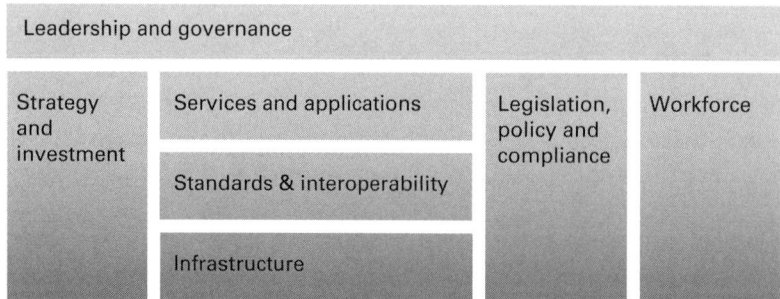

Figure 8.1
Seven major eHealth components from the WHO-ITU National eHealth Strategy Toolkit.

country-wide eHealth implementations are complex and require large investments with far-reaching multisectoral impact, they should be supported by a robust and internationally accepted IT governance framework.

Presently, there are only two IT governance frameworks available as reference to countries planning on carrying out their national eHealth strategy: ISO 38500 and COBIT 5. ISO 38500 [16], or "corporate governance of information technology," is available at the www.iso.ch website. COBIT5 [17] is a "business framework for the governance and management of enterprise IT." It is freely available at www.isaca.org and published by the IT Governance Institute.

ISO 38500 supports top-level decision makers (board of directors, executive, senior managers), while COBIT5 addresses the needs of the same but also extends to IT management and operations. ISO 38500 "sets out six principles for good corporate governance of IT that express preferred behavior to guide decision making: responsibility, strategy, acquisition, performance, conformance, and human behavior." COBIT5, on the other hand, has five domains divided into two main areas: governance and management of enterprise IT. Governance advises the highest decision-making body to "evaluate, direct, and monitor (EDM); while management should "align, plan, organize (APO); build, acquire, implement (BAI); deliver, service, support (DSS), and monitor, evaluate, and assess (MEA)." In terms of scope, COBIT5 is larger than ISO 38500, since the former encompasses both governance and management.

Enterprise Architecture

Leadership and governance covers all components of the WHO-ITU Toolkit (see figure 8.1), such as "strategy and investment," "legislation, policy, and compliance," and "workforce," but a special stack of components ("services and applications" that run on top of "standards and interoperability" over an "infrastructure") require an organized way to keep these different components working together at optimal state. To keep this stack aligned, an enterprise architecture is needed to serve as the blueprint documenting how the health and business priorities of a country can be translated into technology solutions, and how they relate with each other [18].

Managing the enterprise architecture is a key process in COBIT5. This process ensures there is a disciplined approach to ensuring the business architecture and requirements are aligned with the data, application, and technology architectures. The overarching architecture then becomes a guide for all components regarding how they will fit within the national eHealth implementation framework.

One of the key functions of governance is to define and mandate an enterprise architecture for the national eHealth strategy. This architecture serves as a reference point for many stakeholders in the health sector, giving them confidence that compliance with it will ensure they will benefit from participating in the national eHealth program. Thus, it is highly advisable that a clear and published process for defining the EA is adopted and followed.

There are presently four major enterprise architecture frameworks. The United States Federal Enterprise Architecture Framework [19] is one of the most complete in terms of taxonomy and methodology, and is especially constructed to be responsive to the needs of the United States government. The Gartner enterprise architecture [20] is defined by specialists. Zachman's enterprise architecture [21] is a taxonomy of artifacts that describes what documents and policies must be available for each type of stakeholder to ensure there is a well-described architecture for the enterprise. Lastly, the Open Group Architecture Framework [22] provides an architecture development methodology to assist enterprises with crafting and maintaining their enterprise architecture.

Using any of these frameworks, or a combination of them, countries will be able to describe how their services and applications can adapt standards for interoperability and run on defined infrastructure. Access to the architecture by as many stakeholders as possible enhances its ability to guide civil society on how to participate in the national eHealth strategy and how they can leverage their innovations toward a common goal. More details on enterprise architecture can be found in chapter 14.

Standards and Interoperability

Once the architecture is defined, it can now be populated with architectural artifacts that will become the basis for the selection or creation of solutions. These artifacts serve as building blocks that inform implementers how to configure their solutions to become compliant with the business, data, application, and technology constraints of the national eHealth strategy. Since compliant solutions must adopt the same standards, the potential for interoperability is present. In practice, however, there are other issues, such as trust and financing, that can influence standardization and interoperability [23]. Implementers should be aware of such issues, which have proved very challenging in countries like the United States with many proprietary legacy systems. More on standards and interoperability can be found in chapter 12.

Program Management

Beyond the architecture and standards are the actual details involved in managing country-wide eHealth solutions. Program management is a key capability for national eHealth strategy implementations, and inadequacy in this area can stifle benefit delivery. Fortunately, there are programs that can build capacity for program management, such as Project Management Professional [24] and Projects in Controlled Environments (PRINCE2) [25]. Program management experience and continuous quality improvement are keys to ensuring progress in implementation. It should be noted, however, that studies have shown these programs are merely enablers and do not guarantee success. [26].

Monitoring and Evaluation

Monitoring and evaluation are important aspects of program implementation, since they provide feedback to implementers on the status of activities and their affinity to the original objectives set at the start of the project. An effective monitoring and evaluation system aligned with the expectations of the top-level governance body is important in ensuring investments are optimally used. This monitoring must be directly embedded within program management operations and validated through periodic and independent evaluation by third parties. It is through this learning cycle that the processes and tasks involved with national eHealth programs can be optimized for delivering the benefits expected by the principals. More on monitoring and evaluation can be found in chapter 24.

Conclusion

Health information systems are usually dependent on several components and are difficult to implement even in a single facility setup. This complexity increases exponentially in multistakeholder, country-wide implementations. With the scarcity of human resources experienced in developing and implementing national-scale health information systems, it is likely that most eHealth projects will fail to scale.

Because every country will have specific health issues that need to be addressed, a comprehensive, evidence-based national health strategy can help guide and provide input to the national eHealth strategy. The WHO-ITU National eHealth Strategy Toolkit offers a stepwise approach to crafting the national eHealth strategy from a set of objectives. It guides countries to the proper organizational and functional requirements to deliver the eHealth strategy [27].

Thereafter, keys to success are a governance framework, an enterprise architecture, and program management capability in support of the strategy, along with capacity building in policy, design, software development, implementation, and evaluation. It is only through continuous monitoring and evaluation fed back to the governance structure that the projected benefits of a national eHealth program can be definitively demonstrated.

Questions for Discussion

- Why are national health information systems difficult to establish?
- What is the role of information technology governance in national eHealth programs?

References

1. See http://www.who.int/topics/ehealth/en/.

2. See http://www.who.int/goe/en/.

3. World Health Organization. 2014. Atlas of eHealth country profiles 2013. http://apps. who.int/iris/bitstream/10665/112761/1/9789241507288_eng.pdf?ua=1.

4. Littlejohns P, Wyatt JC, Garvican L. 2003. Evaluating computerised health information systems: Hard lessons still to be learnt. *BMJ* 326(7394): 860–863. doi:10.1136/bmj.326.7394.860.

5. Bréant C. 2008. Health information systems: Current challenges and developments. *Yearb Med Inform* 52–54.

6. Luna A, Almerares A, Mayan JC 3rd, González Bernaldo de Quirós F, Otero C. 2014. Health informatics in developing countries: Going beyond pilot practices to sustainable implementations: A review of the current challenges. *Healthc Inform Res* 20(1): 3–10.

7. Heeks R, Mundy D, Salazar A. 1999. Why healthcare information systems succeed or fail. Information systems for public sector management working paper series. Institute for Development Policy and Management, University of Manchester, Manchester UK.

8. See http://www.aehin.org.

9. Kimaro H, Nhampossa J. The challenges of sustainability of health information systems in developing countries: Comparative case studies of Mozambique and Tanzania. *J Health Inform Dev Ctries* 1(1).

10. World Health Organization. 2011. Country health information systems: A review of the current situation and trends.

11. Department of Health, Republic of the Philippines. National Objectives for Health 2011–2016. http://www.doh.gov.ph/sites/default/files/publications/noh2016.pdf.

12. Department of Health. 2010. Kalusugang Pangkalahatan Execution Plan and Implementation Arrangements. Republic of the Philippines.

13. Scott RE, Mars M. 2013. Principles and framework for eHealth strategy. *J Med Internet Res* 15(7):e155.

14. Hamilton C. 2013. The WHO-ITU national eHealth strategy toolkit as an effective approach to national strategy development and implementation. *Stud Health Technol Inform* 192: 913–916.

15. International Standards Organization. Corporate governance of information technology. ISO/IEC 38500:2015.

16. http://www.isaca.org/cobit.

17. Hsieh SL, Lai F, Cheng PH, Chen JL, Lee HH, Tsai WN, et al. 2006. An integrated healthcare enterprise information portal and healthcare information system framework. *IEEE Eng Med Biol Soc* 1: 4731–4734. doi:10.1109/IEMBS.2006.260715.

18. See http://www.whitehouse.gov/omb/e-gov/fea.

19. See http://www.gartner.com/technology/consulting/enterprise-architecture.jsp.

20. See http://www.zachman.com.

21. See http://www.opengroup.org/togaf.

22. Geissbuhler A. 2013. Lessons learned implementing a regional health information exchange in Geneva as a pilot for the Swiss national eHealth strategy. *Int J Med Inform* 82(5): e118–e124.

23. See http://www.pmi.org.

24. See http://www.axelos.com/prince2.

25. Silva de Araujo CC, Pedron CD. Date unknown. IT Project Management Success: The influence of project manager competencies. https://www.academia.edu/7277111/IT_Project_Management_Success_the_influence_of_project_manager_competencies_and_team_commitment.

26. Riazi H, Jafarpour M, Bitaraf E. 2014. Toward national eHealth implementation—a comparative study on WHO/ITU national eHealth strategy toolkit in Iran. *Stud Health Technol Inform* 205: 246–250.

27. Hamilton C. 2013. The WHO-ITU national eHealth strategy toolkit as an effective approach to national strategy development and implementation. *Stud Health Technol Inform* 192: 913–916.

9 Databases and Registries

Mujeeb A. Basit and Susana Vieira

Take-Home Messages

- Data is an essential part of medical care, research, and business in general. The organization and effective use of data is necessary for efficiency and success.
- Two common uses of databases in health care are electronic health records and registries, both of which use clinical information, but registries are population-focused, while electronic health records are focused on the collection and use of an individual's health-related information.
- With the variety of large, unstructured, complex data, the choices in database technology have expanded from relational to NoSQL and NewSQL, which perform the functions of data integrity, consistency, and concurrency that allow high-level systems to work efficiently.

Introduction

Databases were first proposed in the 1960s with the advent of random access storage. They were originally used only for very specialized applications due to their cost and complexity. Today, they are ubiquitous in all aspects of our daily interactions with computer systems. Whether we are doing banking, checking social media, reading articles, or even playing a game, we are interacting with a database that stores and manages our data. Today's databases are significantly larger and faster than anything imagined at that time. The rate of data growth and size has exceeded most expectations. Therefore, database technology has continued to grow and expand to accommodate new forms of data and the different requirements these systems place on the databases.

The first databases were navigational databases, which then evolved into hierarchical databases. These databases required significant custom coding and

were difficult to analyze. The advancement of relational databases introduced more functionality into the database, creating an explosion of database technology. These systems
maintain the integrity and access to complex data in a multi-user environment. They
handle the complex task of data management so that developers can handle the higher-
level systems. Today, a greater variety of databases are tailored to a greater variety of
problems. In this chapter we will cover an overview of databases and key features, including the main types and the use of SQL for relational databases.

What Is a Database?

A database is a structured collection of information, records, or data that is stored in a
computer system. Databases usually contain structured data, including text and numbers,
and frequently they also hold still images, sounds and video, or film clips. In order for a
database to be truly functional, it must not only store large amounts of records in an
effective way, but it must also be easily accessed and added to. In order to have a highly
efficient database system, a program that manages queries and information stored on the
system must be incorporated. This is usually referred to as database management system
(DBMS), and allows users to interact with one or more databases, providing access to all
of the data contained in the database. The DBMS provides various functions that allow
entry, storage, and retrieval of large quantities of information as well as ways to manage
how that information is organized. Both a database and its DBMS conform to the principles of a particular database model. "Database system" refers collectively to the database model, database management system, and database. Physically, database servers are
dedicated computers that hold the actual databases and run the DBMS and related
software. All databases that are created should be built with high data integrity and the
ability to recover data if hardware fails.

Databases and DBMSs can be categorized according to the database model that they
support (such as relational or hierarchal), the type of computer they run on (from a server
cluster to a mobile phone), the query language used to access the database (such as SQL
or Xquery), and their internal engineering, which affects performance, scalability, resil-
ience, and security.

Types

Modern databases are subdivided into three major categories: relational, NoSQL, and
NewSQL. Technically, for example, simple text files ("flat" files) can be considered a
database, as they can meet the definition as stated above. However, they lack some key
features to provide efficient, reliable, convenient, and safe multi-user storage of and access
to massive amounts of persistent data. For example, two users are editing the same file,
and both save it at the same time. Whose changes survive? This is unknown when dealing

with flat files but is something that a database management system guarantees. A sophisticated DBMS can even handle a power outage during the above save, when a simple flat file gives highly variable results.

By far the most popular database type is the relational database. E. F. Codd at IBM initially proposed it in 1970. He introduced the term in his seminal paper, "A Relational Model of Data for Large Shared Data Banks." In this and subsequent papers, he defined key rules and mathematical principals that defined this new database methodology. Codd went on to define 13 rules (numbered zero to 12), which define what it means to be a relational database. Two key rules are: (1) rule 0, the foundation rule, that a relational DBMS (RDBMS) must manage its stored data using only relational capabilities and (2) rule 12, the nonsubversion rule, that a system that provides a low-level (record-at-a-time) interface cannot use that interface to bypass a relational security or integrity constraint. Following the popularity of relational DBMS systems came structured query language, or SQL. SQL is prevalent and easy to use, but difficult to master. The following section will cover SQL in greater detail.

At the time, relational databases had significant advantages over the prior most popular database models, such as graph or hierarchical databases. Graph databases allowed data elements to connect to other database elements via edges. Hierarchical databases were graph databases that only allowed an element to have one parent. These databases were very fast but required more coding for analysis and aggregate statistics. However, these database strategies are again becoming popular as systems are being developed that push the boundaries of RDBMSs.

The RDBMS provided transactional guarantees, known as the ACID principles. ACID stands for atomicity, consistency, isolation, and durability. Atomicity requires that each transaction be "all or nothing": if one part of the transaction fails, the entire transaction fails, and the database state is left unchanged. The consistency property ensures that any transaction will bring the database from one valid state to another. The isolation characteristic ensures that the concurrent execution of transactions results in a system state that would be obtained if transactions were executed serially (i.e., one after the other). Durability means that once a transaction has been committed, it will remain so, even in the event of a power loss, crashes, or errors. In a relational database, for instance, once a group of SQL statements execute, the results need to be stored permanently (even if the database crashes immediately thereafter). To defend against power loss, transactions or their effects must be ultimately recorded in a nonvolatile memory. Each one of these principles is very difficult to implement but provide invaluable benefit during development. These principles are also crucial to the integrity of medical data and protect users from actions that would cause errors in the stored data or inadvertently destroy relationships in the data. A lack of such rules and integrity checks is what makes spreadsheets like Microsoft Excel such poor tools for data storage and management (as opposed to analysis), resulting in frequent data corruption and loss.

Applications in Health

Medical databases serve a critical function in health care, including the areas of patient care, administration, research, and education. The quality and breadth of information collected into existing databases varies tremendously between databases, institutions, and national boundaries. The field of critical care medicine, for example, could be advanced substantially by the development of comprehensive and accurate databases.

Accurate and comprehensive health care data are vitally important for a variety of purposes, as clearly stated in the newly released article examining diagnostic coding in intensive care patients [1]. These data may be used for local assessments or evaluations within a health care system, such as for specific outpatient conditions or inpatient hospital events. The data may also be used regionally or nationally for assessing performance within or across health care systems. In addition, while comparisons between countries become enormously difficult, administrative data may be used for comparison across national boundaries to assess international differences in health care and disease.

Administrative health care databases are valuable in epidemiological studies of disease, particularly for studying the incidence or outcome of rare diseases that are impossible to study locally or within traditional cohort studies [2]. Such data are also uniquely suited to understanding secular trends in disease and examining health care resource consumption for planning the future of health care with respect to diseases and financial allocations.

Health care research databases are most frequently developed for the purpose of assessing the quality of health care, often for a specific disease or within a specific health care delivery system. In the field of critical care medicine, there are databases such as Project Impact Critical Care Medicine (PICCM); the Acute Physiology and Chronic Health Evaluation (APACHE) system; the French intensive care databases Collège des Utilisateurs de Bases de données en Réanimation (Cub-Réa); OutcomeRea; the UK Intensive Care National Audit and Research Centre (ICNARC) Case Mix Program Database; and the MIMIC-II project (Multiparameter Intelligent Monitoring in Intensive Care) database, which contain physiologic signals and vital-sign time series captured from patient monitors and comprehensive clinical data obtained from hospital medical information systems for tens of thousands of intensive care unit patients [3]. Condition-specific registries have been developed with some success, such as with the US National Registry of Cardiopulmonary Resuscitation [4]; the PROGRESS sepsis registry [5], and the institutional Harborview Medical Center ARDS Registry [6].

Outside critical care, there are data collected for primarily administrative purposes, such as the Medicare Provider Analysis and Review database (MedPAR); the Hospital Discharge Survey (NHDS), or the Health Care Cost and Utilization Project (HCUP)–all set by the US government—or databases maintained by the University Health Care

Consortium and Kaiser-Permanente, to mention just a few. As a general rule, in the US corporate databases are proprietary, while government data are publicly available, with some corporations offering the ability to combine regional and national health care system data into a unified database [7]. In countries like the United Kingdom, national health data is publically owned even if collected in proprietary systems, allowing researchers access to data and the ability to link several databases with careful ethical oversight. Recent European community rules may make access to patient data more difficult, however.

Health care databases have been an essential component of understanding and improving critical care worldwide. Investigators have utilized primary administrative data to increase our knowledge of specific diseases, particularly through epidemiological studies. In addition, the development of the APACHE score, the Simplified Acute Physiology Score, and the Mortality Probability Model have permitted determination of risk-adjusted outcomes for critically ill patients and are now routinely utilized for assessing health care quality. As with many health care databases, their use has expanded from the original intent to permit novel research investigations for important areas in health care. For example, the APACHE database has permitted examination of the relationship between hospital volume and outcomes of mechanically ventilated patients [8], the HCUP databases have permitted examination of longitudinal trends in pulmonary artery catheterization [9], and the ICNARC, Cub-Réa, and NHDS databases have provided important information regarding sepsis and factors that influence its incidence and outcome [10–17].

While both electronic health records (EHRs) and registries use clinical information at the patient level, registries are population-focused, purpose driven, and designed to derive information on health outcomes defined before the data are collected and analyzed. On the other hand, EHRs are focused on the collection and use of an individual patient's health-related information. While in practice there may be some overlap in functionality between EHRs and registries, their roles are distinct, and both are very important to the health care system.

Electronic Health Records

An EHR is the systemic collection of the electronic health information of an individual patient or population. EHRs can be comprehensive systems that manage both clinical and administrative data; for example, an EHR may collect medical histories, demographics, laboratory data, and physician notes, and may assist with billing, interpractice referrals, appointment scheduling, and prescription refills. The system is designed to represent data that capture the state of the patient at all times. It is possible to view an entire patient history without the need to track down the patient's previous medical record volume, and EHRs assist in ensuring data is accurate, appropriate, and legible.

According to the Institute of Medicine, an EHR has four core functionalities: health information and data, results management, order entry and support, and decision support [18]. Since all the information is in a single system, it is much more effective when extracting medical data for the examination of possible trends and long-term changes in the patient.

The true promise of EHRs in evidence development is in facilitating the achievement of a practical, scalable, and efficient means of collecting, analyzing, and disseminating evidence. Digitizing information can dramatically reduce many of the scalability constraints of patient registries and other clinical research activities. Paper records are inherently limited because of the difficulty of systematically finding or sampling eligible patients for research activities and the effort required to re-enter information into a database. Digitized information has the capacity to improve both of these requirements for registries, enabling larger, more diverse patient populations, and avoiding duplication of effort for participating clinicians and patients. However, duplication of effort can be reduced only to the extent that EHRs capture data elements and outcomes with specific, consistent, and interoperable definitions—or that data can be found and transformed by other processes and technologies (e.g., natural language processing) into standardized medical ontologies. Besides enabling health care information to be more readily available for registries and other evidence-development purposes, bidirectionally interoperable EHRs may also serve an efferent role in delivering relevant information from a registry back to a clinician (e.g., information about natural history of disease, safety, effectiveness, and quality) [19]. A comprehensive discussion on EHRs is found in chapter 10.

Registries

A registry is an organized system that uses observational study methods to collect uniform data (clinical and otherwise) to evaluate specified outcomes for a population defined by a particular disease, condition, or exposure, and that serves one or more predetermined scientific, clinical, or policy purposes. Registries are focused on populations and are designed to fulfill specific purposes defined before the data are collected and analyzed. EHRs are patient-centric and are designed to collect, share, and use that information for the benefit of an individual.

Other terms also used to refer to patient registries include clinical registries, clinical data registries, disease registries, and outcomes registries [23,24].

A patient registry can be a powerful tool to observe the course of disease; understand variations in treatment and outcomes; examine factors that influence prognosis and quality of life; describe care patterns, including appropriateness of care and disparities in the delivery of care; assess effectiveness; monitor safety and harm; and measure quality of care. Through functionalities such as feedback of data, registries are also being used to study quality improvement [20].

E. M. Brooke, in a 1974 publication of the World Health Organization, further delineated registries in health information systems as "a file of documents containing uniform information about individual persons, collected in a systematic and comprehensive way, in order to serve a predetermined purpose" [21].

The National Committee on Vital and Health Statistics describes registries used for a broad range of purposes in public health and medicine as "an organized system for the collection, storage, retrieval, analysis, and dissemination of information on individual persons who have either a particular disease, a condition (e.g., a risk factor) that predisposes [them] to the occurrence of a health-related event, or prior exposure to substances (or circumstances) known or suspected to cause adverse health effects" [22].

A well-established data registry is the Nacional Cardiovascular Data Registry (NCDR). The American College of Cardiology developed NCDR in 1997 as an exploration into strategies for improving cardiovascular care through the use and application of clinical data. Today, the NCDR is a reputable and dependable quality improvement resource that continues to evolve to meet the demands of the changing health care environment.

One of their success registries is an implantable cardioverter defibrillator (ICD) and lead registry. The ICD Registry establishes a US standard for understanding treatment patterns, clinical outcomes, device safety, and the overall quality of care provided to ICD patients. As the Centers for Medicare and Medicaid Services (CMS)-mandated registry for hospitals that perform ICD implantation procedures, the ICD Registry plays an important role in determining the association between evidence-based treatment strategies and clinical outcomes.

SQL Overview

Structured query language (SQL) is a special-purpose programming language for interacting with and extracting data from relational databases. Due to the popularity of relational database systems, SQL has become the most popular data query language in the world. In 1986, SQL became a standard of the American National Standards Institute. It has undergone multiple revisions, most recently in 2011. Although it is a standard, most database systems create additional commands, which differ across platforms. We will only discuss standard commands in this section.

Tables and relationships define the core data in a relational database (figure 9.1). Each table comprises multiple columns, with each row representing a record called tuple in technical documents. Each column has a specific data type and attributes. SQL data types support multiple data formats, including exact and approximate numeric data, date and time, character or string data, and binary large objects, or BLOBs. Along with the data type, attributes such as allow null, default value, length, precision, scale, and integrity are associated with the data. The entirety of this information comprises the database metadata and improves the efficient operation of the database.

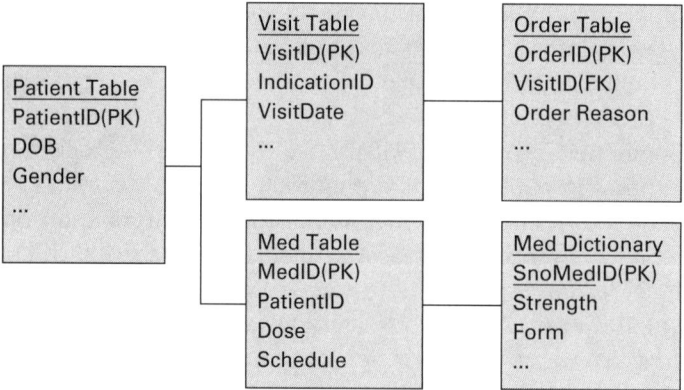

Figure 9.1
Example of a relational database.

SQL is an interpreted language with relatively few commands that can be executed directly or embedded in an application or website. It extends the work by Codd's relational model published in 1970 with a foundation in relational algebra. D. D. Chamberlin and R. F. Boyce originally developed SQL in the 1970s while at IBM. The language is easy to learn, but hard to master. It provides the core commands to perform all CRUD operations; CRUD stands for create, read, update, and delete. The standard SQL commands to interact with relational databases are *create*, *select*, *insert*, *update*, *delete*, and *drop*. These commands can be classified into groups based on their core functions. The data-definition language groups of commands includes *create*, which is used to build new tables, views, and other objects; *alter*, which changes existing database objects; and *drop*, which deletes database tables, views, or other structures. These commands are very powerful and generally not reversible, so extreme caution should be exercised with their use.

The data-manipulation commands are used to interact with data within the database instead of the structure itself. *Select* retrieves certain records from one or more tables; *insert* is used to create a record; *update* changes an existing record; and *delete* removes one or more records. There are also data-control commands that are beyond the scope of this book.

A SQL expression is constructed by unique set of rules and guidelines to make the command unambiguous and easily understandable by the DBMS. The command is constructed similar to an English sentence, with a verb, expression, predicate, and joining elements. In addition, SQL operators allow relatively complex Boolean or arrhythmic functions.

Select Statement

The most frequently used SQL statement is the *select* statement. The SQL *select* statement is used to query or retrieve data from a table in the database. A query may retrieve information from specified columns or from all of the columns in a table. To create a simple *select* statement, you must specify the column(s) name and the table name. The whole query is called the SQL *select* statement:

```
SELECT column list FROM table-name
     [WHERE Clause]
     [GROUP BY clause]
     [HAVING clause]
     [ORDER BY clause];
```

Here, table-name is the name of the table from which the information is retrieved, and column list includes one or more columns from which data is retrieved. The code within the brackets is optional. A very simple select statement example is:

```
SELECT DEXA.TotPFat
FROM DEXA;
```

This query returns all the total percent fat from the DEXA scan table. Although interesting, it would be more interesting to compare this percent body fat to the cholesterol level from the chemistry table. To include two elements from two different tables, the addition of a join operation is needed. The above example expands to the following select statement:

```
SELECT DEXA.TotPFat, Chem24.Chol
FROM DEXA INNER JOIN
Chem24 ON
DEXA.SubjectID = Chem24.SubjectID;
```

The example selects the total percent fat from the table DEXA results and combines it with the cholesterol results from the chemistry 24 table based on subject ID as the common element. The first few results of this query are shown in the table below.

TotPFat	Chol
35.12888344	202
30.08782107	229
27.95192733	192
...	...

Complex questions can be answered by joining multiple tables to create a composite result. The power of relational algebra takes an easy-to-use language and makes it a powerful analytic and data extraction tool. Even with few unique commands in SQL, their combinations make them infinitely useful.

There exist today multiple wonderful resources to learn more about SQL and other programming languages. A good online resource is w3schools.com, which includes a nice SQL section. Other options include SQLZoo (http://sqlzoo.net/); SQL Problems and Solutions (https://sqlandsql.wordpress.com/); and Envato's Tuts+ SQL for Beginners (http://code.tutsplus.com/articles/sql-for-beginners--net-8200). For even more in-depth database information, several college courses are available online for free, such as Database Systems at MIT OpenCourseWare (http://ocw.mit.edu/) and Introduction to Databases from Stanford University (https://lagunita.stanford.edu/).

Future of Databases

SQL and relational databases make for a very powerful database architecture. However, their Achilles' heel is the significant overhead in performing ACID transactions. Maintaining integrity requires additional computational time and processing power. Therefore, larger and larger servers and mainframes have been created to handle these demands. There are limits based on current technology to build ever-larger servers. To scale beyond these limitations, design methodologies have come into or back into fashion. New database architecture known as NoSQL became popular. These systems do not have anything to do with SQL, but loosen the restriction of ACID. Instead, they use the more relaxed BASE principle. (BASE stands for basically available, soft state, and eventual consistency.) Unlike ACID, the system sacrifices consistency for greater availability and scalability.

These compromises are reasonable for handling the large volume of unstructured and semistructured data. As the Internet and all connected systems deal with the continuing growth of the test files, log files, blogs, tweets, audio, pictures, and video, these NoSQL databases and BASE principle serve as a cornerstone of the data-management architecture. In medicine particularly, we deal with the onslaught of multidimensional images and genetic results from radiology, pathology, gynecology, and cardiology. These nontraditional databases are optimized to handle such diverse and unstructured data formats.

NoSQL

NoSQL has very little, if anything, to do with SQL, but refers to the loosening of some of the restrictions that RDBMS imposes such as ACID. NoSQL, more accurately, means not only SQL. These newer systems relax the ACID criteria and focus more on data availability, scaling, and eventual consistency. A traditional RDBMS works best on predictable, structured data. RDBMSs scale well vertically (with a larger machine) but struggle at horizontal (multiple machines) expansion with increasing data size and complexity. Therefore, RDBMSs can become very challenging to manage as the amount of data being stored grows. An alternative, more cloud-friendly approach is to use one of the many NoSQL solutions. A NoSQL database is precisely the type of database that can handle unstructured, complex, and unpredictable data that can scale effectively.

The NoSQL systems comprise four major types: key-value store, column-oriented store, document store, and graph database.

Key-value stores are a simple, high-performance, two-column database. The first column is the key, and the second column is the value. The value can be any data, from a simple number to a large video.

Column-oriented stores are generally a very wide data table, but optimize the organization or the columns so that related columns are stored on the same server. Therefore, transactions do not have to span multiple servers often.

Document stores are similar to key-value stores, but with the additional restriction that the value is an XML hierarchical document. The document is self-describing, so that all or part of the document can be searched and modified.

Graph databases are the most primitive of all database designs, dating back to the 1960s. They store nodes and edges, where either element can have parameters. Nodes represent entities such as "Dr. Brown," "surgery," and "BIDMC" in the example in figure 9.2. Edges are the connection between the nodes, such as "specialist," "department of," and "work at." Navigating graph databases is very fast, and users can analyze the complex relationships to glean knowledge from social networks.

NoSQL offers significant performance improvements with greater scalability when compared to traditional RDBMS. However, it lacks consistency and requires more development to handle those situations.

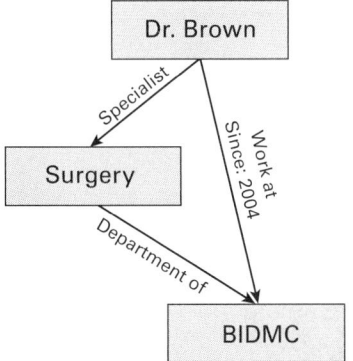

Figure 9.2
Example of a simple graph database.

NewSQL

As the variety of data in medicine has increased with the advent of complex testing such as genome sequencing and expression arrays, the need for different data stores has also grown. However, unlike NoSQL databases, which sacrifice consistency for scalability and availability, medical systems need new solutions, which guarantee ACID constraints. These new systems are called NewSQL, and they guarantee consistency while being optimized for distribution across multiple servers and the handling of large, complex data. They are best for systems with a large number of transactions that are short-lived, touch a small subset of data using primarily index lookups, and are repetitive.

These systems loosely divide in three major categories of new architectures, SQL engines, and transparent sharding. New architecture systems are completely new designs optimized for large, distributed clusters. Examples are Google Spanner, Clustrix, and VoltDB. SQL engines are optimized storage engines for existing database systems. An example is TokuDB, which uses fractal trees to improve scalability of relational database systems. Transparent sharding is a middleware architecture, a layer of code between the server and the application that automatically splits the database across multiple different servers. Examples of this type include dbShards and ScaleBase.

Selection Criteria for Choosing Database Types

Table 9.1
Characteristics of Key Database Types

	Relational	**NoSQL**	**NewSQL**
Structured data	+++	+	++
Schema-less		+++	++
ACID transaction	+++		++
Horizontal scalability	+	+++	++
Performance/big volume	+	+++	++
SQL	+++		++
Advanced analysts	++	+++	++

Open-Source Database Options

There exist several solutions on the market that are very expensive and tailored to the enterprise solution market (table 9.1). However, there are also many powerful open-source, GNU public-license solutions. Currently, the most popular and very powerful solution is MySQL (http://www.mysql.com/). It is currently implemented on multiple platforms, including Windows, OS X, Linux, UNIX, z/OS, and Android, to name a few. It supports ACID transactions, partial referential integrity, two stage commit for transactions, complex joins, and row-level locking. Support for unlimited database sizes and large tables can be implemented with alternative data stores. For example, a table up to 256 TB can be stored using MyISAM. This is a powerful solution that can be used for many implementations. Like most current, well-adopted open-source solutions, there is a secondary industry that offers consulting and enterprise solutions. There are other well-known open-source SQL databases including PostgreSQL (www.postgresql.org).

For NoSQL solutions, there exist even more options. Examples include MongoDB, Redis, Apache Cassandra, CouchDB, and HBase. Please see table 9.2 for a description and key features of these solutions. Examples of NewSQL open-source solutions include

Table 9.2
Examples of Open-Source Databases

Database	Type	Website	Description
MySQL	Relational	www.mysql.com	Relational database implementation with multiple data-store options and extensions. Very popular, with multiple support and consulting options. Acquired by Oracle after it purchased Sun Microsystems.
MariaDB	Relational	http://mariadb.org	A branch of MySQL that became popular after Oracle acquired MySQL. The group's goal is to import all MySQL new code and make it more stable.
PostgreSQL	Object-relational	www.postgresql.org	Object-relational database that supports most standard SQL functions. It allows for definition of custom data types.
MongoDB	Document	www.mongodb.org	Document database similar to CouchDB that supports multiple platforms and is easy to set up for beginners.
Redis	Key value	https://redis.io	Primarily an in-memory, key-value hash and store, but manages persistence by dumping dataset to disk. Persistence can be disabled for better performance.
CouchDB	Document	http://couchdb.apache.org	Document store with advanced document management function. Includes fault tolerance, transformation, and notifications.
Cassandra	Column-oriented	http://cassandra.apache.org	Developed by Facebook as hybrid key value and column-oriented. Used for very large datasets that cannot be stored on one server.
HBase	Column-oriented	http://hbase.apache.org	BigTable implementation that is the native database in Hadoop.
VoltDB	NewSQL	https://www.voltdb.com	In-memory, ACID-compliant RDBMS with shared-nothing architecture.
TokuDB	NewSQL	https://www.percona.com/software/mysql-database/percona-tokudb	High-performance storage engine for MySQL or MariaDB that uses fractal trees to improve performance and horizontal scaling.

the VoldDB community edition and TokuDB. NewSQL solutions serve a much harder problem domain, and therefore require more complex and more expansive options. Therefore, if one needs a NewSQL solution, expect significant hardware, software, and implementation costs.

Conclusion

Data is an essential part of medical care, research, and business in general. The organization and effective use of data is necessary for efficiency and success. The selection of data model and implementation used to be a very simple decision. One would choose either a relational, or in a few cases, a hierarchical database. However, now, with the variety of data, especially unstructured, large, and complex data, the choices in database technology have expanded. What was old, such as graph databases, has become new again. With that come new challenges and new opportunities. These systems are used throughout health care, from primary care of patients to billing and even research and registries. These databases are complex and perform the functions of data integrity, consistency, and concurrency that allow high-level systems to work efficiently. Understanding of data and database systems is necessary for the success and advancement of medicine. Health care providers and administrators are some of the most ravenous consumers of data who need information at the right time, at the right place, and for the right person to make life and death decisions.

Questions for Discussion

- What important factors should one consider when deciding on what database technology to use?
- What are three strengths and limitation of relational database systems? Is there a problem, from your experience, that would benefit from NoSQL or NewSQL technologies?
- What other types of database system are widely used in medicine, and what are the advantages and disadvantages of them?

References

1. Misset B, Nakache D, Vesin A, Darmon M, Garrouste-Orgeas M, Mourvillier B, et al. 2008. Reliability of diagnostic coding in intensive care patients. *Crit Care* 12: R95. doi:10.1186/cc6969.

2. Martin GS. 2006. Epidemiology studies in critical care. *Crit Care* 10: 136–137. doi:10.1186/cc4897.

3. Saeed M, Villarroel M, Reisner AT, Clifford G, Lehman LW, Moody G, Heldt T, Kyaw TH, Moody B, Mark RG. 2011. Multiparameter Intelligent Monitoring in Intensive Care II (MIMIC-II): A public-access intensive care unit database *Crit Care Med* 39: 952–960.

4. US National Registry of Cardiopulmonary Resuscitation; see http://www.nrcpr.org.

5. Vincent JL, Laterre PF, Decruyenaere J, Spapen H, Raemaekers J, Damas F, et al. 2008. A registry of patients treated with drotrecogin alfa (activated) in Belgian intensive care units — an observational study. *Acta Clin Belg* 63: 25–30.

6. Milberg JA, Davis DR, Steinberg KP, Hudson LD. 1995. Improved survival of patients with acute respiratory distress syndrome (ARDS): 1983–1993. *JAMA* 273: 306–309. doi:10.1001/jama.273.4.306.

7. Premier; see http://www.premierinc.com.

8. Kahn JM, Goss CH, Heagerty PJ, Kramer AA, O'Brien CR, Rubenfeld GD. 2006. Hospital volume and the outcomes of mechanical ventilation. *N Engl J Med* 355: 41–50. doi:10.1056/NEJMsa053993.

9. Wiener RS, Welch HG. 2007. Trends in the use of the pulmonary artery catheter in the United States, 1993–2004. *JAMA* 298: 423–429. doi:10.1001/jama.298.4.423.

10. Padkin A, Goldfrad C, Brady AR, Young D, Black N, Rowan K. 2003. Epidemiology of severe sepsis occurring in the first 24 hrs in intensive care units in England, Wales, and Northern Ireland. *Crit Care Med* 31: 2332–2338. doi:10.1097/01.CCM.0000085141 .75513.2B.

11. Harrison DA, Welch CA, Eddleston JM. 2006. The epidemiology of severe sepsis in England, Wales and Northern Ireland, 1996 to 2004: Secondary analysis of a high quality clinical database, the ICNARC Case Mix Programme Database. *Crit Care* 10: R42. doi:10.1186/cc4854.

12. Annane D, Aegerter P, Jars-Guincestre MC, Guidet B. 2003. CUB-Réa Network. Current epidemiology of septic shock: The CUB-Réa Network. *Am J Respir Crit Care Med* 168: 165–172. doi:10.1164/rccm.2201087.

13. Martin GS, Mannino DM, Eaton S, Moss M. 2003. The epidemiology of sepsis in the United States from 1979 through 2000. *N Engl J Med* 348: 1546–1554. doi:10.1056/ NEJMoa022139.

14. Esper AM, Moss M, Lewis CA, Nisbet R, Mannino DM, Martin GS. 2006. The role of infection and comorbidity: Factors that influence disparities in sepsis. *Crit Care Med* 34: 2576–2582. doi:10.1097/01.CCM.0000239114.50519.0E.

15. Danai PA, Moss M, Mannino DM, Martin GS. 2006. The epidemiology of sepsis in patients with malignancy. *Chest* 129: 1432–1440. doi:10.1378/chest.129.6.1432.

16. Martin GS, Mannino DM, Moss M. 2006. The effect of age on the development and outcome of adult sepsis. *Crit Care Med* 34:15–21. doi:10.1097/01.CCM.0000194535.82812. BA.

17. Danai PA, Sinha S, Moss M, Haber MJ, Martin GS. 2007. Seasonal variation in the epidemiology of sepsis. *Crit Care Med* 35: 410–415. doi:10.1097/01.CCM.0000253405 .17038.43.

18. Institute of Medicine. *Key Capabilities of an Electronic Health Record System.* Washington DC: National Academies Press; 2003.

19. Gliklich RE, Dreyer NA, Leavy MB, eds. *Registries for Evaluating Patient Outcomes: A User's Guide* 3rd ed. Rockville, MD: Agency for Healthcare Research and Quality; 2014. http://www.ncbi.nlm.nih.gov/books/NBK208616/.

20. LaBresh KA, Gliklich R, Liljestrand J, Peto R, Ellrodt AG. 2003. Using "get with the guidelines" to improve cardiovascular secondary prevention. *Jt Comm J Qual Saf* 29(10): 539–550.

21. Brooke EM. 1974. The current and future use of registers in health information systems. Publication no. 8. Geneva: World Health Organization.

22. National Committee on Vital and Health Statistics. Frequently asked questions about medical and public health registries. August 14, 2012. http://ncvhs.hhs.gov/9701138b .htm.

23. Dokholyan RS, Muhlbaier LH, Falletta JM, Jacobs JP, Shahian D, Haan CK. 2009. Regulatory and ethical considerations for linking clinical and administrative databases. *Am Heart J* 157(6): 971–982.

24. Hammill BG, Hernandez AF, Peterson ED, Fonarow GC, Schulman KA, Curtis LH. 2009. Linking inpatient clinical registry data to Medicare claims data using indirect identifiers. *Am Heart J* 157(6): 995–1000.

10 Electronic Health Records

Hamish S. F. Fraser and Foster Kerrison

Take-Home Messages

For people planning to develop or implement electronic health record systems in low- and middle-income countries, important lessons from the many years of experience around the world include the following.

- Pay close attention to the use cases and workflow of existing clinical processes and record keeping.

- Try to focus on specific, high value clinical problems first to simplify the initial implementation and build confidence and understanding of the users and organization. At the same time, use an open and flexible design that is not tied to one disease or environment.

- Keep a strong focus on data quality before, during, and after implementation.

- Do not start "from scratch." There are many systems, designs, and lessons learned from previous implementations. Ideally, do not build your own system, but modify and improve on existing ones. This is facilitated by the use of open-source software and modular architectures.

- Carry out evaluations of the system at each stage, especially during the first implementation and if scaling up to larger numbers of users and sites.

- Plan for interoperability and sharing of data between systems, and ensure the use of open standards for coding and data exchange.

- Ensure confidentiality of clinical data by good design and frequent testing of security, by training and supervision of all users, and by clearly informing patients of how their data is used and allowing them to "opt out" of data sharing.

Introduction

This chapter is intended for people who are potentially building, deploying, or evaluating eHealth systems in Low and Middle Income Countries (LMICs), including any electronic system supporting clinical care. To do so requires understanding what an Electronic Health Record (EHR) is, what it does, and the core functionality required for managing clinical data electronically. These issues are relevant for all clinical data-management systems, whether or not the system is called an EHR. In the context of this book, we will treat electronic health records and electronic medical records as equivalent; however, readers should be aware that some definitions treat EHRs as having more comprehensive functionality, including interoperability with other eHealth systems.

At the outset of this chapter, we discuss a brief history of EHRs in LMIC. Then, we discuss the core principles and functionality of EHR systems. Next, we focus on types of EHRs and wider perspectives on EHR use. Finally, we provide a brief discussion of lessons learned in low- and middle-income countries (LMIC).

Evolution of EHRs in Global eHealth: A Brief History

New technologies have driven the increasingly rapid expansion of eHealth on a global scale. Back in the late 1990s, desktop PCs were starting to be seen in hospitals and clinics in low-income countries. Some were meant to assist managers, and a few had applications to help in the delivery of care- but they tended to end up on the desk of the senior manager either way. Out of that era came EPINFO [1], with its tools for medical research data collection and management, which came to be used in low-income countries like Haiti for collecting data for programmatic management and clinical research. In the late 1990s, floppy disk drives were being used for data storage, and the first affordable consumer digital cameras became available with 1-megapixel resolution. Combined with dial-up e-mail, this led to the first boom in store-and-forward telemedicine [2].

A great challenge was affording, shipping, and supporting desktop PCs in low-income settings, which proved very difficult and expensive. Local collection and storage of data was vulnerable to crashes and theft, and the high power usage of PCs prevented most smaller clinics from running them reliably, particularly given the high price of solar power systems then. The Boabab Health system in Malawi was perhaps the first successful attempt to circumvent these challenges in a systematic way and provide energy-efficient systems and cost-effective and well-engineered power backups [3]. Connectivity outside of cities in those days was rare and almost exclusively from satellite Internet connections—expensive, slow, with long latency and prone to technical problems.

An early example of a successful EHR system in use in a low-income environment was the Mosoriot Medical Record System developed in Eldoret, Kenya, in 2000. This was designed to support primary care in the rural Mosoriot Medical Center and developed with Microsoft Access. Patients who were seen at the clinic had a form filled out by the registration staff and clinician, then took that form to the pharmacy if they had a prescription for medications. The forms were entered into the EHR before the patients left the clinic. This system greatly improved the quality and timeliness of documentation and allowed clinical and Ministry of Health reports to be generated, as well as research on public health issues such as sexually transmitted diseases and road traffic accidents [4].

The big technology change began around 2000 with the spread of web-based technologies, including database-backed websites. The first simple web-based EHR systems were starting to be rolled out in the United States. At the same time, dial-up Internet plus some broadband connectivity were spreading fast in Latin American countries like Peru. The logical next step was to use a web-based EHR design for managing clinical data in LMICs. The scale-up of treatment of multidrug-resistant TB (MDR-TB) in Peru, funded by the Gates Foundation, provided an early example. This led to the Partners In Health EMR (PIH-EMR) in 2001, an early "cloud-based" system that had a server based in Boston, and initially dial-up Internet access from two clinics in Peru. There were great benefits in this arrangement in allowing the server to be supported and the system upgraded regularly, with the improvements immediately available to the users. Security was managed centrally, accompanied by local staff training and supervision to protect passwords to and teach the principles of data security to staff. Along with site visits, early Internet-based video conferencing was used to train and support the team and co-design improvements.

Other projects were also addressing eHealth issues over the last 15 years. Baobab Health, in Malawi, discussed earlier, is one key example, and Care2X is an open-source EHR project for hospitals that has been deployed in Tanzania and other countries for more than a decade [5]. Other EHR systems inspired by Care2X have sprung up in Tanzania, such as Afya Pro [6], developed by a local programming company with support from the Dutch government. A number of these systems and their designs are discussed in detail here [7].

Paper versus Electronic Records

Paper medical records or charts have been around for more than a century, and will likely still be in use for many years. There are many practical advantages of paper records, including low cost; the speed and simplicity of creating a basic record; minimal training requirements; no power requirements; flexibility of recording, including diagrams and summaries; ability to create a narrative story; and general ability of staff to navigate a book-like structure. The downsides of paper records are well known: potentially illegible handwriting; lack of standard structure to data collection and analysis, which can make finding key information difficult; difficulty in copying records, resulting in frequent cases of missing records; difficulty in analyzing and summarizing records for clinical care, disease surviellance or research; and difficulty in managing large records for patients with complex or chronic diseases. In high-income countries, paper records have been updated and improved over the last few decades, particularly with the introduction of the problem-oriented medical record. This includes four key sections: history (*s*ubjective), examination (*o*bjective), *a*ssessment, and *p*lan—called a SOAP note in the United States [8]. The key clinical problems identified in the patient, such as presenting complaints, diagnoses, and social circumstances are threads that run through each of the four sections. Some paper records use templates to encourage or mandate collection of key data items in a structured fashion.

An EHR is not just an electronic version of a paper medical record. Instead, an EHR has expanded capabilities, which include the facility to collect, store, analyze, and report clinical data. While these individual capabilities form the core of an EHR, an integrated system typically includes a number of other functions. In 2003, the Institute of Medicine in the United States issued a recommendation that an EHR have eight core functions [9], as follows:

1. health information and data (collection and management)
2. result management (e.g., laboratory tests)
3. order management (e.g., drug orders)
4. decision support
5. electronic communication and connectivity
6. patient support (e.g., patient info sheets, patient portal to access part of their record)
7. administrative processes and reporting
8. public health reporting (e.g., generating lists of notifiable diseases).

An important function of EHRs is the ability to summarize and visualize clinical data in a wide variety of formats. These summaries are typically tailored to specific problem areas and help to pull together the key information in an easily accessible manner to aid clinical decision making. Chronic disease management requires a long-term record of the patient's diagnoses, investigations, clinical course, and treatments. Such data can be difficult to assemble and visualize from paper records (even in well-run hospitals in high-income countries), but EHRs have the advantage being able to generate longitudinal perspectives for subsequent review. This was a major driving force for the development of EHRs to support HIV care in African and other low-income countries like Haiti [10].

Another key benefit of EHRs compared to paper records is the ability to scale up to large quantities of data in each record and to large numbers of patients. Managing such large record libraries in high-income hospitals is an expensive and complex process, and many low-income countries do not have traditions of effective paper medical record keeping. Implementation of an EHR may be the first time effective records have been kept, making the process especially challenging but potentially more acceptable in the longer run.

An extensive list of EHR functions is included in a vendor guideline checklist produced by the US National Learning Consortium [11], but for a first-time implementation we recommend concentrating on the core functions first, then expanding on those as an EHR system becomes established.

Core Principles and Functionality

Planning for EHR Implementation

One of the key tasks *prior* to making an implementation decision is to carefully plan for it. This is a detail-oriented task and should be described in a way that illustrates the strategic and tactical benefits of the proposed implementation to the practice, clinic, or hospital [12]. Especially with a new EHR system, it is important to carry out a formative evaluation of the proposed implementation (which is undertaken before full implementation; see chapter 24 for details). This should include a "reality check" on what is involved, how well it is functioning, and how it will improve care and administration. Generally speaking, there has been insufficient attention paid to pre-implementation planning for EHRs, with few implementations including a formative evaluation or ensuring that lessons learned are incorporated in the implementation process.

Planning reviews, according to E. Coiera, should include both design and evaluation, as follows (adapted from [13]).

1. *Requirements analysis.* What problem is being addressed by what users in what context? Include the roles of different users, use cases, and success metrics.

2. *Functional specification.* Convert contextual requirements into formal technical and functional specification documents, often including user interface designs.

3. *Architectural design.* Develop an architectural design describing how system components interact with each other, including hardware, software, and organizational processes (which may be called enterprise architecture).

4. *System build.* Selection of hardware and programming language and translation of architectural design into functional code to control the operation of each step in the system.

5. *Unit test.* Ensuring that each component is functioning as intended and works correctly with others including creating test cases.

6. *System integration.* Different units that need to share data may need interfaces to be developed. These interfaces and their interactions need to be tested in an integrated manner.

7. *Acceptance test.* After bench tests, a system needs to be field tested with users in a formal, documented evaluation (similar to a formative evaluation; see chapter 24).

8. *User training.* Training is an essential part of an implementation.

9. *Outcome assessment.* Once implemented, systems should be evaluated against the success metrics—in a summative evaluation—to ensure that the original objectives are being met (see chapter 24). This only needs to occur in a few sites generally.

This planning process is complex and combines social, professional, and technical needs, inputs, and outputs. Consequently, planning for EHR implementation requires inputs and reviews from a wide variety of users. Recognizing their diverse and unique needs is challenging to do well. For example, the way a physician interacts with a system compared to how a patient interacts are very different and complicated by their relative situations (age, comfort with technology, technical training, urgency of need, and so on). In LMICs, this problem can be compounded by major differences in infrastructure, health systems, culture, disease burden, staff training, and availability.

Usability Principles

Good usability of EHR systems is essential to helping clinical staff to access them quickly and accurately, and ultimately is an important factor in the success or failure of a project. In 2013, the American Medical Informatics Association issued a list of 14 usability principles for EHRs [14], as follows.

1. Consistency: design consistency and standards utilization.

2. Visibility: system state visibility.

3. Match: system and world match, is it appropriate for the clinical situation?

4. Minimalism: minimalist design, avoiding clutter.

5. Memory: memory load minimization for users.

6. Feedback: informative feedback to users.

7. Flexibility: flexible and customizable systems, ideally avoiding the need for advanced technical skills.

8. Message: useful error messages.

9. Error: use error prevention techniques such as checking data type.

10. Closure: clear closure.

11. Reversibility: reversible actions (until the entry is complete, after which changes must be audited against the user login ID).

12. Language: user language utilization.

13. Control: user control.

14. Documentation: help and documentation.

While these recommendations are primarily written for functional EHRs in a developed health care system and may not always be appropriate in an LMIC context, they provide a development framework. Basic principles exist for design and testing of user interfaces, and these need to be part of the development of any EHR system. As with other aspects of EHR development, it is important to learn from the experience of existing projects with user interface development and testing, minimize the complexity and need for expertise in each project, and maximize performance potential. Chapter 21 discusses user design in more detail.

Patient and Clinical Data Capture

Data on patient demographics and clinical status and care are the primary resource for any EHR Accurate capture, input, updating, and comprehensive retention of historical patient data in a safe, secure, culturally and socially appropriate manner is a fundamental requirement. To operate effectively, the EHR will always require data that identifies the patient (demographics); and typically includes name (four names required in many countries); gender; address; phone number (increasingly patients in LMIC have mobile phones); date of birth; marital status; and other identifiers used to verify that the patient is the correct patient. Some systems will include other patient identifiers (such as tax numbers, etc.), and these data require special treatment because misuse may transgress privacy and security policies and practices. See chapter 13 for a discussion on data security.

Patient data is often collected from handwritten forms or as spoken by a patient and transcribed into EHRs. This can be prone to error, and identifying and correcting errors is typically difficult and time-consuming, so first-time data entry accuracy is critically important. In the past, insufficient emphasis has been placed on the issue of data quality in EHR systems worldwide but new initiatives are working to address that [15]. Speed and accuracy of patient identification is important for staff and patients [16], and a dedicated identification application such as a master patient index is typically a component of an eHealth architecture (see chapters 9 and 14).

Clinical data capture and entry is at the core of every EHR system. Clinical data includes the presenting complaint, diagnoses, vital signs, prescriptions, drug interactions, test results, and treatment plans and orders. The accuracy of these data is vital to the patient record and subsequent physician review. Where feasible, these data should be collected in a structured and coded form to allow use for quality improvement, analysis, and decision support. Free text data, while valuable for direct patient care and to create the clinical "story," are difficult to analyze, except to a limited extent with natural language processing software.

EHRs are particularly useful in prescribing and in maintaining the accuracy of pharmacy data, since many now contain registries of formularies, drug strengths, generic alternatives, adverse reactions, and so on. These can be called up in order entry systems, thus reducing the dangers of inaccurate prescribing, adverse drug events, and improper recording and their associated risk. Modular input devices such as bar-code scanners enhance accuracy, ensuring that the correct patients get the medication prescribed at the appropriate time and manner. Scanning of patient ID bracelets to confirm identity each time medications are given has been shown to reduce medical errors [17], and is feasible even in LMICs. See chapter 26, "Clinical Decision Support," for a more in-depth discussion of drug ordering and reducing errors.

Clinical Decision Support

Management of complex conditions can be assisted by the application of a clinical decision-support system (CDSS). These are usually based on rules that allow comparison of patient data and determine if certain actions are required by clinicians. A CDSS can warn of inappropriate treatment, inaccurate diagnoses, the potential for adverse drug reactions, or incompatible drug prescribing, for example. Designing accurate and useful alerts and reminders in an EHR system is difficult, and these notifications can be a source of clinician fatigue and distraction, resulting high levels of overriding [18–21]. Analysis of alert overrides typically show that high alert rejection rates are based on reasonable clinical judgment and often related to missing or inaccurate data [22], suggesting that there is a need to improve alert specificity and data quality. It is important to recognize that clinicians are trained to make clinical and medical treatment decisions, and, therefore, CDSS recommendations are considered supportive in nature to the clinician in charge. If less highly trained staff, such as community health care workers, use a CDSS, the responsibility for accurate and safe advice should potentially fall more on the system developers and the health system. These issues are described in more detail in chapter 26.

Standardization of Coding and Data Use

Standardization of data input maximizes the system capability of an EHR. A paper record, on the other hand, has limited capacity for structured systematic input, and retrieval of data depends entirely on a manual review of prior notes. These are typically unstructured, and consequently prone to error and misunderstanding, although some paper notes make good use of structured forms. Standardized clinical codes that represent diagnoses and treatment decisions enhance the capability to share data among clinicians and specialists, and this key attribute reduces ambiguity and misunderstanding. Alignment to the service-delivery model is also improved through use of EHR technology and standardization [23].

Standard diagnostic and treatment codes are the cornerstone of information gathering, reporting, and analysis. This is the core capability of an EHR in constructing a longitudinal patient record, which illustrates trends and interrelationships that would be inefficient or impossible to recreate from a paper-based record. However, accurate and specific coding of clinical data is a skilled and time-consuming task.

Interoperability describes the capability to transmit patient data to other clinical sites; for example, an emergency room sending a discharge notice to a primary care physician for follow-up, or a laboratory sending results back to the EHR. This is facilitated by standardized codes and structures, allowing the data to be integrated into the patient record in both locations and ensuring the meaning of data is equivalent in each site, a process described as "semantic interoperability." Coding, interoperability, and eHealth architectures are described in detail in chapters 12 and 14.

With increasing EHR penetration, more clinical data has become available, which is leading to an increase in calls for data by the research community and research funding agencies. Because of the standardization of data elements, EHR data can be more compatible with research protocols than paper-based records. However, a major concern is ensuring patient data is subjected to privacy and access constraints, irrespective of whether it is paper-based or in an EHR (see chapter 22).

A valuable capacity of EHRs is to generate follow-up lists for patients with chronic illness. Physicians can set outcome targets for each patient as a useful tool for emotional, aspirational, and motivational use. Care outcomes can be measured more effectively and quickly with EHR systems than on paper, and as payment models move from treatment activity to patient outcomes in the United States and some other countries, this will become increasingly important.

EHR systems can be used to improve a number of other nonclinical requirements; for example, the ability to identify use of resources and supplies and conduct supply chain management (including medications, surgical supplies, food, energy, facilities, etc.). Clinical data in EHR systems has been shown to improve drug requirement forecasting [24,25] (also see chapters 27 and 34). Other benefits include assisting with human resource management.

EHR Choices and Constraints

Making good choices in EHR selection is critical to the ultimate success of an EHR implementation project. It is also important to recognize that implementation requires a significant human resource commitment in design, implementation, and training. There is a strong argument in favor of well-structured evaluations being undertaken before choosing a system. In a survey of nearly 17,000 EHR users in 2013 by Black Book Rankings, 31% stated they would like to change EHR vendors and that 17% would change systems in the next 12 months [26]. This implies a significant additional and unnecessary cost in financial and human resources, and also suggests that implementers did not undertake a good assessment of requirements before implementing their system or a formative evaluation.

Once implemented, an EHR tends to lead initially to a loss of physician productivity, partly due to the structured application of the system, which is often disruptive to workflow. In addition, some patients have reported that they feel that they are not part of the process any longer, so the choice of system also needs to consider workflow integration. Failure to rapidly deliver appropriate and accurate data to the clinician at the point of care affects the clinician's work practice. A 2012 study of nurses in Turkey indicated that a high proportion of nurses felt "EHR systems were not well integrated into their workflow" [27]. It is likely that in the longer term, the ability to find key data in longitudinal EHR records and improve diagnosis, patient tracking, and laboratory data management will lead to productivity gains, but these are harder to measure than the immediate extra workload of data entry for clinicians. In addition, some well-designed applications reduce clinician workload, such as a system for collecting vital signs data in hospitals in Oxford, UK, which reduced nursing time for this activity by 20% [D. Wong, personal communication]. There is also evidence that more effective patient registration and labeling of laboratory samples in Malawi can save clinician time and lab resources [28].

Lack of system support and upgrades are often a source of concern to physicians and health systems. If a vendor goes out of business or is acquired by another business, that can lead to a significant change in that vendor's business relationship, often affecting system upgrades, customization, and so on. Vendors and their systems should be included in evaluations. Use of EHRs based on open-source software can reduce the risks from vendors failing, dropping support for a product, or increasing prices, a particular concern in LMICs, which typically lack resources to pay for replacement systems.

Wider EHR Perspectives

Primary Care EHR systems

Many countries in Europe as well as Australia and New Zealand have developed primary care EHR systems that are very widely used. In the United Kingdom, for example, virtually 100% of 64 million citizens have records in such EHRs, with early versions going back more than two decades. Currently two systems, both web-based, SystmOne and EMIS, cover almost 57 million patients in England and Wales. SystmOne allows local practices to configure forms and reports without requiring programming. Patient data can be downloaded from one primary care EHR system in the United Kingdom and uploaded to another, but in many cases it is just a question of the system administrator (e.g., SystmOne) changing permissions to allow a different primary care physician access. Increasingly, laboratory data is sent electronically to the EHR systems in the

United Kingdom and automatically uploaded. These EHR system have successfully overcome the challenges to achieve widespread usage and high levels of clinician satisfaction, which is likely due in part to the long experience of EHR systems in UK primary care [29].

Personal Health Records

Patients are concerned about *their* health more than aggregation of health outcomes or treatment, so in principle, systems that recognize and service personal needs should be popular. Personal health records (PHRs) can be grouped into those that provide access to the patient's EHR record managed by a hospital through a web portal, and those that allow patients to enter their own data. Some systems combine both functions, such as the pioneering INDIVO system [30]. PHRs have been slow to take off, although some organizations have achieved high uptake of patient portals, such as the US government's Veterans Administration with their open-source VistA system [31]. There are a growing number of personal mHealth applications, particularly for topics like weight management and exercise. The integration of patient information is an important function of EHRs, and as patients become more familiar with EHRs, they will likely demand more effective integration of their information into their official EHR and the ability to view it themselves. Some systems allow patients (or the parents of pediatric patients) to enter data into the hospital EHR via specialized paper or electronic forms. These have proved useful in improving completeness of data and speeding up consultations [32]. In low-income settings, some initiatives are giving patients access to key data, such as laboratory results [33]. In Jordan, a number of hospitals now use the VistA EHR system and are implementing a PHR component.

Telehealth and Telemedicine

Many LMIC have populations in remote and hard-to-reach areas, but these areas increasingly have access to the Internet via mobile phones, satellite, or broadband. In addition, there is increasing availability of image- and data-capture devices (photographic, standalone, or wearable devices such as heart-rate and blood-pressure monitors, etc.), offering opportunities for telehealth. Telereferral and consultation from remote locations is frequently a viable option—particularly when specialist medical resources are not available locally. This can best be accomplished as part of an integrated web-based EHR. When there is likely to be a need, telehealth should be considered in the planning process for an EHR implementation, as opposed to setting up a standalone telemedicine system. A trial of sharing primary care records with hospital specialists is currently underway in the United Kingdom with SystmOne in the city of Bradford [34]. A related project allows the sharing of the primary care record between the doctor and the nurses looking after patients in care homes [35]. In both cases, the patients have to consent to the record being shared.

Image-intensive telemedicine applications, such as in radiology reporting, dermatology, and ophthalmology, have had an impact on care processes. In addition, there is some evidence of improvements in quality of care and health-service utilization in high-income countries [36], particularly for more seriously ill patients, but overall there is limited rigorous evidence of benefits from telehealth in LMICs to date. Chapter 25 discusses telemedicine in more detail.

Lessons Learned and Case Studies

In this section, we discuss challenges and learning points from the development and implementation of the PIH-EMR to support MDR-TB and HIV care mentioned at the beginning of this chapter. The PIH-EMR was designed to support several functions:

- Clinical care, through direct use by clinicians and through analysis and reports on quality of care
- Reports to Ministry of Health and funders
- Logistics and supply-chain management
- Clinical research.

The system provided a platform for implementation of important informatics innovations in a new environment. Figure 10.1 shows the different data types collected in the system.

Fraser and colleagues [37] described the different applications developed in the early stages of the project. As shown in figure 10.1, an mHealth component was also added that collected laboratory data in over 100 small health centers using Palm Pilots [38]. Despite the older technologies involved, the basic principles and many of the problems are the same for EHR systems and implementations used in LMICs today.

Data quality and completeness were the biggest challenge, and remain so for most projects today. A range of tools for data validation and reports of data quality were implemented with some success, but training and direct "buy in" by users was and remains critical. The system provided data for several highly influential studies on MDR-TB [39] but that data set had to be very extensively "cleaned," another lesson on the importance of monitoring data quality and completeness early and often. Another challenge was local IT and software support once the system was established—this slowly took place through training of local programmers. In another paper, Fraser and colleagues describe the work on MDR-TB and how it has been taken forward into current projects [40].

The next step in the PIH-EMR project was to implement the system in 2002 in Haiti to support the care of HIV patients. This required extensive modification of the system

PIH-EMR Data

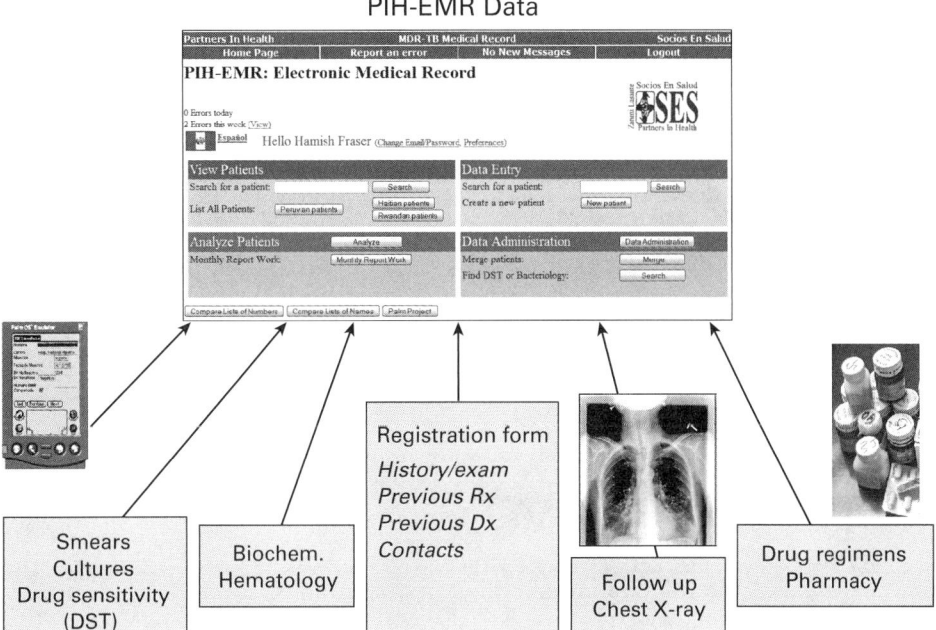

Figure 10.1
PIH-EMR data. Copyright H. Fraser.

and translation into French. The biggest challenge then (and in many sites to this day) was poor infrastructure and unreliable power and Internet connectivity. This was a critical issue for the cloud-based design and required the development of a simple offline application that allowed offline viewing of a limited subset of patient's records and the entry of follow-up forms. This data was then synchronized with the EHR web server when the Internet was available [41].

Another important lesson was the importance of collection and use of laboratory data for both MDR-TB and HIV. In Haiti, CD4 counts (an indicator of the condition of the immune system in HIV patients) were entered into the EHR in the lab, and alerts and reminders were generated for abnormal results. Figure 10.2 shows an example of CD4 count alerts in an e-mail generated by the system and sent daily to the clinical team since 2003. The e-mails are especially intended to flag patients who do not yet have an antiretroviral therapy regimen for HIV entered into the system—a critical quality-of-care issue.

Although simple in principle, this form of decision support (originally designed with P. Farmer at Partners In Health) has been heavily used and often initiates clinical discussions in e-mail exchanges. This illustrates a critical function of an EHR: the need for a place where all the key clinical data can be brought together and analyzed. While in this case

Site = Cange							
EMR ID	Previous CD4	Previous CD4 Date	Last CD4	Last CD4 Date	Change in CD4	Current ARV Regimen	Phone
5002	625	20/MAY/2015	898	05/MAY/2016	+43.7%	3TC, AZT, NVP	N/A
94085	N/A	N/A	1057	19/APR/2016	N/A	N/A	N/A

Site = Lascahobas							
EMR ID	Previous CD4	Previous CD4 Date	Last CD4	Last CD4 Date	Change in CD4	Current ARV Regimen	Phone
4352	436	07/SEP/2015	309	02/JUN/2016	-29.1%	N/A	N/A
92407	400	14/OCT/2015	369	02/JUN/2016	-7.8%	3TC, EFV, Tenofovir	N/A
5586	454	18/JAN/2016	429	02/JUN/2016	-5.5%	AZT/3TC, NVP	N/A
23397	769	05/JAN/2016	850	02/JUN/2016	+10.5%	AZT/3TC, NVP	N/A
768	953	09/JUL/2015	1589	02/JUN/2016	+66.7%	AZT/3TC, NVP	N/A

Site = Petite Rivière							
EMR ID	Previous CD4	Previous CD4 Date	Last CD4	Last CD4 Date	Change in CD4	Current ARV Regimen	Phone
23893	216	22/DEC/2014	11	07/JUN/2016	-94.9%	3TC, EFV, Tenofovir	N/A
91467	188	23/DEC/2015	150	07/JUN/2016	-20.2%	3TC, EFV, Tenofovir	N/A
68374	267	14/MAY/2015	168	07/JUN/2016	-37.1%	N/A	N/A
45154	153	10/DEC/2015	187	07/JUN/2016	+22.2%	3TC, NVP, Tenofovir	N/A
92831	551	15/DEC/2015	333	07/JUN/2016	-39.6%	3TC, EFV, Tenofovir	N/A
29046	573	17/DEC/2015	425	07/JUN/2016	-25.8%	N/A	N/A
31531	519	08/DEC/2015	436	07/JUN/2016	-16.0%	3TC, EFV, Tenofovir	N/A
92832	942	24/NOV/2015	466	07/JUN/2016	-50.5%	AZT/3TC, NVP	N/A
91115	776	28/DEC/2015	553	07/JUN/2016	-28.7%	3TC, EFV, Tenofovir	N/A

Figure 10.2
Example of clinical alerts generated for CD4 counts on patients in Haiti. Copyright PIH with permission.

specific EHR software was developed by the PIH team, a "virtual EHR" can be any database or other program to store and compare data. For example, mHealth applications typically have a database with a web interface where data can be downloaded and analyzed. This need to bring data together is also the key motivation for interoperability and eHealth architecture projects–allowing feeds of clinical data in a timely fashion to be combined in one place for viewing, alerting, and analysis (chapter 14).

Figure 10.3 shows how a range of clinical data from a clinic or hospital can be linked to an EHR—in this case, the open-source OpenMRS system. In principle, all the tools and the components to achieve this interoperability are available and functioning in a number of projects in LMIC, but architectures like the one shown here are just starting to happen.

Many other projects have used simpler, Microsoft Access–based, "home-developed" EHR systems (similar to the Mosoriot Medical Record System) successfully in individual sites in LMICs. Some systems based on Access or FileMaker Pro have been scaled to large numbers of sites, such as IQChart [42]; however, these simple database tools lack many sophisticated functions like decision support, use of open data-coding standards, and interoperability.

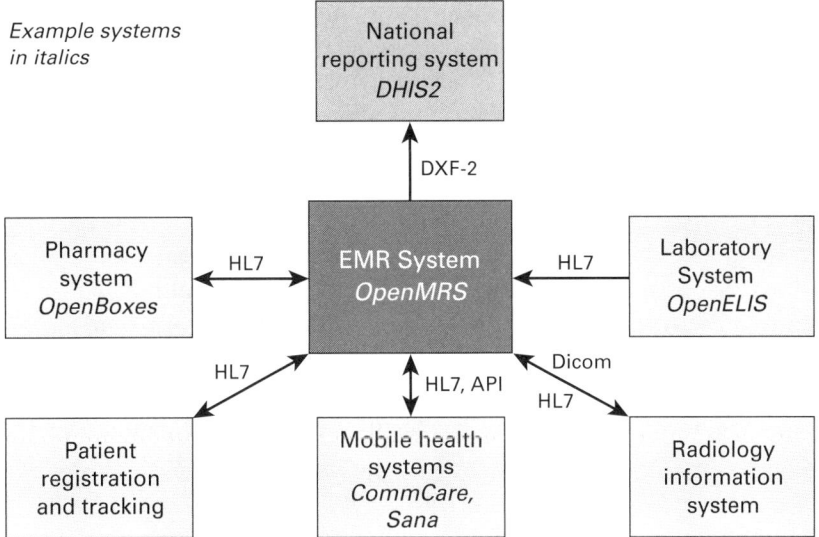

Figure 10.3
Interoperable hospital information systems. Copyright H. Fraser.

The design principles, examples, and lessons learned presented in this chapter should help decision makers make good choices from available EHR systems, or, if a new system must be developed, to do so based on existing best practices and wherever possible using existing frameworks and components. We believe that the time, effort, expense, and associated risk in attempting to build a home-grown EHR "from scratch" is simply not worthwhile today unless an organization is very strong technically and has unique requirements. There are a number of reputable open-source EHR systems available that have extensive support networks and user communities and companies with practical experience in adapting and implementing them, such as OpenMRS, Baobab Health, iSante, VistA, and others. Chapter 40 is a detailed case study of OpenMRS.

Conclusion

EHR systems have become a core technology for modern health care, with most high-income countries, such as the United Kingdom, moving to near 100% usage in primary care. Many key clinical and management activities are facilitated by such systems, and they allow additional functionality, including reporting on quality of care and other clinical activities; decision-support tools such as alerts and reminders; and the ability to visualize trends in clinical data. EHRs are also the key tools for the collection, storage, coding, and transmission of clinical data.

We have outlined a variety of uses, benefits, and issues with EHRs in this chapter, but in a short overview of this type it is not possible to cover every possible issue. It is important to emphasize that an EHR is a key element in global eHealth initiatives, but its effective use is very much a social and clinical process. Consequently, readers are encouraged to think in a wider interpersonal and sociotechnical context about how an EHR can be used to improve health and well-being in any location. Celi and colleagues give a vision for a new EHR paradigm that facilitates clinical data collection and data integration via monitoring devices, and organizes this data to help clinicians to focus on aspects most relevant to the patient [43]. In September 2015, the World Health Organization published a planning guide to scaling up mHealth systems, "The MAPS Toolkit mHealth Assessment and Planning for Scale" [44], which is very relevant for a range of eHealth projects, including EHRs. Fritz et al. [45] studied success criteria in a systematic review of EHR implementations in LMICs. They identify "highly reliable data handling methods, human resources and effective project management, as well as technical architecture and infrastructure" as key success factors. Extensive additional information on EHR systems is available in a variety of texts, such as Coiera [46].

New initiatives are focusing on the wider sharing of key data to improve clinical care, such as eConsultations in the United Kingdom using SystmOne, and health information exchanges in the United States and several African and Asian countries. Despite this progress, there are still high numbers of users, especially physicians and nurses, who express concerns with the usability of systems, their match to the clinical workflow, and the time taken to enter data. Much more effective design, workflow mapping, and usability testing are required. The quality of clinical data remains a major concern that limits the effective use of systems for clinical care, and research in particular, and this issue requires a much higher profile.

Finally, these concerns and initiatives are equally relevant around the world. LMICs have the opportunity to learn lessons from high income countries to build effective, easy to use, and interoperable systems, ideally using open-source and modular systems. Such EHRs can fulfill the promise of supporting clinicians' workflow, providing targeted decision support, improving reporting and analytics, automating disease surveillance, and improving clinical outcomes.

Questions for Discussion

- What are the benefits of using an electronic health record (EHR) system over paper records? When might paper records be better? How can clinics in low- and middle-income countries best move to EHR systems if they have poor infrastructure and access to power?

- What are the most important challenges to effective use of decision-support tools in an EHR?

• Consider different eHealth applications, such as laboratory information systems, pharmacy systems, and disease surveillance systems. What features of an EHR does each one rely on for optimal functioning? What are the benefits and disadvantages of using independent, stand-alone systems for each function?

• What are the potential benefits of using an EHR for noncommunicable diseases like heart failure and cancer? What aspects of care might be enhanced?

• What are the likely benefits of eHealth architecture approaches, as opposed to building and implementing one integrated system for all functions?

References

1. Centers for Disease Control and Prevention. Epi Info software. https://wwwn.cdc
.gov/epiinfo/. Accessed October 25, 2015.

2. Fraser HSF, McGrath JD. 2000. Information technology and telemedicine in Sub-Saharan Africa. *BMJ* 321(7259): 465–466.

3. Douglas GP, Gadabu OJ, Joukes S, Mumba S, McKay MV, Ben-Smith A, et al. 2010. Using touchscreen electronic medical record systems to support and monitor national scale-up of antiretroviral therapy in Malawi. *PLoS Med* 7(8): E1000319. doi:10.1371/journal.pmed.1000319.

4. Rotich JK, Hannan TJ, Smith FE, Bii J, Odero WW, Vu N, et al. 2003. Installing and implementing a computer-based patient record system in sub-Saharan Africa: The Mosoriot medical record system. *J Am Med Inform Assoc* 10(4): 295–303.

5. Care2x. http://www.care2x.org. Accessed October 25, 2015.

6. Christian Social Services Commission. 2014. Afya Pro software. http://www.cssc.or.tz/node/404. Accessed October 25, 2015.

7. Fraser HSF, Biondich P, Moodley D, Choi S, Mamlin B, Szolovits P. 2005. Implementing electronic medical record systems in developing countries. *Inform Prim Care* 13: 83–95.

8. Weed LL. 1968. Medical records that guide and teach. *N Engl J Med* 278: 593–600. doi:10.1056/NEJM196803142781105.

9. Agency for Healthcare Research and Quality. 2003. Key capabilities of an electronic health record system. http://iom.nationalacademies.org/Reports/2003/Key-Capabilities-of-an-Electronic-Health-Record-System.aspx. Accessed July 2015.

10. Fraser HSF, Jazayeri D, Nevil P, Karacaoglu Y, Farmer PE, Lyon E, Smith-Fawzi MK, Leandre F, Choi S, Mukherjee JS. 2004. An information system and medical record to support HIV treatment in rural Haiti. *BMJ* 329: 1142–1146.

11. National Learning Consortium. 2012. Contracting guidelines and checklist for electronic health record vendor selection. http://webcache.googleusercontent.com/sear ch?q=cache:fc18bBrfY5IJ:https://www.healthit.gov/sites/default/files/contracting -guidelines-and-checklist-for-ehr-vendor-selection.docx+&cd=1&hl=en&ct=clnk&gl =us. Accessed July 28, 2016.

12. Coiera E. *Guide to Health Informatics.* 3rd ed. Boca Raton, FL: CRC Press; 2015: 154–158.

13. Coiera E. 2015. *Guide to Health Informatics.* 3rd ed. CRC Press; 2015.

14. Middleton B, Bloomrosen M, Dente MA, Hashmat B, Koppel R, Overhage JM, et al. 2013. Enhancing patient safety and quality of care by improving the usability of electronic health record systems: Recommendations from AMIA. *J Am Med Inform Assoc* 0: 1–7. doi:10.1136/amiajnl-2012-001458.

15. Liaw S-T, Rahimi A, Ray P, Taggart J, Dennis S, de Lusignan S, et al. 2013. Towards an ontology for data quality in integrated chronic disease management: A realist review of the literature. *Int J Med Inform* 82(1): 10–24.

16. Douglas GP, Gadabu OJ, Joukes S, Mumba S, McKay MV, Ben-Smith A, et al. 2010. Using touchscreen electronic medical record systems to support and monitor national scale-up of antiretroviral therapy in Malawi. *PLoS Med* 7(8): E1000319. doi:10.1371/ journal.pmed.1000319.

17. Poon EG, Keohane CA, Yoon CS, Ditmore M, Bane A, Levtzion-Korach O, et al. 2010. Effect of bar-code technology on the safety of medication administration. *N Engl J Med* 362(18): 1698–1707.

18. Kerrison F, Fraser HSF. 2008. The impact of uncertain diagnostic results on responses to a decision support system for TB drug prescribing. AMIA Annu Symp Proc, November 6, 949.

19. Fraser HS, Habib A, Goodrich M, Thomas D, Blaya JA, Fils-Aime JR, et al. 2013. E-health systems for management of MDR-TB in resource-poor environments: A decade of experience and recommendations for future work. *Stud Health Technol Inform* 192: 627–631.

20. Weingart SN, Massagli M, Cyrulik A, Isaac T, Morway L, Sands DZ, Weissman JS. 2009. Assessing the value of electronic prescribing in ambulatory care: A focus group study. *Int J Med Inform* 78(9): 571–578.

21. Carspecken CW, Sharek PJ, Longhurst C, Pageler, NM. 2013. A clinical case of electronic health record drug alert fatigue: Consequences for patient outcome. *Pediatrics* 131(6): e1970–e19703.

22. Bryant AD, Fletcher GS, Payne TH. 2014. Drug interaction alert override rates in the meaningful use era. *Appl Clin Inform* 5(3): 802–813.

23. Bauer AM, Thielke SM, Katon W, Unützer J, Areán P. 2014. Aligning health information technologies with effective service delivery models to improve chronic disease care. *Prev Med* 66: 167–172.

24. Berger L, Jazayeri D, Sauveur M, Manasse J, Plancher I, Fiefe M. 2007. Implementation and evaluation of a web based system for pharmacy stock management in rural Haiti. *Proc AMIA Symp* 46–50.

25. Yamanija J, Durand R, Bayona J, Blaya J, Jazayeri D, Fraser H. 2006. Comparing actual medication consumption against the quantities ordered and a prediction using an information system. *Int J Tuberc Lung Dis* 10: S69–S70.

26. Adler KG. 2014. EHR dissatisfaction: Is it time to switch your EHR? *Fam Pract Manag* 21(4): 6.

27. Top M, Gider O. 2012. Nurses' views on electronic medical records (EMR) in Turkey: An analysis according to use, quality and user satisfaction. *J Med Syst* 36(3): 1979–1988.

28. Driessen J, Cioffi M, Alide N, Landis-Lewis Z, Gamadzi G, Gadabu OJ, et al. 2013. Modeling return on investment for an electronic medical record system in Lilongwe, Malawi. *J Am Med Inform Assoc* 20(4): 743–748.

29. Schoen C, Osborn R, Huynh PT, Doty M, Peugh J, Zapert K. 2006. On the front lines of care: Primary care doctors' office systems, experiences, and views in seven countries. *Health Aff* 25(6): W555–w571.

30. Mandl KD, Simons WW, Crawford WCR, Abbett JM. 2007. Indivo: A personally controlled health record for health information exchange and communication. *BMC Med Inform Decis Mak* 7: 25.

31. Nazi KM. 2010. Veterans' voices: Use of the American Customer Satisfaction Index (ACSI) survey to identify My HealtheVet personal health record users' characteristics, needs, and preferences. *J Am Med Inform Assoc* 17(2): 203–211.

32. Carroll AE, Biondich PG, Anand V, Dugan TM, Sheley ME, Xu SZ, et al. 2011. Targeted screening for pediatric conditions with the CHICA system. *J Am Med Inform Assoc* 18(4): 485–490.

33. Siedner MJ, Lankowski AJ, Kanyesigye M, Bwana MB, Haberer JE, Bangsberg DR. 2015. A combination SMS and transportation reimbursement intervention to improve HIV care following abnormal CD4 test results in rural Uganda: A prospective observational cohort study. *BMC Med* 13(1): 160.

34. Vimalananda VG, Gupte G, Seraj SM, Orlander J, Berlowitz D, Fincke BG, et al. 2015. Electronic consultations (e-consults) to improve access to specialty care: A systematic review and narrative synthesis. *J Telemed Telecare* 21(6). doi:1357633X15582108.

35. Pope R, Muchan M, Malin R, Binks R, Wagner A. 2013. The results of 24 hr tele-consultation with people at home and in residential care settings. *Int J Integr Care* 13(7). doi:http://doi.org/ 10.5334/ijic.1421.

36. McLean S, Sheikh A, Cresswell K, Nurmatov U, Mukherjee M, Hemmi A, Pagliari C. 2013. The impact of telehealthcare on the quality and safety of care: A systematic overview. *PLoS One* 8(8): E71238.

37. Fraser HSF, Jazayeri D, Mitnick CD, Mukherjee JS, Bayona J. 2002. Informatics tools to monitor progress and outcomes of patients with drug resistant tuberculosis in Perú. *Proc AMIA Symp* 270–274.

38. Blaya JA, Cohen T, Rodríguez P, Kim J, Fraser HSF. 2009. PDAs to collect tuberculosis bacteriology data in Peru reduce delays, errors, workload, and are acceptable to users: Cluster randomized controlled trial. *Int J Infect Dis* 13(3): 410–418.

39. Mitnick CD, Shin SS, Seung KJ, Rich ML, Atwood SS, Furin JJ, et al. 2008. Comprehensive treatment of extensively drug-resistant tuberculosis. *N Engl J Med* 359(6): 563–574.

40. Fraser HS, Habib A, Goodrich M, et al. 2013. E-health systems for management of MDR-TB in resource-poor environments: A decade of experience and recommendations for future work. *Stud Health Technol Inform* 192: 627–631.

41. Fraser HSF, Jazayeri D, Nevil P, Karacaoglu Y, Farmer PE, Lyon E, Smith-Fawzi MK, Leandre F, Choi S, Mukherjee JS. 2004. An information system and medical record to support HIV treatment in rural Haiti. *BMJ* 329: 1142–1146.

42. IQ Chart. http://www.iqstrategy.net/products/iqchart/. Accessed October 25, 2015.

43. Celi LA, Marshall JD, Lai Y, Stone DJ. 2015. Disrupting electronic health records systems: The next generation. *JMIR Medical Informatics* 3(4).

44. World Health Organization. 2015. The MAPS toolkit: MHealth assessment and planning for scale. http://apps.who.int/iris/bitstream/10665/185238/1/9789241509510_eng.pdf. Accessed July 28, 2016.

45. Fritz F, Tilahun G, Dugas M. 2015. Success criteria for electronic medical record implementations in low-resource settings: A systematic review. *J Am Med Inform Assoc* 22: 479–488.

46. Coiera E. *Guide to Health Informatics.* 3rd ed. CRC Press; 2015: 173–193.

11 Communication Networks and Global Health

Mengling Feng and Mohammad Ghassemi

Take-Home Messages

- Mobile data connections in the developing world are often more reliable than physical connections, which can deteriorate if not maintained or be harmed as a result of instability.
- Mobile deployment must consider practical limitations on the ground and be tailored to constraints including access speeds, cost, and coverage.
- The constraints may be used to leverage participants, establish collaborations, and attract early adopters through the provision of free or low-cost Internet connections.

Any set of two of more entities that can exchange information with one another, be they human, machine, animal, or otherwise, are part of a communication network. Communication networks have always been an important part of human survival and success, be it coordinating a hunt on the savanna or planning out a defensive strategy during a sports match. As technology has developed, however, people and machines are now communicating in unprecedented volumes, over incredible distances, and in a multiplicity of forms ranging from simple text to live video streams. Indeed, one might argue that the digital components of communication are becoming even more critical to human interaction and progress than the traditional face-to-face mode.

Given its clear importance, this chapter will describe the two most heavily utilized faces of digital communication networks: (1) the Internet and (2) the mobile cellular network. More specifically, this chapter will elucidate the technical fundamentals facilitating these two modes of communication, review the availability of services in low- and middle-income countries, and discuss the utility of these networks in the context of global health.

Internet

With over 2.92 billion users, the Internet is so widely used that it hardy needs an introduction. Indeed, anyone who has used Google, Facebook, YouTube, or Wikipedia knows the practical reality of the world's most powerful and ever-evolving communication network far better than any verbal description could do justice. The Internet has come a long way since its humble beginnings as a communication network for researchers [1,2]. From 1993 till the present, the Internet has transformed from carrying a mere 1% of the world's digital communication to a staggering 97% [3,4].

Yet while many have mastered the World Wide Web, many are unfamiliar with what exactly the Internet is and what is going on behind the scenes. How does Google know what website to direct you to? What is the difference between the World Wide Web and the Internet? Where are websites stored? How do all the computers in the world send and receive the millions of e-mail messages sent daily? In this section, we introduce the Internet from the inside out.

Connection to the Internet

At its core, the Internet is simply a massive global system of interconnected computers. Just like a human network, computers need a common language to understand one another. The language that is used by computers to communicate over the Internet is called the transmission control protocol/Internet protocol (TCP/IP). TCP/IP allows any device to remotely connect to any other device from around the world.

There are two ways to connect to the Internet: (1) through a fixed broadband connection and (2) via a mobile broadband connection. Figure 11.1(a) illustrates Internet access volumes across the world using fixed broadband connections. Importantly, the figure illustrates that while Internet access is common in developed countries, it is still fairly scarce in the developing world. In particular, there is a paucity of access in sub-Saharan Africa and central Asia. Figure 11.1(b) illustrates access volumes using mobile broadband connections. Note that the access volumes using mobile connections differ from those shown in figure 11.1(a). In the developed countries, we see that high volumes of fixed connections tend to correlate well with high volumes of mobile connections. In the developing world, however, areas with low volumes of fixed connections often exhibit higher volumes of mobile access. This interesting result is a consequence of the reality that developing countries often lack the infrastructure to install and maintain fixed connections, while mobile solutions are cheaper and often easier to deploy. A single cell phone tower can provide service to hundreds of customers and requires little maintenance. In Egypt, for instance, only 2.7% of the population has fixed broadband service at home, but nearly 10 times as many Egyptians have Internet access using a cell phone. The story is similar in Ghana, Uzbekistan, Indonesia, South Africa, and Nigeria [6].

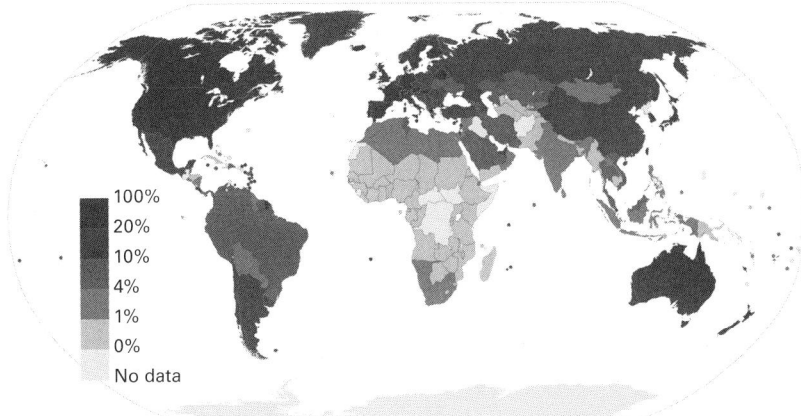

(a) Popularity of fixed broadband Internet access

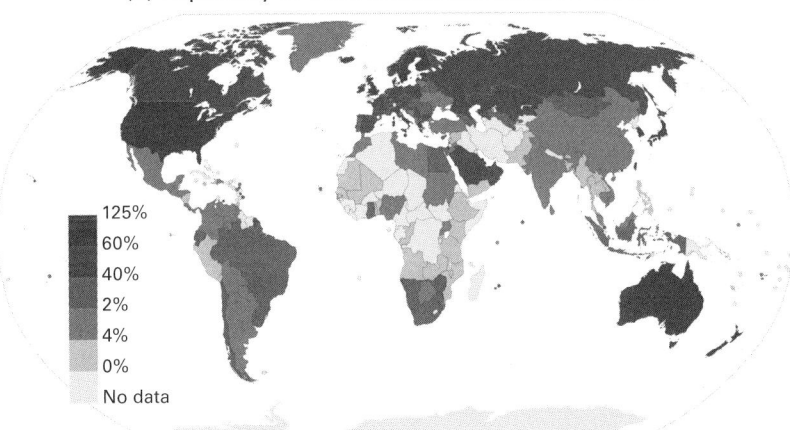

(b) Popularity of mobile broadband Internet access

Figure 11.1
Popularity of fixed and mobile broadband Internet access around the world. The legend indicates the percentage of people in the country with a particular form of access. In some cases, this may be over 100% when, on average, there is more than one access point per person. Data source: International Telecommunications Union [5].

Yet despite the relative advantages of the mobile solution over fixed broadband, many developing areas still lack access to the Internet. The issue is not one of demand nor one of supply, since many individuals in the developing world are eager to get connected, and many telecom carriers or service providers would love to set up the fixed or mobile broadband connection infrastructures in these untapped markets [7]. Issues ranging from political instability to infrastructure have kept access limited. Most of all, it has been shown that approaches that provide full coverage are not economically feasible in low-density areas [8]. One potential solution is the deployment of wireless local area networks (known as WLAN, or wireless LAN).

A LAN simply refers to a network of computers or other devices that share a common communication protocol (such as TCP/IP, in the case of the Internet). WLAN refers to a network that allows connection via wireless technology. Wi-Fi, short for wireless fidelity, is just one instance of WLAN that uses the IEEE 802.11 wireless protocol. Wi-Fi is relatively quick and cheap to deploy, and is therefore particularly well suited for areas where there isn't an incentive to build new cellular towers. Wi-Fi also has the advantage being an open and unlicensed spectrum, which allows grassroots organizations to set up Wi-Fi networks with very low capital investments and avoid dependence on a telecommunications carrier. Additionally, Wi-Fi cards are cheap and highly available, enjoying economies of scale. The cost of a long-distance Wi-Fi link has been estimated as approximately US$800 (excluding the cost of tower) with no recurring cost. Hence, Wi-Fi can be deployed in areas with low population density, such as rural villages, where connectivity is required by employing long-distance point-to-point Wi-Fi links.

Capacity and Cost of Internet

The supply of international connectivity has expanded dramatically since 2009, when several submarine fiber cables came online to connect even the poorest countries in Africa to the Internet. As shown in figure 11.1, with only a few exceptions, nearly every developing country now has some form of competitive market for broadband services. Nevertheless, one should not easily conclude that the differences in connectivity are narrowing between developed and developing countries. To have a more complete understanding of the current connectivity status of developing regions, we need to take into consideration the connection capacity (or bandwidth) and costs.

In 2011, Hilbert et al. conducted a survey [9] to compare the differences in connectivity between developed and developing countries over the last decade. The OECD (Organization for Economic Co-operation and Development) countries [10] were selected to represent the developed countries, which were then compared against the rest. Network connectivity was measured both in terms of the subscription rate per capita and the network capacity (in kilobits per second) per capita. As demonstrated in figure 11.2, the

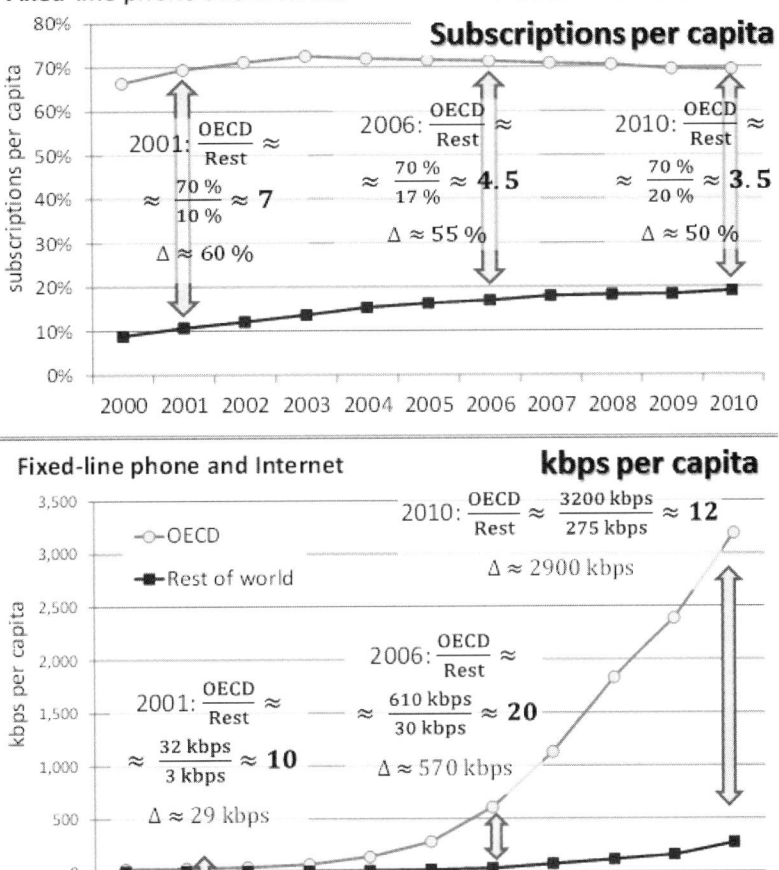

Figure 11.2
Connectivity differences between developed countries (OECD) and developing countries measured in subscription per capita and capacity (kbps) per capita [14].

gap in subscription rate has been closing over the years. On the other hand, the gap in capacity per capita has increased exponentially.

In addition to the constrained capacity, cost is another barrier for populations in developing regions to get connected to the Internet. As defined by the UN Broadband Commission, an affordable entry-level Internet service should be priced at less than 5% of average monthly income. According to The Affordability Report [11] by the Alliance for Affordable Internet (A4AI), only a small number of developing countries are close to achieving the UN Broadband Commission standard. In 50 of the studied countries, the cost of entry-level Internet services were priced at more than 40% of the populations' average monthly income, and in some cases the cost exceeded 80% of monthly income.

Low capacity and high cost of Internet services are difficulties that need to be addressed to facilitate the deployment of mobile health technologies in developing regions. However, we may also make use of these constraints to test collaborations and attract participants and early adopters by providing them with free or low-cost Internet connections.

Services on the Internet

The World Wide Web, or web, is easily the most popular Internet service in existence. The web is so widely used that people will often mistake it for the Internet in its entirety. In reality, the web is just one of the many Internet services that allows the sharing of text, image, and video information. The web supports many applications that can help to address the challenges in global health. It is an effective channel to distribute health care information, such as educational materials on infectious diseases and tips on how one may avoid exposure to diseases. The web can also serve as an interface for a back-end electronic health record (EHR) system and allow clinicians and health care workers to document and archive patients' information. Some existing web applications already allow health care workers to report local activities of infectious disease.

In addition to the web, the Internet provides many services that are useful for global health problems. For example, e-mail services facilitate nonurgent exchange of information between local health care and social workers with remotely sited physicians. The voiceover Internet protocol (VOIP) service, together with video-streaming and file-sharing services, can make telemedicine more effective in rural and resource-limited regions.

Many information technology companies have already realized that wider Internet coverage, particularly in rural areas, can provide value to developing countries in both the economic and health care domains [12]. Google and Facebook are two representative examples. In 2013, Google launched Project Loon, which aims to provide free wireless Internet coverage to developing countries through the use of hot air balloons. Facebook has also established a global partnership called Internet.org for the purpose of providing low-cost Internet access in the developing world.

Mobile Cellular Network

The mobile cellular network is a wireless network distributed over land areas called cells, where each cell (as shown in figure 11.3) is served by at least one fixed-location transceiver, known as the base station. A transceiver is a device that contains both a transmitter, which sends data, and a receiver, which receives data. Radio waves are used to transmit signals between the mobile phones, the receivers, and the base stations. The transmitting radio-frequency bands are a limited, shared resource. To allow multiple

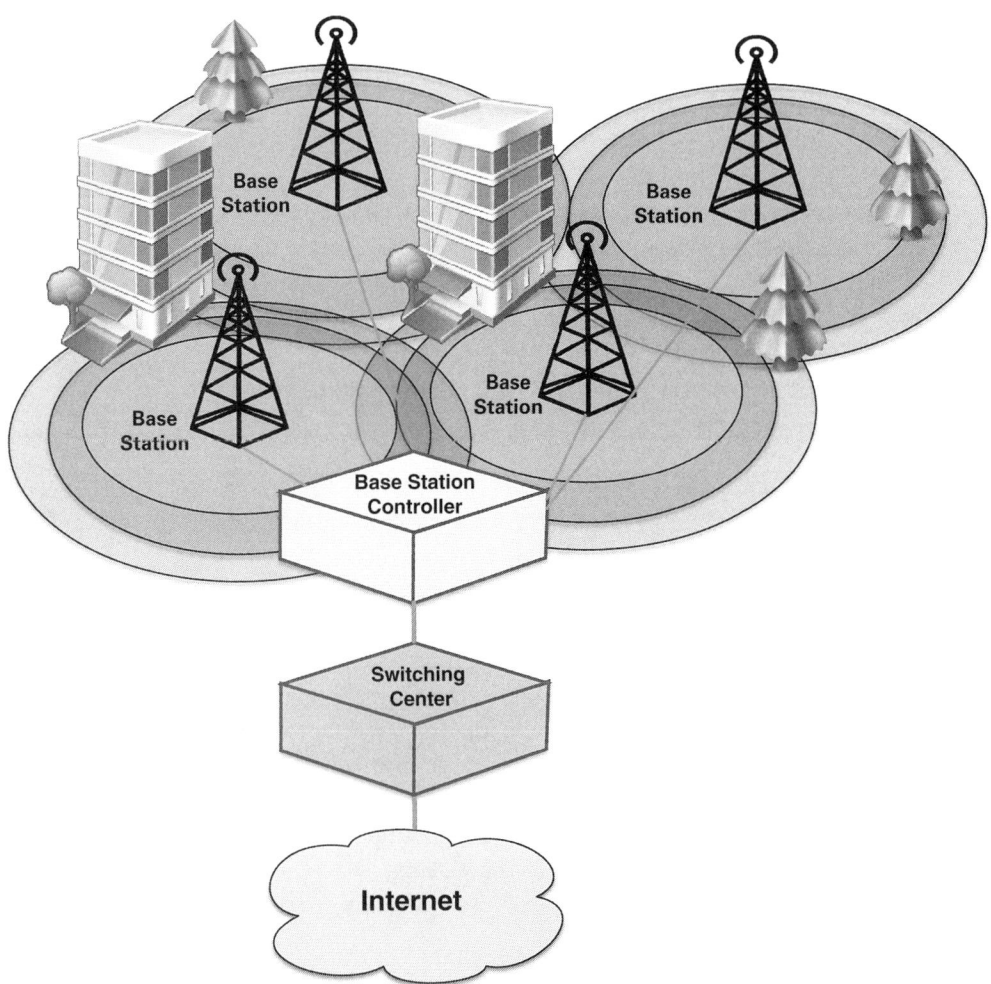

Figure 11.3
Infrastructure of mobile cellular network [13].

callers to use the limited bandwidth of radio with minimum interference, low-power transmitters are used. Not surprisingly, transmitters and receivers have limitations as to the volume of data they can send and receive. To solve this issue, packet or circuit switching is employed. In packet switching, messages are collected from several transmitters, broken into small chunks, and transited as packets for reassembly on the receiver end. In circuit switching, a transmitter waits in a queue with other transmitters on the network to establish a dedicated connection with the receiver, then sends all the data at once. A standard mobile cellular network consists of the following main components:

• a network of radio base stations forming the base station subsystem

• the core circuit-switched network for handling voice calls and text

• a packet-switched network for handling mobile data

• the telephone network to connect subscribers to the wider telephony network.

The voice call functionality of the mobile cellular network is, in general, well understood by the public. Therefore, in the following section, we further investigate the text-messaging aspect of the mobile network.

Short Message Service

Short message service (SMS) is a text-messaging service component of the mobile network. It uses standardized communications protocols to allow mobile phone devices to exchange short text messages with each other [14]. The SMS service can be a useful component of global health solutions.

The SMS messages are very small data packages that require minimum bandwidth to transmit. SMS services are also much cheaper to transmit compared to mobile voice calls. It follows that SMS is a highly feasible communication channel in areas where network bandwidth is limited and unstable. Importantly, the SMS messaging service is an attractive option for health care applications, including follow-up appointment and medication reminders, transmitting short health records, and brief health care consultancy.

Yet, despite the potential of SMS as part of a health care solution, it is worth bearing in mind the limitations of the SMS service.

First, SMS supports a limited message size. Each message carries a maximum of 140 bytes of data. Messages exceeding the quota are broken down into multiple segments for transmissions. If long messages are expected in an application, one needs to incorporate a message reassembling function in the message receivers.

Secondly, SMS message delivery is not guaranteed, and many implementations provide no mechanism through which a sender can determine whether an SMS message has been delivered in a timely manner. Furthermore, SMS messages are generally treated as lower-priority traffic compared to voice messages. Various studies have shown that around 1%

to 5% of messages are lost entirely, even during normal operation conditions, and others may not be delivered until long after their relevance has passed [14]. Thus, SMS may be suboptimal in the case of emergency or time-sensitive health care situations.

Thirdly, security vulnerabilities are a prominent weakness for SMS. In the Global System for Mobile (GSM) communications [13], the airway traffic between the mobile station and the base station is optionally encrypted and may be easily broken with a stream cipher. The authentication is unilateral and also vulnerable. Such vulnerabilities are inherent to SMS as one of the superior and well-tried services with a global availability in the GSM networks. SMS messaging has some extra security vulnerabilities due to its store-and-forward feature as well [15,16]. As a result, additional encryption mechanisms are necessary if protected health information is to be transmitted through SMS.

Advanced Topics and Further Information

Mobile connectivity has transformed the way we work, socialize, and organize our lives around the world. The 2014 GSMA Mobile Economy Report estimates that mobile technologies will be responsible for over 5% of the global GDP by 2020. The utility of mobile networks in the developed world is due to broad and affordable access to fast and efficient 3G or 4G networks. What makes these technologies so special? 3G and 4G are the third and fourth generation of mobile communication technology according to the standards set forth by the International Telecommunications Union. For a system to be rated as 3G, it must be capable of providing data at a kilobit speed, whereas 4G systems often operate at gigabit speeds. With significantly more bits per second, 4G networks can handle large volumes of data, at far faster speeds than 3G.

Unfortunately, the same accessibility to high-speed networks cannot be said of mobile connections in much of the developing world. According to the same report, only one-third of global mobile connections in 2013 were made on 3G or 4G networks, and by 2020, one-third of the world's mobile users will still not have access to 3G or 4G. It follows that the design of mobile health solutions for deployment in the developing world must be highly sensitive to slow transmission rates and provide services that minimize information transmitted while maximizing value.

For additional information on networks, please refer to the video "Introduction to Networks," available at https://www.youtube.com/watch?v=psMhKIWvFjU.

Questions for Discussion

- Does the deployment of wireless technologies in underdeveloped areas decrease incentives for the deployment of more permanent and larger bandwidth technologies such as fiber optics?

- Keeping global health in mind, what are the advantages and challenges of each networking paradigm discussed in the chapter (Wi-Fi, LAN, WAN, 4G, etc.) with respect to promoting stability, cost, security, and efficiency?
- What are the trade-offs between security, reliability, and cost for the SMS platform as it pertains to global health?

References

1. Hafner K. *Where Wizards Stay Up Late: The Origins Of The Internet.* Simon & Schuster; 1998.

2. Peter I. 2004. So, who really did invent the Internet?. http://www.nethistory.info/History%20of%20the%20Internet/origins.html. Accessed November 27, 2014.

3. Hilbert M, López P. 2011. The world's technological capacity to store, communicate, and compute information. *Science* 332(6025): 60–65.

4. Miniwatts Marketing Group. 2011. World internet users and population stats. June 22. http://www.internetworldstats.com/stats.htm. Accessed June 23, 2011.

5. International Telecommunications Union. 2013. Percentage of individuals using the Internet 2000–2012. http://www.itu.int/en/ITU-D/Statistics/Documents/statistics/2014/Individuals_Internet_2000-2013.xls. Accessed June 22, 2013.

6. Lee TB. 2014. 40 maps that explain the internet. Vox. June 2 http://www.vox.com/a/internet-maps.

7. Mishra SM, Hwang J, Filippini D, Du T, Moazzami R, Subramanian L. 2005. Lecture Notes in Computer Science, vol. 3828, 184-194. 1st International Workshop on Internet and Network Economics, Hong Kong. doi:10.1007/11600930_19.

8. Subramanian L. 2006. Rethinking wireless in the developing world. Proceedings of the 5th Workshop on Hot Topics in Networks (HotNets), University of California, Irvine, Irvine, CA, November 29–30. http://www.read.cs.ucla.edu/hotnets5/program.pdf.

9. Hilbert M. 2011. Mapping the dimensions and characteristics of the world's technological communication capacity during the period of digitization (1986–2007/2010). Document INF/15-E. Presented at the 9th World Telecommunication/ICT Indicators Meeting, Mauritius, December 7–9. https://www.itu.int/ITU-D/ict/wtim11/documents/inf/015INF-E.pdf.

10. Organisation for Economic Co-operation and Development. 2015. List of OECD countries. http://www.oecd.org/about/membersandpartners/list-oecd-member-countries.htm. Accessed February 15, 2015.

11. A4AI Affordable Report. 2013. http://a4ai.org/category/policy-research/a4airesearch-policy/. Accessed February 15, 2015.

12. World-wide Wi-Fi: Why Google and Facebook are providing free wireless to developing countries. Accessed November 27, 2014.

13. Mobile Technology GSM. http://www.etsi.org/technologies-clusters/technologies/mobile/gsm. Accessed July 25, 2016.

14. Kelly H. 2012. OMG, the text message turns 20. But has SMS peaked? CNN, December 3. http://www.cnn.com/2012/12/03/tech/mobile/sms-text-message-20/. Accessed December 15, 2014.

15. Traynor P. 2011. Characterizing the security implications of third-party EAS over cellular text messaging services. *IEEE Trans Mobile Comput* 11(6): 983–994.

16. Toorani M. 2008. Solutions to the GSM security weaknesses. Proceedings of the 2nd IEEE International Conference on Next Generation Mobile Applications, Services, and Technologies, 576–581. doi:10.1109/NGMAST.2008.88.

12 Health Information Standards and Interoperability

Boonchai Kijsanayotin and Win Min Thit

Take-Home Message

- To achieve interoperability, all stakeholders need to agree on the use of the same data standards to enable different information systems to exchange data and be able to use that exchanged data. There are many layers of health information standards. It is not as easy as it seems to develop, maintain, and implement standards. Standards and systems interoperability are essential for the development of integrated health information systems that serve the ultimate goal of achieving better health.

Introduction

In this chapter, we first discuss global eHealth development, and then define interoperability and standards in general. The important concept of interoperability in health care, and benefits and challenges of interoperability, are explained. Furthermore, we discuss the landscape of health data standards. In the last part of the chapter, we present Thailand's health information standards development as an example of a country's health information standards evolution.

eHealth, Information Standards, and Interoperability

Information and communication technology (ICT) has been changing education, economic development, rural development, and health care. The World Health Organization (WHO) defines eHealth as the use of ICT for health [1]. The European Commission refers to eHealth as ICT tools and services that can improve prevention, diagnosis, treatment, monitoring, and management [2]. The use of ICT in health and health care has enormous potential to increase health care efficiency, improve quality of life, and reduce soaring health expenditures [3]. While eHealth has been a prominent topic in health care in recent years, the use of ICT in health has lagged compared to other industries.

In 2005, at the Fifty-Eighth World Health Assembly (WHA), the WHA 58.28 resolution recognized the importance of ICT in health. The resolution urged member countries to draw up a long-term strategic plan for developing and implementing eHealth services, develop eHealth infrastructure, and build closer collaboration between the public and private sectors on eHealth [4]. Since then, many countries have been working on utilizing ICT to improve national health information systems, but they also have been facing several challenges to build effective and functional eHealth. One big implementation challenge is the development of interoperable eHealth systems and lack of national health information standards. In 2013, WHA resolution 66.24 urged member states to draw up a road map for implementation of eHealth and health data standards at national and subnational levels and to develop policies and legislative mechanisms linked to an overall national eHealth strategy in order to ensure compliance in the adoption of eHealth and health data standards [5]. Resolution WHA 66.24 focuses on improving quality of health information on the Internet and recognizes the necessity of ensuring secure online management of health data and increasing trust in eHealth tools and health services. Moreover, the International Telecommunication Union (ITU) has stated that advancements in eHealth will be only accomplished through ICT standards efforts that facilitate interoperability among systems and devices, provide unqualified privacy and security, address the unique needs of the developing world, and leverage existing ubiquitous technologies such as social media applications and mobile devices. In 2012, WHO and ITU, working together, published a National eHealth Strategy Toolkit responding to the needs of countries at every level of development who seek to adapt and employ eHealth [6].

eHealth Components

The WHO-ITU National eHealth Strategy Toolkit identifies seven important building blocks or components that must be in place to realize the national eHealth vision (see figure 12.1). The seven components are (1) leadership and governance; (2) strategy and investment; (3) legislation policy and compliance; (4) workforce; (5) infrastructure; (6) service and applications; and (7) standards and interoperability. Interoperability of various health information systems and health data standards are essential for comprehensive and integrated health information, which is primary for effective decision making of all health-related stakeholders, from policy makers and health care providers to the general public.

In general, the integrated information needed at point-of-care services includes who received services; who provided them; where; and what type of services were provided. Figure 12.2 shows an architectural model of the health information exchange

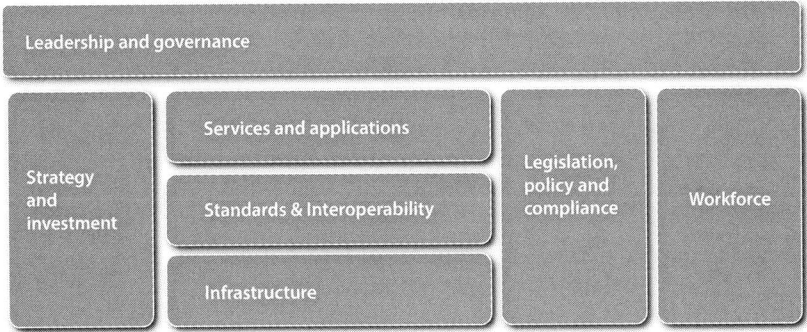

Figure 12.1
eHealth Components (WHO-ITU model).

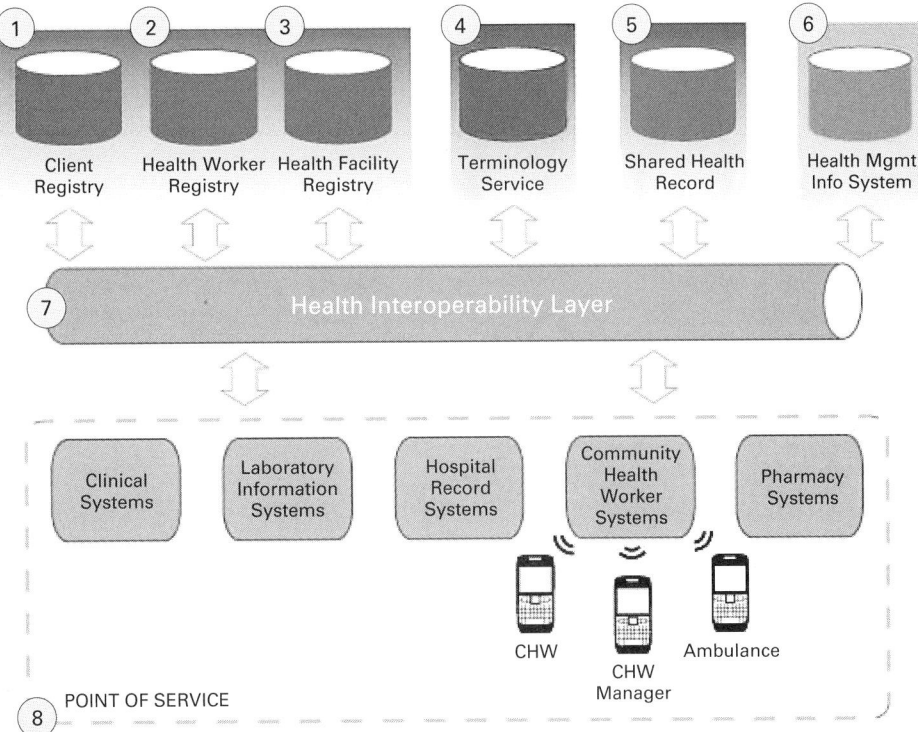

Figure 12.2
The health information exchange architecture or the eHealth blueprint: model representation of the eHealth system that should be built. The structures numbered 1–6 are the shared assets of the system. The health interoperability layer (structure number 7), which connects with health data standard components (the shared assets), is the shared service for all applications (number 8). As a result, health information in the application level is exchangeable.

(HIE), presented by the OpenHIE group, which is an enabler of health information integration [7]. HIE refers to the technology, standards, and governance that enable the exchange of data between the information systems of various health care stakeholders [8]. The OpenHIE architecture demonstrates the importance of interoperability and standardization in identifying people, providers, and types of medical services to ensure that the meaning of medical concepts is interpreted in the same way by different applications.

Interoperability

Health information should be seamlessly shared among medical devices and enterprise systems to optimize health care, and meaningfully used to serve health care delivery systems, personal health, and the health of the population. The information should meet the requirements of both health care services and public health functions, and such information should be comprehensive, integrated, and of good quality. In addition, patient health information should be exchanged between providers and authorized agencies, and should be available to the right people at the right time and the right place. To achieve this, different health information systems, both inside and outside the organization, must be interoperable. Interoperability is important to patient care, since patients' vital data can be shared among stakeholders, which will lead to fewer medical errors and unnecessary tests and more efficient decision making.

The Healthcare Information Management Systems Society (HIMSS) has stated that interoperability describes the extent to which systems and devices can exchange data and interpret that shared data. For two systems to be interoperable, they must be able to exchange data and subsequently present that data such that it can be understood and used by a user [9]. The Institute of Electrical and Electronics Engineers (IEEE) defines interoperability as the ability of a system or a product to work with other systems or products without special effort on the part of the user. Another definition from ISO/IEC 2382–01 for interoperability is "the capability to communicate, execute programs, or transfer data among various functional units in a manner that requires the user to have little or no knowledge of the unique characteristics of those units."

In health care, interoperability is the ability of different information technology (IT) systems and software applications to communicate, to exchange data accurately, effectively, and consistently, and to use the information that has been exchanged. To say that two or more information systems are interoperable is to say that they not only have the ability to exchange information, but that they can also use the exchanged information. Interoperability requires standards to ensure data being shared in health systems is available and retains the same meaning and context throughout different processes of clinical care. Interoperability is made possible by the implementation of standards.

Level of Interoperability

There are multiple levels of interoperability, from the basic level, at which systems can only exchange messages without knowing the meaning of the message—for example, that a person who only knows the English language can receive an e-mail written in Thai—to the highest level of interoperability, in which the disparate systems not only understand the messages but also work together seamlessly with a common business model. Figure 12.3 describes the multiple levels of interoperability. The first level is technical interoperability, which refers to the ability to move data from system A to system B, neutralizing the effects of distance. Technical interoperability is domain-independent. It does not know or care about the meaning of what is exchanged. Structural interoperability means that the systems can exchange messages based on an agreed dataset. It is the standardization

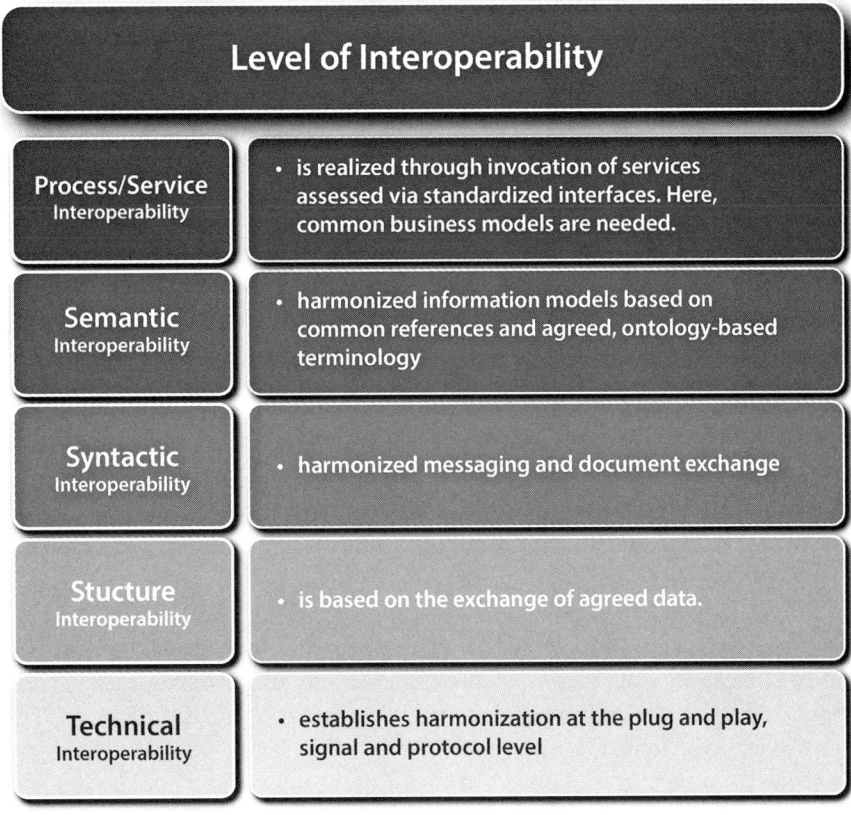

Figure 12.3
Levels of interoperability.

of data content. Syntactic interoperability is the level at which various systems adopt the same standards of syntax or format for the exchanged messages. Semantic interoperability ensures that sender and recipient understand the same data in the same way and allows computers to share, understand, interpret, and use data without ambiguity. Semantic interoperability usually involves the use of codes and identifiers that are based on common references and agreed terminology. Process interoperability is achieved when human beings share a common understanding across a network, business systems interoperate, and work processes are coordinated.

In this chapter, we focus on three levels of interoperability: structural, syntactic, and semantic interoperability.

Standards

Interoperability needs standards. A standard is a definition, a set of rules or guidelines, a format, or a document that establishes uniform engineering or technical specifications, criteria, methods, processes, or practices. In addition, it has to be approved by a recognized standards-development organization or have been accepted by the industry. The eHealth Initiative defines a standard as a well-defined approach that supports a business process, has been agreed upon by a group of experts, and has been publicly vetted.

Standards are basically universally agreed-upon ways to handle data to ensure interoperability. Standards can also be described as a group of guidelines concerning the essential requirements that a certain process, product, or service must meet in order to attain quality objectives. Standards allow data to be shared across systems and across stakeholders, regardless of the application. In fact, standards are the foundations of interoperability; it is not possible to build interoperable systems without them. Standardization is a process of agreeing upon the standards that represent the common language allowing the exchange of data between disparate data systems. The goals of standardization include achieving comparability, compatibility, and interoperability between independent systems; ensure data compatibility; and reducing duplication of effort and redundancies.

Why Do We Need Standards?

The issues of health data standards and interoperability are not trivial. Many health IT projects, regardless of size, have failed in many countries because health IT services and applications were not interoperable. Information exchange is difficult to achieve in health care systems due to an absence of standards. Studies indicate that lack of standards create a barrier for people to effectively collaborate because their information systems are not interoperable, making it difficult for them to share or interpret data across systems.

For different systems to integrate health information, the information needs to be transferred from one system to another through interfaces. The formula $N^2 - N/2$

demonstrates that the interfaces needed to connect N systems increases exponentially [10]. For example, in a general hospital IT environment, there are around a hundred applications. The number of interfaces that need to be communicated between those systems is almost 5,000 (figure 12.4). If the number of systems increases, the number of interfaces will also increase.

The star in the center of the right figure replaces the 15 separate specifications described in the left figure (figure 12.5). The diagram illustrates how much wasted time, resources, and effort we expend if standards are not deployed [10]. The benefit of standards

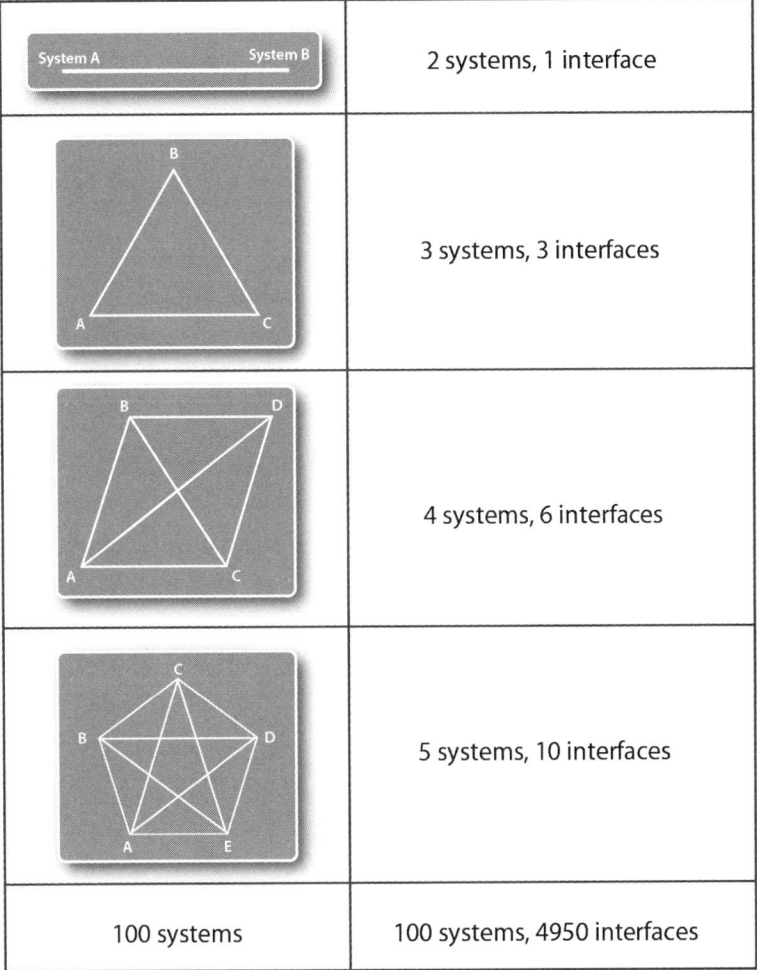

System A System B	2 systems, 1 interface
B / A C (triangle)	3 systems, 3 interfaces
B D / A C (quadrilateral)	4 systems, 6 interfaces
C / B D / A E (pentagon)	5 systems, 10 interfaces
100 systems	100 systems, 4950 interfaces

Figure 12.4
Number of interfaces needed for the interoperability of systems without standards.

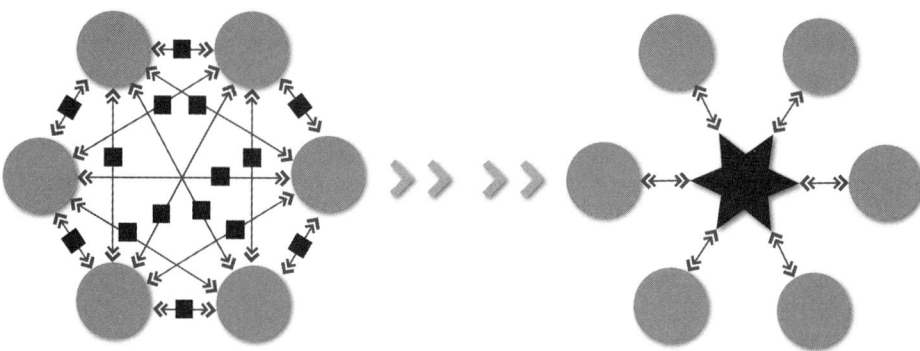

Figure 12.5
The benefits of the implementation of standards.

is that they enable interoperability and may also allow innovation based on common foundation.

Categorizing Different Standards

There are many types and levels of health information standards. Figure 12.6 shows the landscape of the standards that are needed to serve systems interoperability. In health care, we need different types of health data standards to support systems interoperability. In order to share data across health care institutions, exchanged data must hold similar data elements, use similar terminology, and use an agreed-upon messaging format.

We can simplify numbers of health information standards by categorizing them into four major groups (figure 12.7): content exchange standards; semantic or vocabularies standards; syntactic or messaging standards; and privacy and security standards.

1. *Content exchange standards,* or the standards dataset, are the set of data parties have agreed to exchange (e.g., datasets for billing or continuity of care documents).

2. *Semantic standards,* or standard vocabularies, are the standards of meanings. Sometimes a term may mean different things or represent different concepts; for example, the term "cold" in one circumstance means a respiratory infection disease, and in another means the feeling people get when exposed to low temperature. Sometimes, different terms may represent the same concept; for example, the terms "heart attack" and "myocardial infarction" represent the same meaning: "death of cardiac muscle." As a result, we need standardized ways to represent concepts. There are several coding systems that represent meaning in several aspects in medicine. Examples of semantic standards are patient identifier, provider identifier, ICD, SNOMED CT, and LOINC. They have different objectives, and are all important in a HIE. Internationally, there

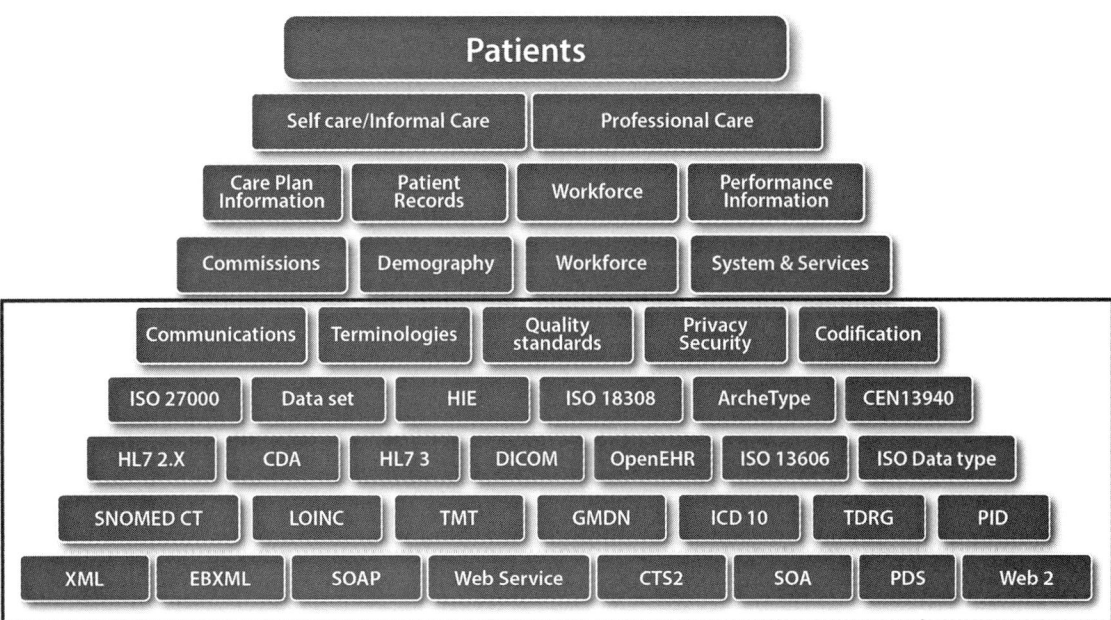

Figure 12.6
Health information standards landscape. The lower five stacks are different types of standards needed for health information exchange.

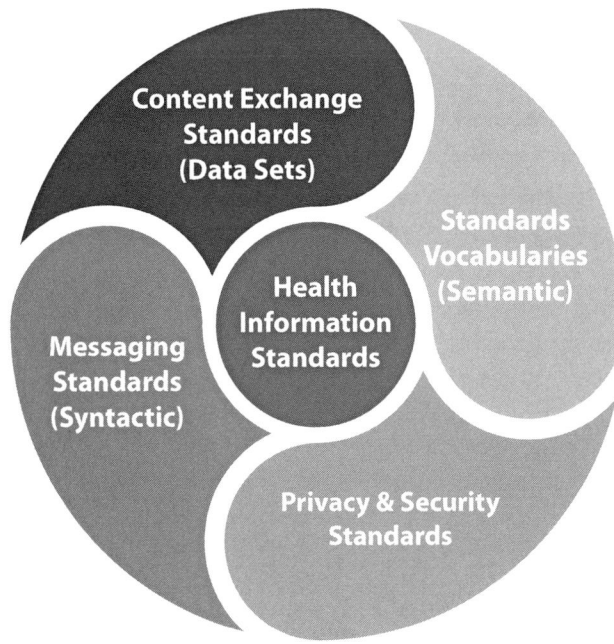

Figure 12.7
Categories of health information standards.

is a range of core semantic standards used to represent clinical findings, diseases, laboratory results, and clinical observations. The following are some important examples.

- The International Classification of Diseases (ICD) system [11] is the classification of diseases and related health problems. Its main objective is disease statistical reports and epidemiological data, as well as administrative reimbursement. It is also the standard diagnostic tool for epidemiology, health management, and clinical purposes. ICD is developed and maintained by the WHO in Geneva, Switzerland.

- Logical Observation Identifiers Names and Codes (LOINC) [12] is a standard used for identifying laboratory and clinical observations. The LOINC database, developed and maintained by the Regenstrief Institute in Indianapolis in the United States, provides a set of universal names and identification codes for identifying laboratory and clinical test results.

- The Systematized Nomenclature of Medicine Clinical Terms (SNOMED CT) is a detailed clinical terminology maintained and distributed by the International Health Terminology Standards Development Organization (IHTSDO), the not-for-profit organization based in Copenhagen, Denmark. SNOMED CT is considered to be the most comprehensive, multilingual health care terminology in the world. It was created as a result of the merger of SNOMED Reference Terminology and NHS Clinical Terms Version 3. SNOMED CT provides core general terminology and contains more than 300,000 active concepts with unique meanings and formal logic-based definitions organized into hierarchies [13]. SNOMED CT is being used around the world in several domains such as academic research; health information exchange; clinical decision support; clinical documentation and electronic health record. [14].

- The Diagnosis-Related Group (DRG), a case mix system, is a statistical system of classifying a hospital's acute care patients into groups, which is used for a prospective payment system [8].

3. *Syntactic or messaging standards* are an agreed-upon format specifying the grammar of messages. The most popular messaging standard is the HL7 V2.x. standard. This standard, developed and maintained by the Health Level Seven International (HL7) organization, primarily defines specifications for exchange of health informatics data between health care IT applications. The Digital Imaging and Communication in Medicine standard, or DICOM, handles storing, printing, and transmitting information in medical imaging.

4. *Security and privacy standards* include rules and regulations to keep patient information secure. Examples include public key infrastructure, SSL, and Digital Signature, which is a system for creating, storing, and distributing digital certificates, which are used to verify that a particular public key belongs to a certain entity.

There are many health information standards that cannot simply be grouped into one of the above categories. For example, the HL7 CDA (Clinical Document Architecture) is a model for exchange of clinical documents like discharge summaries and prescriptions, and aims to cater to the needs of an actual electronic medical record. CDA uses the XML document format and is based on HL7 v3 RIM (Reference Information Model) and its vocabularies to represent content data. Thus, CDA makes the documents both machine-readable and human-readable. The HL7 and Continuity of Care Document (CCD) is the standard that represents health care information in document format. CCD uses the vocabulary defined by the HL7 CDA standard and uses HL7 v3 messaging specifications for transmitting documents over a network [8,10,15].

Implementing Interoperability and Standards Is Hard

Having interoperability and achieving standardization is easier to say than to implement. For example, the worldwide use of electric sockets is supposed to be one standard but in the real world, it is not. Figure 12.8 shows a variety of electric sockets currently used in various countries. Imagine how convenient and effective it would be if only one standard were adopted across the world.

Health information standards are complex. Many standards are needed to make different systems interoperate. Although there are many international standards developed and ready for implementation, countries need capacity to know which standards to choose and how to use and customize the standards to suit the country context. Health information standards implementation takes time and investment, and Interoperability benefits will not prevail until the majority adopts these standards. Unfortunately, this capacity and investment are usually lacking in the lower- and middle-income countries (LMIC). Commitment from all stakeholders, the development and establishment of a good governing body, and having a clear roadmap for which standards to implement to achieve interoperability in health care systems are also of importance. There is no silver bullet or best answer for how LMIC should make systems interoperable or implement health information standards.

However, having knowledge of a country's current eHealth situation, learning from other country experiences, and working together among LMIC through networking will help. In Asia, a group of health IT/eHealth professionals from South and Southeast Asia countries have formed a health IT/eHealth peer-to-peer and learning network called the Asia eHealth Information Network (AeHIN) [16]. Composed of members from ministries of health, academia, nongovernmental organizations, and international development partners such as WHO, ADB, UNICEF, GIZ, and others, it promotes better use of ICT to achieve improved health through peer-to-peer assistance, knowledge sharing, and learning via a regional approach. The network works on eHealth governance, enterprise architecture, and standards and interoperability within and across countries.

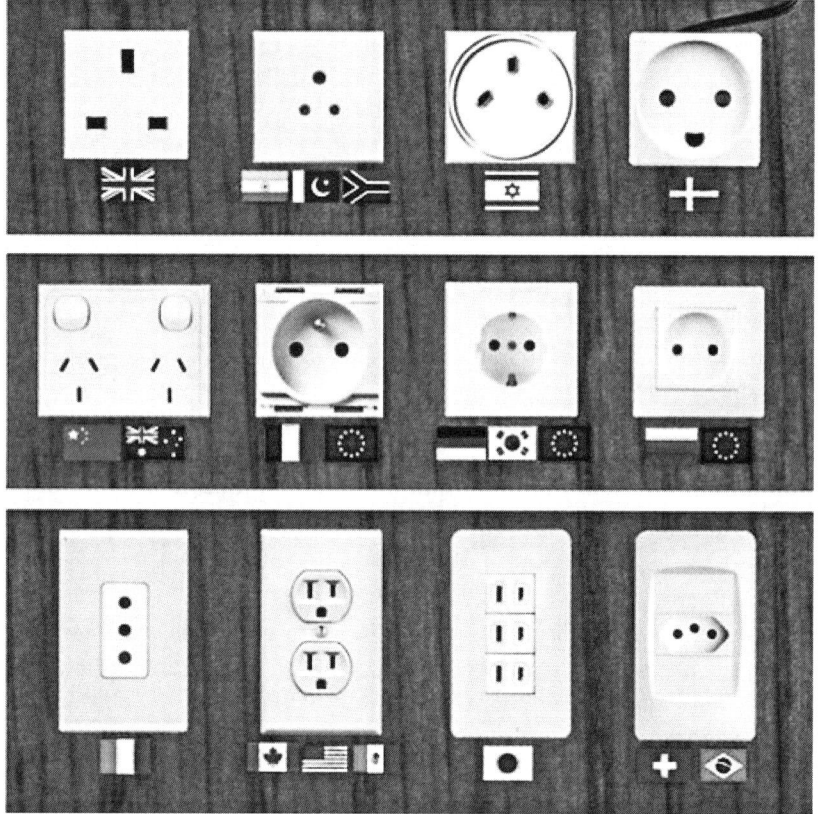

Figure 12.8
Variety of electric sockets.

Thailand Health Information Standards: Current and Future

To provide an example of health information standards development in LMIC, we explain health information standards in Thailand. At the national level, Thailand had adopted ICD 10 since its inception more than a decade ago; its main use is for public health reports and reimbursements. The ICD10-TM (Thai modification) and ICD9-CM (clinical modification) are used for coding diagnosis and health service interventions, respectively. Thailand developed and implemented a citizen identification number more than three decades ago [17]. Every Thai citizen has their unique 13-digit identification number. It is also used as patient identifier. There are two national minimal health dataset standards developed for administrative purposes. They are (1) standard datasets for health insurance, known as the 12-file dataset; and (2) standard datasets for health centers, known as the 18-file dataset. They are used mainly for health insurance payment and health care activities reports [18]. A national drug code, known as the Thai Medicine Terminology (TMT), is also being developed and implemented. The code is a SNOMED CT extension for medicinal products used in Thai health care. National health care providers' facility identifier is also available for health information exchange.

HL7 messaging and LOINC standards are implemented in a few large hospitals. They are not the national standards. DICOM is used in many health facilities in the country, usually where PACS (picture archiving and communication system) are implemented. However, it is not instituted as a national standard.

Thailand is employing more health information standards to serve clinical needs and continuity of care, and considering adopting several international standards for clinical care, such as LOINC, SNOMED CT, and HL7 CDA, as its national health information standards.

Conclusion

The use of ICT in health care, or eHealth, has enormous potential to increase health care efficiency, improve quality of life, and reduce health care costs. WHO and ITU are encouraging and supporting countries to develop national eHealth roadmaps and strategies. Health information standards and interoperability are one of the seven essential eHealth components. Interoperability of ICT-enabled solutions and of data exchange are preconditions for better coordination and integration across the entire chain of health care delivery and health data exchange. Interoperability of health information systems needs health information standards. They are many health information standards. The adoption and implementation of standards is one of the big challenges in developing a national eHealth strategy.

Questions for Discussion

- How are standards developed and maintained?
- What major challenges do you think influence the adoption of health information standards?
- There are many health data standards from which to choose. If you were a national decision maker, how would you decide what standards are suitable for your country?

Recommended Web Links

Most of the sites listed below have substantial information on stated standards. They are regularly updated and provide educational content.

- https://loinc.org/
- http://www.searo.who.int/entity/health_situation_trends/topics/health_data_standrads/en/
- http://www.ihtsdo.org/snomed-ct
- http://www.himss.org/
- http://www.himss.org/library/interoperability-standards
- http://www.imia-medinfo.org/new2/
- https://www.amia.org/

References

1. World Health Organization. *Building Foundations for eHealth: Progress of Member States: Report of the Global Observatory for eHealth with CD-ROM, 1 Pap/Cdr.* World Health Organization; 2006.

2. European Commission. eHealth Policy—European Commission. http://ec.europa.eu/health/ehealth/policy/index_en.htm. Accessed October 13, 2014.

3. President's Council of Advisors on Science and Technology. 2010. Report to the President realizing the full potential of health information technology to improve healthcare for Americans the path forward. Washington, DC: Executive Office of the President, President's Council of Advisors on Science and Technology.

4. World Health Organization. 2005. World Health Assembly Resolution WHA58.28. World Health Organization.

5. World Health Organization. 2013. World Health Assembly Resolution WHA66.24. World Health Organization.

6. World Health Organization and International Telecommunication Union. 2012. National eHealth strategy toolkit. Geneva, Switzerland: World Health Organization, International Telecommunication Union.

7. OpenHIE architecture [website]. http://ohie.org/architecture/. Accessed October 1, 2014.

8. Wager KA, Lee FW, Glaser JP. *Health Care Information Systems: A Practical Approach for Health Care Management.* 2nd ed. San Francisco, CA: Jossey-Bass; 2009.

9. Healthcare Information and Management Systems Society. What is interoperability? http://www.himss.org/library/interoperability-standards/what-is. Accessed October 13, 2014.

10. Benson T. *Principles of Health Interoperability HL7 and SNOMED.* 2nd ed. Dordrecht, The Netherlands: Springer; 2012.

11. World Health Organization. 1992. International statistical classification of diseases and related health problems. WHO Collaborating Centres for Classification of Diseases, and International Conference for the Tenth Revision of the International Classification of Diseases. Geneva: World Health Organization.

12. Regenstrief Institute. Logical Observation Identifiers Names and Codes (LOINC®). http://loinc.org/. Accessed October 14, 2011.

13. International Health Standards Development Organization. About SNOMED CT. http://www.ihtsdo.org/snomed-ct/. Accessed October 12, 2014.

14. International Health Terminology Standards Development Organisation. SNOMED In Action. SNOMED CT: The global language of healthcare. http://snomedinaction.org/listing-plain-heading/. Accessed November 5, 2015.

15. Sinha PK. *Electronic Health Records Standards, Coding Systems, Frameworks, and Infrastructures.* Hoboken, N.J.: John Wiley & Sons; 2012.

16. Asia eHealth Information Network. Home page. http://aehin.org/. Accessed November 5, 2015.

17. Kijsanayotin B, Ingun P, Sumputtanon K, and Thai Health Information Standards Development Center. *Review of national civil registration and vital statistics systems: A case study of Thailand.* Nonthaburi, Thailand: Thai Health Information Standards Development Center; 2013.

18. Kijsanayotin B, Kasitipradith N, Pannarunothai S. 2010. eHealth in Thailand: The current status. *Studies in Health Technology and Informatics* 160(Pt 1): 376–380.

13 Data Security for Mobile Health Care

Tyrone Grandison

Take-Home Messages

- There is an ecosystem of business, legislative, societal, and technical issues that security must be aware of and complement.
- The constraints placed on a system running in a mobile environment limit the controls available and introduce interesting new concerns.
- Mobile Security Reference Architecture provides a framework for thinking about and examining the security issues in a mobile health care system.

The Foundation

At the core, mobile health care solutions are constrained and are critical computer solutions with a set of business, legal, technology, and social concerns that need to be navigated. In this context, the word "constrained" refers to the fact that their processing power and storage or memory footprint is lower than contemporary computers. The word "critical" means that these solutions have the potential for far more severe consequences, by the nature of the domain and the data, than systems from other industries.

All computer solutions are a combination of hardware and software elements operating within a specific context.

Business concerns dictate the technological assumptions that must be made, whether implicitly or explicitly, to execute on a profitable business model. For example, if a company's business model is to package and resell user data, then the company would be resistant to include security and privacy controls that make it more difficult for this to easily happen.

Legal directives or mandates define the parameters within which these solutions must operate to be in compliance or face legislative penalty. A prime example of this is the OECD Data Protection Guidelines [1], which are the common starting point for privacy and security legislation across the globe and describe seven principles that must be employed when protecting personal data. Laws—such as HIPAA [2] in the United States, the Privacy Act [3] in Australia, the Personal Data Protection Act [4] of Argentina, PIPEDA [5] in Canada, and the other privacy laws worldwide [6]—instantiate these principles and create a compliance framework for health care solutions. Recognizing that the mobile sector requires special and specific guidance, there are some entities that have started the discussion on the precise legal environment for mobile devices. The production of mobile app guidelines [7] by the attorney general of California is an example of one such initiative.

The technology environment defines the set of tools that can be used and drives the expected user experience. For example, medical and financial software in the early 1980s would most likely be written in a procedural manner using the COBOL, Pascal, or Ada programming languages. Today's systems are expected to be asynchronous, responsive, and web-enabled. Thus, the current technology toolkit includes Python, Ruby on Rails, and Java.

Social or societal concerns encapsulate the attitudes, beliefs, and assumptions made by common users when they interact with computing solutions. More often than not, patients assume that medical computer systems will be extensions of or proxies supporting their relationship with their primary care provider [8]. The divide between this perception and the reality of the company that produces these systems is an area that must be managed well and that also requires acute focus by health care practitioners and solution builders.

The prior discussion provides a common platform from which we can have a meaningful (and holistic) conversation on security.

The Security Dimension

Computer security is normally defined as the ability of a computer system to protect information and system resources [9]. This protection is typically focused on several dimensions, described below.

- *Confidentiality:* ensuring information is not accessed by unauthorized persons.
- *Integrity:* ensuring information is not altered by unauthorized persons in a way that is not detectable by authorized users.
- *Authentication:* ensuring users are the persons they claim to be.
- *Access control:* ensuring users access only those resources and services they are entitled to access and that qualified users are not denied access to services they legitimately expect to receive.
- *Nonrepudiation:* ensuring the originator of a message cannot deny that they in fact sent the message.
- *Availability:* ensuring that a system is operational and functional at a given moment.

For each of these elements, there is a wealth of tools and research on how to achieve each goal. However, it must be mentioned again that a computer system is not a singular entity, but a coordinated integration of hardware and software layers (firmware, operating system, and applications) linked via an interconnected network infrastructure. This means that the set of threats one has to guard against, and the security mechanisms to be built, must focus on the physical system components (i.e., hardware); the persistent code built into the start-up process (i.e., firmware); the code that makes the device useful (i.e., operating system); the software on the operating system that makes our lives easier (i.e., applications); and the network and networking resources that enable systems to communicate (i.e., network traffic, which includes API use).

This creates a complex landscape to traverse. Fortunately, a lot of work has gone into solving a lot of these issues at all levels. With this information, one can see that the constrained nature of a mobile system creates an interesting challenge.

The Mobile Platform

The sensitivity of the data and the interactions on mobile health care devices and solutions, as well as the relevant legal mandates that have to be complied with, typically means that developers of mobile apps for health should build systems that (1) securely access medical data from a secured back-end database, (2) do not store personally identifiable information (or any medical data that may be sensitive in the future) on the device, and (3) ensure that the hardware and software of the mobile device are secure.

This third requirement is the most intense of all. It requires safeguarding the mobile stack from missing passwords (i.e., lack of authentication); poorly implemented authentication (i.e., the nonuse of two-factor, or higher, authentication); application misconfigurations; malware; operating system holes; unauthorized modifications; and so on. Fortunately, there is prior work in the space.

In May of 2013, the US Federal CIO Council and the US Department of Homeland Security produced the Mobile Security Reference Architecture (MSRA) [2], which provides a solid architectural pattern for developers of mobile solutions to allow them to ensure the confidentiality, integrity, and availability of data accessed through a mobile computing solution.

The MSRA (figure 13.1) assumes an enterprise back end. However, a mobile health solution developer should interpret this as the cloud or server infrastructure they will be using. MSRA consists of the following conceptual components, discussed further below:

- virtual private network
- mobile device management
- mobile application management
- identity and access management

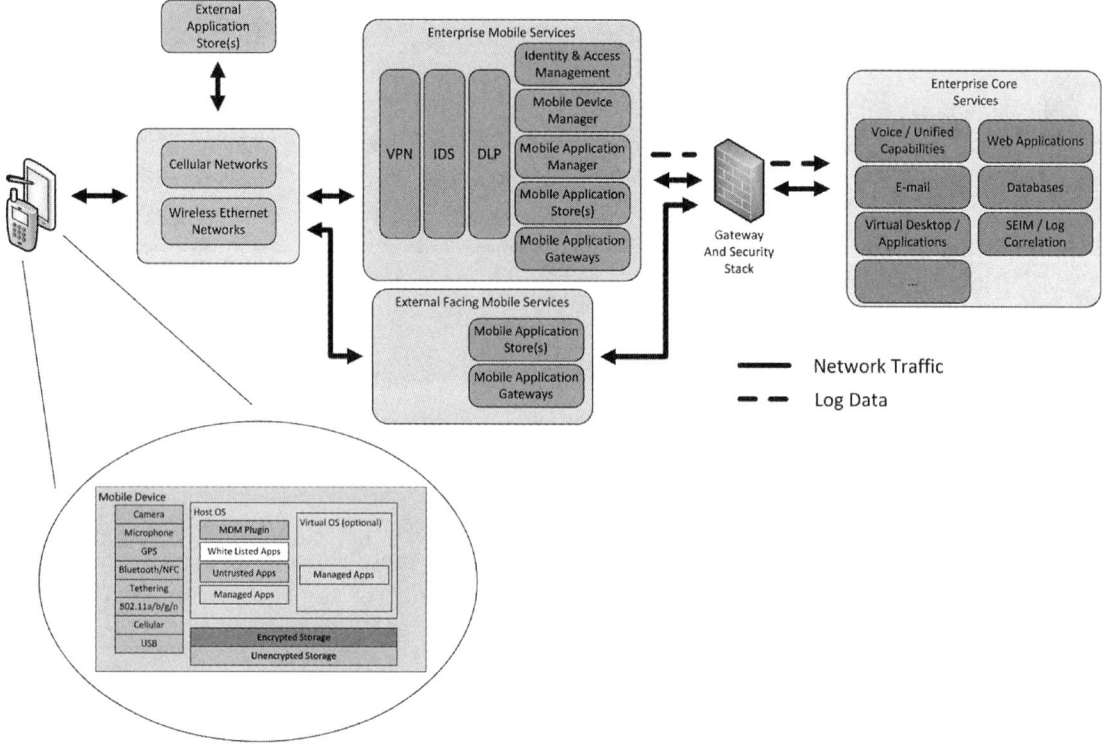

Figure 13.1
The Mobile Security Reference Architecture. Source: Federal CIO Council and DHS 2013.

- mobile application store
- mobile application gateway
- data loss prevention
- intrusion detection system
- gateway and security stack.

Virtual Private Networks

Virtual private networks are a method for creating secure connections between mobile devices and the back end while using public, often unsecured networks. For the mobile app developer, this is similar to always using a secure channel, with a strong encryption key, to communicate with the back end.

Mobile Device Management

Mobile device management refers to administration and supervision of the applications, data, and configuration settings on a mobile device. It seeks to centralize and optimize the functionality and security management of mobile communications.

Mobile Application Management

Mobile application management functionality provides a subset of the operations provided by mobile device management. It provides in-depth distribution, configuration, data control, and lifecycle management for specific mobile applications.

Identity and Access Management

Identity and access management systems are used to integrate and coordinate services such as authentication and authorization across the mobile solution to form a cohesive security profile for each user.

Mobile Application Store

A mobile application store is a repository of mobile applications. Examples include external application stores like Google Play and Apple's App Store. Since this repository provides a selection of approved applications that can be downloaded and installed on the device, one can limit the damage done from malicious apps by managing the store.

Mobile Application Gateway

A mobile application gateway is a piece of software that provides application-specific network security for mobile application infrastructures. Its purpose is to act as a network proxy, accepting connections on behalf of the application's network infrastructure, filtering the traffic, and relaying the traffic to mobile application servers. Mobile application gateways are often used in place of traditional network protections, such as intrusion detection systems, when application traffic is encrypted or opaque in structure.

Data Loss Prevention

Data loss prevention focuses on preventing restricted information from being transmitted to mobile devices, or from mobile devices to unauthorized locations outside the organization. A data loss prevention solution monitors all traffic flowing to mobile devices from the organizational infrastructure, validating the traffic against a set of predefined words, phrases, images, and patterns that are considered too sensitive to leave the enterprise boundary.

Intrusion Detection System

An intrusion detection system is a network appliance that uses a set of heuristics to match known attack signatures against incoming network traffic, and raises alerts when suspicious traffic is seen.

Gateway and Security Stack

Mobile devices, like almost all computing devices, have the capacity to be used to attack other networked devices. The unique, dual-connected nature (cellular and wireless Ethernet) of mobile devices makes them ideal platforms for circumventing traditional network-security boundary protections. To prevent damage to the back end from a compromised mobile device, access to the enterprise must be restricted through one or more known network routes (i.e., gateways), and inspected by standard network defenses such as stateful packet inspection, intrusion detection, and application protocols.

It should also be noted that all data-storage mechanisms must conform to FIPS requirements, specifically FIPS 199, FIPS 200, and FIPS 140.

This design and articulation of the high-level constructs that should be considered when building mobile solutions is very useful to help developers grasp the issues. Their environments do not have to be as robust as the one proposed in the MSRA. However, developers should be able to say they have broadly addressed the particular concern in those specific areas.

For a more grounded set of existing tools that can be utilized to address each of these concerns, the interested user may peruse the mobile-platform-specific information at Prism-Break.org [10].

The Future

In a resource-strained environment such as mHealth, where security is a concern, the emphasis should be on cloud-based services served through secure HTML5 apps. As the promise of emerging security technologies, like homomorphic encryption (which allows computations to be performed on encrypted data without decrypting it), comes closer to reality, their application to mHealth systems through cloud-based configurations will be seamless.

Questions for Discussion

- What additional risks are faced in mobile environments that do not exist in nonmobile settings?
- What security features complement the business, social, and legal frameworks of the United States?
- What security features complement the business, social, and legal frameworks of Europe?
- What are the differences in implementing Mobile Security Reference Architecture (MSRA) in the United States versus in Europe, given the differing legal frameworks (i.e., HIPAA versus the EU Data Protection Directive)?
- What challenges or threats are not addressed by the MSRA?

References

1. Organisation for Economic Co-operation and Development. 1980. Recommendations of the council concerning guidelines governing the protection of privacy and trans-border flows of personal data. http://www.oecd.org/internet/ieconomy/oecdguide linesontheprotectionofprivacyandtransborderflowsofpersonaldata.htm. Accessed October 7, 2014.

2. U.S. Department of Health and Human Services Office for Civil Rights. 2013. HIPAA Administrative Simplification. http://www.hhs.gov/ocr/privacy/hipaa/administrative/combined/hipaa-simplification-201303.pdf. Accessed August 27, 2014.

3. Office of the Australian Information Commissioner. 1988. The Privacy Act. http://www.oaic.gov.au/privacy/privacy-act/the-privacy-act. Accessed October 7, 2014.

4. Government of Argentina. 2000. Argentina Personal Data Protection Act. http://unpan1.un.org/intradoc/groups/public/documents/un-dpadm/unpan044147.pdf. Accessed October 7, 2014.

5. Office of the Privacy Commissioner of Canada. 2011. The Personal Information Protection and Electronic Documents Act. http://laws-lois.justice.gc.ca/PDF/P-8.6.pdf. Accessed August 27, 2014.

6. Information Shield. International Privacy Laws. October 7, 2014. http://www .informationshield.com/intprivacylaws.html. Accessed October 7, 2014.

7. Harris K. Privacy on the go: Recommendations for the mobile ecosystem. January 1, 2013. http://oag.ca.gov/sites/all/files/agweb/pdfs/privacy/privacy_on_the_go.pdf. Accessed October 7, 2014.

8. Meingast M, Roosta T, Sastry S. 2006. Security and privacy issues with health care information technology. 28th Annual International Conference of the IEEE Engineering in Medicine and Biology Society. *Conf Proc IEEE Eng Med Biol Soc* 1: 5453–5458.

9. Ross ST. *Unix System Security Tools.* New York, NY: McGraw-Hill; 1999.

10. Zhong P. 2014. Prism-Break.org.

14 Enterprise Architectures for Digital Health

Christopher J. Seebregts, Anban Pillay, Ryan Crichton, Sagree Singh, and Deshendran Moodley

Take-Home Messages

- Developing digital health system components using a "bottom-up" approach helps to ensure they match the real needs of users and the health system, but this approach can contribute to fragmentation of systems.
- Enterprise architectures (EA) take a more "top-down" approach to designing the components of larger-scale digital health systems and their interactions.
- EA provides a methodology and reusable "architectural assets" that can assist in the development of complex, large-scale systems systematically and holistically, and can potentially create reusable architecture components for global health projects.
- Several different paradigms and standards exist for creating digital health architectures that are mostly complementary, but sometimes contradictory.
- The potential benefits of using EA approaches and tools are that they help to ensure the appropriate use of standards for interoperability and data storage and exchange, and encourage the creation of reusable software components and metadata.

Introduction

As we have seen in earlier chapters, health information systems (HISs) are increasing in functionality and use in low-resource settings. However, they are generally fragmented and lack coordination in terms of their design and operation. This is a result of the fact that they are usually developed through a succession of uncoordinated projects that are not harmonized with the public health system of the country. This fragmentation can also result, in part, from an appropriate "bottom-up" approach to designing and implementing systems, as discussed elsewhere in this book. There needs to also be a "top-down" approach. Enterprise architecture (EA) is a common approach to developing systems that are more coordinated and integrated at a systems level. It can also help to address the challenges that have arisen with closed, proprietary, monolithic, nonstandardized systems with an emphasis on more open, collaborative, and rigorous approaches that are more amenable to an architectural approach.

EA has been described as "a well-defined practice for conducting enterprise analysis, design, planning, and implementation, using a holistic approach at all times, for the successful development and execution of strategy."[1] EA offers a methodology and reusable architectural assets to assist in approaching the development of complex, large-scale systems systematically and holistically, and potentially creating a set of health architecture components that can be reused globally, as shown by Mwanyika and colleagues [1].

EA has been proposed as a possible approach to designing and developing national HISs for global health [2]. The rationale is that the tools and techniques included in the EA approach will help address certain design issues currently limiting the application of HIS in low-resource settings, including:

1. lack of standardization, including the use of standards for data storage and interoperability [3]

2. minimal interoperability between individual applications developed for single solutions [4]

3. limited reuse of existing applications that are often engineered around a single application use case [2]

4. lack of data integration as a result of different conceptual frameworks and lack of use of standards [3]

5. poor data quality, often resulting from lack of effective data use locally as well as poor data entry tools and training.

In addition, EA may help achieve some of the internationally endorsed principles for digital development.[2] For example, EA has tools to assist with "understanding the existing ecosystem," and the approach may assist with principles such as "use of open standards, open data, open source, and open innovation."

Enterprise Architecture Frameworks

EA frameworks are central to the EA approach and generally useful to EA development projects. The IEEE-1471 standard [5] separates an architectural description from the architecture itself, and also introduced the notion of architectural viewpoints now widely used to model and illustrate EA designs. The hope is that a standard set of architectural viewpoints will help to understand and reuse EA patterns.

The ISO/IEC/IEEE 42010 standard defines an architecture framework as follows: "architecture framework conventions and common practices for architecture description established within a specific domain or stakeholder community"[3] [6]. Emery and Hilliard have compiled the following definition: "an enterprise architecture framework, or architecture framework for short, is a prefabricated structure that you can use to organize your enterprise architecture into complementary views"[4] [7]. The Generalized Enterprise Reference Architecture and Methodology was an early attempt to create an EA reference framework[5] [8], but has largely been replaced by newer initiatives.

One of the challenges in understanding this terminology is that the term "framework" is significantly overloaded in enterprise architecture, with various authors meaning different things by the term. There are several different EA frameworks which may be better reclassified[6] [9]. For example:

- the Open Group Architecture framework (TOGAF) is better described as a methodology.
- the Zachmann framework [10] is better described as a taxonomy.
- the Federal Enterprise Architecture framework [11] is better described as an example of an EA [9].

The International Organization for Standardization (ISO) has published a useful survey of EA frameworks.[7] Open architectural frameworks have also been proposed for mobile health [12–13].

The Health Metrics Network Framework

The Health Metrics Network (HMN) of the World Health Organization (WHO) was probably the first to systematically apply an architectural approach to national HIS development through its Framework and Standards for Country Health Information Systems [14]. Although version two of the HMN framework does not really meet the criteria of being an EA framework and is oriented mostly toward civil registration and vital statistics systems, along with its associated assessment tools it remains one of the most widely used and applied national HIS architecture design tools (another class of artifact that is useful for creating an EA) in low-resource settings. In a planning document for the third edition that has not yet been published, the HMN also outlined an EA approach [2]. Other authors have suggested an EA approach in civil registration and vital statistics [15] and for national HIS more generally [16], as well as a generic component model for health care [17] and another systematic approach to national HIS development linking public and private health care [18]. The HMN framework is probably better described as a domain architecture and methodology. The online Civil Registration and Vital Statistics Digitization Guidebook applies an EA methodology and the use of reusable artifacts to the work of digitizing CRVS processes in low resource settings [19].

The Open Group Architecture Framework

Of all the current frameworks, the Open Group's TOGAF is probably the most well developed and accessible, possibly due to the fact that it is open and has an associated community. As a result, it has also been able to integrate with other open standards, such as the unified modeling language,[8] business process modeling notation,[9] and ArchiMate[10] [20], all of which are useful to the general process of modeling systems as part of an EA approach. TOGAF is a general approach and oriented toward information technology architecture, but can be adapted and applied to the development of EA for national HIS. In a global health setting, the fact that it is an open standard maintained by an active community is a major advantage.

The core features of TOGAF are summarized in this excerpt from A. Josey [21]:

- The architecture development method is central to TOGAF and is operated by the architecture capability and supported by a number of guidelines and techniques.
- Content produced through execution of the method is stored in the repository which is classified according to the Enterprise Continuum and is initially populated with the TOGAF Reference Models [21]

Enterprise Architecture Standards in Health Care

Standards are fundamentally important to the development and application of an EA approach and EA frameworks, both in terms of an EA framework itself as well as in the development and implementation of specific EAs. In addition to its original standard for systems and software engineering (architecture description) [6], ISO has published two technical reports focusing on a capacity-based digital health architecture roadmap as part of ISO standard 14639.[11] Part 1 of the standard focuses on an overview of national digital health initiatives [22], and part 2 focuses on architectural components and a maturity model [23]. ISO 14639 is more focused on strengthening digital health implementations, particularly in low-resource settings.

A case has also been made for the adoption of standards for interoperability in Africa [24]. South Africa has developed and adopted a Health Normative Standards framework (HNSF) for interoperability in eHealth that specifies various standards and profiles to achieve interoperability in the health domain in South Africa [25]. A readable review of standards with a focus on interoperability between mobile health applications has also been published by the Mobile Health Alliance [26].

Applications of Enterprise Architecture in Global Health

One of the first applications of EA in a low-resource setting in Africa was the development of an enterprise architecture by the Ghana Health Service in 2009 [27]. The Ghana

EA includes an analysis of the current state (at that time), followed by a strengths, weaknesses, opportunities and threats, or SWOT, analysis and a description of a future state. The future EA specified four architectures: business, applications, data, and technical. Security architecture was specified separately, along with an information and communication technology governance model and an EA implementation plan. Although the future EA does not cite any particular methodology, it is similar to many of the steps in the TOGAF architecture development method. However, it doesn't identify any reusable assets that could be used to strengthen the implementation of the architecture. About the same time, a similar initiative was carried out in Mozambique (EuroSIS) and yielded a taxonomy of HIS. One disadvantage of these kinds of initiatives is that they need to be actively maintained in order to remain current.

EA frameworks and architectures have also been applied to global health in other low-resource settings. Perhaps the first scientific publication describing the application of EA described a systematic, architected and rational approach—or SARA—for the design and development of HIS and applications in Tanzania [1]. The study includes several important conclusions, including the following.

1. EA has the potential to reduce the complexity associated with HIS development in low-resource settings.

2. TOGAF is a rich framework, but more work needs to be done to further develop a systematic, architected, and rational approach to HIS design.

3. The approach can be used to create generic requirements.

4. While there is increasing acceptance of EA in low- and middle-income countries (LMIC), more needs to be done to develop a tested methodology that empowers LMIC to use the methodology effectively to strengthen HIS [1].

A study of EA trends has also argued that it is possible EA may be more widely used in low-resource settings as we move toward more patient-centric systems [28].

EA has also been developed in other LMIC, including the Philippines[12] and Cambodia.[13] However, in both of these cases, the architecture appears more like a taxonomy of components making up the health system, with a focus on interoperability between individual components. An EA approach was used to develop the business architecture during the development of the Rwanda Health information Exchange [29]. These initiatives focusing on interoperability are described below.

Interoperability Frameworks and Implementations

Another approach that is closely aligned and often integrated with the EA approach is the development of interoperability frameworks. These frameworks are designed to address a particular problem—namely, to strengthen interoperability between individual digital health applications—and are often aligned with a national digital health strategic plan or an eGovernment initiative. Mozambique was one of the early LMIC to develop an eGovernment interoperability framework [30].

In South Africa, the HNSF was developed and legislated in 2014 [25]. It requires the development of an EA as the next step in the application of the framework, and the development of specific digital health solutions to fit that framework. A technical implementation of the HNSF for mobile maternal health in South Africa in 2013 reused technology from the Rwanda Health Information Exchange [29] as elaborated in the Open Health Information Exchange initiative.[14] Other systems have been implemented, such as the Mobile Technology for Community Health technology suite [31], implemented in Ghana, Bangladesh, and several other LMIC.

Conclusion

Enterprise architectures are a relatively new approach to creating effective interoperable digital health environments at multiple levels in health systems. This coincides with and builds on a move to more standards-based and open-source digital health systems that better support interoperability. digital health is benefitting from several broader software initiatives to improve strategy, planning, and scalability of information systems, such as TOGAF. The WHO's HMN was one of the first groups to develop an digital health architecture for global health with a focus mainly on HIS design tools. These approaches can assist in effective use of data standards, interoperability, and reuse of software designs and actual components. Early initiatives have taken place in Ghana, Rwanda, Kenya, the Philippines, and South Africa with open-source health information exchanges and approaches to implement national shared health records as early successes. More research and evaluation is required to understand which approaches are most effective and useful in the wide variety of health care environments worldwide.

Questions for Discussion

- What are the advantages of using an enterprise architecture (EA) approach for digital health projects in low- and middle-income countries (LMIC)?
- What are the key challenges in applying EA techniques in LMIC?
- Are there likely to be differences in how this approach can be applied in LMIC regarding physical, organizational, or policy environments?
- Chose a project you are familiar with or have studied. What EA approaches are most likely to be useful?

Box 14.1

The Rwanda Health Enterprise Architecture project was implemented in Rwanda over a period of five years. The project used an EA approach to design a system for connecting community-based maternal health systems with facility-based systems. The design included the adoption of interoperability and data standards as well as a health information exchange. The exchange connects central registries and services to community-based and facility-based point-of-care applications through a middleware interoperability application, the Open Health Information Mediator.[15] The Rwanda Health Information Exchange was implemented in the national data center in Kigali and serves 14 sites in one district in Rwanda. The design was generalized to create the Open Health Information Exchange,[16] or OpenHIE.

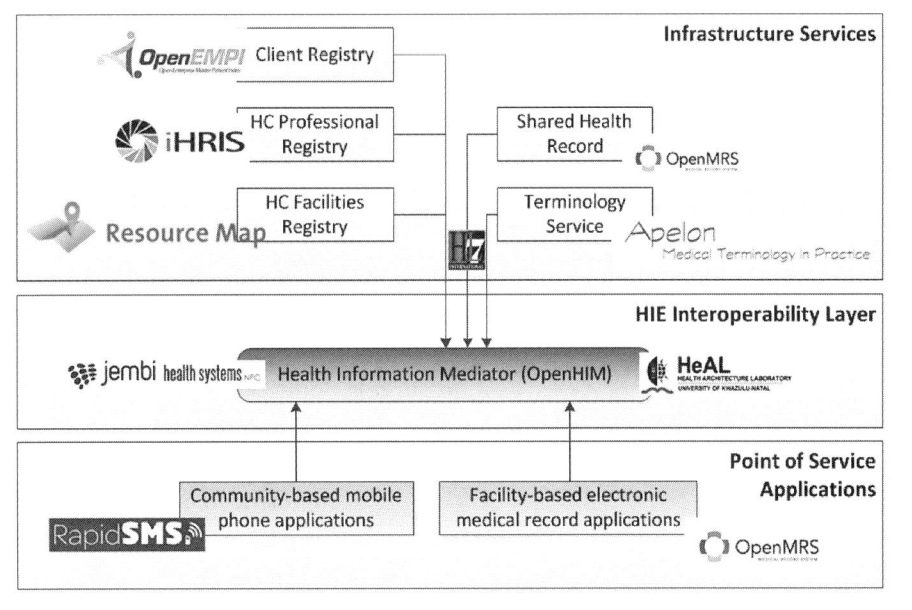

Notes

1. See http://en.wikipedia.org/wiki/Enterprise_architecture/.

2. See http://digitalprinciples.org.

3. See http://www.iso-architecture.org/42010/afs/.

4. See http://www.architectureframework.com/faq/.

5. See http://www.ict.griffith.edu.au/~bernus/taskforce/geram/versions/geram1-6-3/v1.6.3.html.

6. See http://msdn.microsoft.com/en-us/library/bb466232.aspx.

7. See http://www.iso-architecture.org/42010/afs/frameworks-table.html.

8. See http://www.uml.org.

9. See http://www.bpmn.org.

10. See http://www.opengroup.org/subjectareas/enterprise/archimate/.

11. See http://www.iso.org/iso/catalogue_detail?csnumber=54903/.

12. See http://www.doh.gov.ph/sites/default/files/Philippines_eHealthStrategicFrameworkPlan_February02 _2014_Release02.pdf

13. See http://hingx.org/Share/Details/973/.

14. See http://ohie.org.

15. See http://openhim.org.

16. See http://ohie.org.

References

1. Mwanyika H, Lubinski D, Anderson R, Chester K, Makame M, Steele M, et al. 2011. Rational systems design for health information systems in low-income countries: An enterprise architecture approach. *J Enterp Archit* 7(4): 60–69.

2. Stansfield S, Orobaton N, Lubinski D, Uggowitzer S, and Mwanyika H. 2008. The case for a national health information system architecture; a missing link to guiding national development and implementation. http://digital health-connection.org/files/ conf-materials/The%20Case%20for%20a%20National%20Helath%20Info%20 System_0.pdf.

3. Braa J, Hanseth O, Heywood A, Mohammed W, Shaw V. 2007. Developing health information systems in developing countries: The flexible standards strategy. *Manage Inf Syst Q* 31: 1–22.

4. Braa J, Kanter A, Lesh N, Crichton R, Jolliffe B, Sæbø J, et al. 2010. Comprehensive yet scalable health information systems for low resource settings: A collaborative effort in Sierra Leone. AMIA Annu Symp Proc., 372–376.

5. IEEE. 2000. IEEE 1471-2000. IEEE recommended practice for architectural description of software-intensive systems.

6. International Organization for Standardization. 2011. ISO/IEC FDIS 42010 IEEE P42010/D9. Systems and software engineering—architecture description.

7. Emery D, Hilliard R. 2009. Every architecture description needs a framework: Expressing architecture frameworks using ISO/IEC 42010. In 2009 Joint Working IEEE/IFIP Conference on Software Architecture and European Conference on Software Architecture, 31–40.

8. International Federation for Information Processing. 1999. GERAM : Generalised enterprise reference architecture and methodology. Version 1.6.3.

9. Sessions R. 2007. A comparison of the top four enterprise architecture methodologies [white paper].

10. Zachman JA. 1987. A framework for information systems architecture. *IBM Syst J* 26(3): 276–292.

11. Chief Information Officer Council. 2001. A practical guide to federal enterprise architecture. http://www.gao.gov/assets/590/588407.pdf. Government Accounting Office.

12. Estrin D, Sim I. 2010. Health care delivery. Open mHealth architecture: An engine for health care innovation. *Science* 330(6005): 759–760.

13. Chen C, Haddad D, Selsky J, Hoffman JE, Kravitz RL, Estrin DE, et al. 2012. Making sense of mobile health data: An open architecture to improve individual- and population-level health. *J Med Internet Res* 14(4): E112.

14. Health Metrics Network. 2008. *Framework and Standards for Country Health Information Systems* 2nd ed. World Health Organization.

15. World Health Organization. 2013. Civil registration and vital statistics 2013: Challenges, best practice and design principles for modern systems. http://www.who.int/healthinfo/civil_registration/crvs_report_2013.pdf.

16. Braa J, Sahay S. 2012. *Integrated health information architecture: Power to the users. Design, development, and use.* New Delhi, India: Matrix Publishers.

17. Blobel B. 2000. Application of the component paradigm for analysis and design of advanced health system architectures. *Int J Med Inform* 60(3): 281–301.

18. Lopez DM and Blobel BGME. 2007. Connecting public health and clinical information systems by using a standardized methodology. *MEDINFO* 12(1): 132–136.

19. APAI CRVS. 2015. *CRVS Digitisation Guidebook. A Step-by-Step Guide to Digitising Civil Registration and Vital Statistics Processes in Low Resource Settings.* www.crvs-dgb.org.

20. The Open Group. 2012. ArchiMate® 2.0 Specification. The Open Group Standard.

21. Josey A. 2011. TOGAF® Version 9.1 enterprise edition: An introduction. The Open Group.

22. International Organization for Standardization. 2012. Health informatics: Capacity-based digital health architecture roadmap. Part 1: Overview of national digital health initiatives. ISO/TR 14639-1:2012.

23. International Organization for Standardization. 2014. Health informatics: Capacity-based digital health architecture roadmap. Part 2: Architectural components and maturity model. ISO/TR 14639-2:2014.

24. Adebesin F, Foster R, Kotze P, Van Greunen D. 2013. A review of interoperability standards in digital health and imperatives for their adoption in Africa. *South African Comput J* 50: 55–72.

25. National Department of Health and Council for Scientific and Industrial Research. 2014. Health normative standards framework for interoperability in digital health in South Africa. Version 2.0. National Department of Health, South Africa.

26. Payne J. 2013. The state of standards and interoperability for mHealth among low- and middle-income countries. mHealth Alliance. http://www.mhealthknowledge.org/ sites/default/files/12_state_of_standards_report_2013.pdf.

27. Ghana Health Service. 2009. Ghana health service enterprise architecture (the digital health architecture).

28. Mudaly T, Moodley D, Pillay A, Seebregts CJ, Singh S, Seebregts CJ, et al. 2013. Architectural frameworks for developing national health information systems in low and middle income countries. *First Int Conf Enterp Syst* 60–69.

29. Crichton R, Moodley D, Pillay A, Gakuba R, Seebregts CJ. 2013. An architecture and reference implementation of an open health information mediator: Enabling interoperability in the Rwandan health information exchange. *Lecture Notes in Comput Sci* 7789: 87–104.

30. Shvaiko P, Villafiorita A, Zorer A, Chemane L, Fumo T, Hinkkanen J. 2009. EGIF4M: EGovernment interoperability framework for Mozambique. *Lecture Notes in Comput Sci* 5693: 328–340.

31. Macleod B, Phillips J, Stone AE, Walji A, Awoonor-Williams JK. 2012. The architecture of a software system for supporting community-based primary health care with mobile technology: The mobile technology for community health (MoTeCH) initiative in Ghana. *Online J Public Health Inform* 4(1): 1–17.

15 Secondary Data Use

William Perry, Rose Wyber, and Samuel Vaillancourt

Take-Home Messages

- Secondary data use encompasses all analysis beyond the primary intended use. It makes it possible to use information routinely collected to better understand risks and determinants of health for populations and to improve disease management.

- The secondary use of data in low- and middle-income countries has distinctly different dynamics from data use in high-resource settings, and is influenced by different incentives.

- Big data's mechanism of action is magnification; sheer size makes risks and benefits larger. This amplification is greater in low-resource settings, where data is most needed and most vulnerable to fragmentation and misuse.

- There is increasing need for an educated transparent process for data governance on behalf of patients and populations, rather than piecemeal and undecipherable consent protocols that provide little effective choice or protection. Such a process needs to translate societal values and concerns into best practices on complex issues balancing benefits and risks of data use.

Introduction

The primary use of health data is to improve delivery of clinical care to individuals [1]. In high-resource health settings, this is exemplified by the use of electronic medical records (EMRs) to deliver improved services via collating clinical records, generating patient-specific alerts, and automating outputs. In the United States, uptake of EMRs has been promulgated by a 2009 US$27 billion federal government commitment to have EMRs used by hospitals and health care providers [2]. Although there are technical challenges in implementation, adoption of EMRs in primary care is steadily increasing and has been linked to cost savings [3] and improved clinical care [4,5]. However, health records provide only a fragment of information on the determinants of population health. The promise of big data for health is in developing new insights from linking varied sources of information together, a process called secondary data use.

Types of Secondary Data

Secondary data use encompasses all analysis beyond the primary intended use—that is, individual health care delivery, in the case of EMRs. We divide secondary data use into two broad entities [box 15.1]. Direct secondary data in health includes clinical audit, research, and population-level health projects [1]. This data is sourced directly from health records, then collated and analyzed to inform future care at both the individual and population levels. The critical characteristic is the creation of this data during routine provision of individual health care. In contrast, a vast amount of information can be sourced from data not intended for health purposes, such as death certificates, hospital and physician billing data, vehicle registration information, criminal records, public health surveillance, municipal zoning registries, commercial databases, census databases, and so on. When carefully assembled together, these multiple sources of information can be linked to inform population health interventions. This data repurposing is termed indirect secondary data use in health. This data was not initially created for the provision of individual health care, but can be used to inform population health strategy or targeted care delivery.

Secondary data use, whether direct or indirect, makes it possible to use information routinely collected to better understand risks and determinants of health for populations and improve disease management. Thus, secondary data use provides a mechanism to tackle determinants of health status that are unrelated to direct service provision [6]. This chapter outlines the risks and opportunities of secondary uses of data in health. Although we focus primarily on direct secondary data use for health, the principles apply to both direct and indirect uses. The role of secondary data use in high-resource settings is then contrasted with opportunities in low- and middle-income countries (LMIC), before challenges and future steps are discussed.

Box 15.1
Definitions of Secondary Data

Direct secondary data: data sourced directly from health records, created initially in the provision of individual health care.

Indirect secondary data: data accessed from sources that were not initially created for the provision of individual health care.

Secondary Data Use in High-Resource Settings

In high-resource settings, the utility of secondary use of data for health is readily demonstrated. For example, in Franklin County, Ohio, body mass index (BMI) and ZIP code data were extracted from the EMRs of 62,701 people receiving care at an academic medical center [7]. ZIP codes were linked to census and commercial data on infrastructure, such as farmers markets and grocery stores, and to education levels in each ZIP code. This provided new insight into the real-world association between food infrastructure and obesity outcomes. In Durham County, North Carolina, a similar project linked public health surveillance data on blood lead levels with census and tax payments data. This allowed the county to better target its screening efforts to children at higher risk of lead toxicity [8]. EMRs of the future may be able to tap into other databases and repurpose their information for secondary use, allowing, for example, the identification of children at high risk of lead exposure with electronic alerts during routine clinical visits. Increasingly, data collected routinely for administrative or commercial purposes can be harnessed for the improvement of the health of people and straddle the divide between population health and care delivery.

The promise of secondary use of data for health is predicated on access to primary data. This is fraught by confidentiality, security, consent, transferability, ethical, governance, and quality issues. Some of the challenges are illustrated by an Icelandic project in the late 1990s during which health data was declared a national resource and access to individual health records, including genetic data, was provided to private industry without the informed consent of individuals [9]. National and international opposition prevented any data transfer, and by 2003 the project had collapsed [9]. This case highlights the evolving nature of the norms and systems of governance required to harness big data safely and transition it from individual use to use for populations.

Secondary Data Use in Low-Resource Settings

The diffusion of new technology in LMIC is commonly a mix of appropriation, diffusion, and, often, the "leapfrogging" of intermediate development phases. "Leapfrogging" is starkly exemplified by the penetration of mobile phones in low-resource settings over the last 15 years without a preceding period of fixed-line telephone ownership. The use of mobile phones has already provided a pertinent example of indirect secondary data use.

Buckee and colleagues demonstrated how tracking mobile phone use could help fight malaria by revealing where to focus mosquito eradication efforts [10]. They used mobile phone use to analyze the regional travel patterns of nearly 15 million individuals over the course of a year in, and found that people making calls or sending text messages originating at the Kericho tower were three times more likely to visit a region northeast of Lake Victoria, a malaria hot spot. The Kericho tower thus represented a waypoint for transmission of malaria. A similar model has been used in the 2014 Ebola outbreak [11].

The secondary use of data in LMIC has distinctly different dynamics from data use in high-resource settings. Critically, the primary use of physician-held EMRs and health data in LMIC is limited, but the relatively democratized data collection from individuals and communities may be more acceptable. For example, in Kenya, nearly 500 community elders were trained to weigh newborns and report via text messaging birth weights to vital statistics registers [12].

The incentives for collection and use also differ between high- and low-resource settings. Proprietary systems dominate the EMR market in the developed world, and data may be "owned" by health care providers or consortiums. However, different market dynamics in LMIC mean that more mHealth and eHealth projects are conducted by governments and not-for-profit actors. These providers tend to use open-source EMR products [13] and often have a stated goal of improving population outcomes in addition to individual care. However, ad hoc mHealth systems may not follow interoperability standards. This can complicate data linkage and limit analysis.

Indirect use of secondary data is also influenced by differing incentives. In many parts of the world, reliable data may be more likely to be collected by mobile phone operators or banks than government-directed health data sources. However, the private sector may have strikingly different priorities and commercial sensitivities determining the use of data. These issues affect the potential use of indirect secondary data in the interest of humanitarian or public health outcomes. Paradoxically, an uncritical urge to share data of vulnerable populations in order to "do good" can increase the risk of inadequate consultation or unforeseen consequences. Authors of a London School of Economic report caution that "the challenge for developing countries and humanitarian operations is that we have a tendency to think and act on behalf of the citizens and patients"; they call for a rights-based approach to data sharing and collection [14].

The staggering pace of primary and secondary data use for health in LMIC may offer novel opportunities to embed appropriate mechanisms for secondary health data use in first-generation platforms. One of the most promising opportunities for big data in global health can be seen in India's ambitious personal identification program. In 2010, the government of India began issuing "Aadhaar" cards with unique identifying numbers to all 1.2 billion of its citizens [15]. Biometric identification captured through fingerprints and iris identification offers the opportunity for generating and monitoring health and social data [16]. Use of Aadhaar linked to immunization records could help ensure individual children receive the appropriate vaccine according to national schedules. Furthermore, secondary analysis of de-identified data may make it possible to identify areas with low immunization rates for targeted immunization campaigns.

One of the greatest challenges in fulfilling the potential of secondary use of data in resource-limited settings is the ability to analyze quantitative outputs. The uptake of mHealth in LMIC reflects low barriers to entry; namely, widespread mobile phone ownership and the rapidly appreciable utility of text messages or other tangible rewards for participation [17]. In contrast, the value of the secondary use of health data resides in centralizing and linking datasets, which requires technical skills, specialized equipment, interoperability standards, coherent collection, analytical systems, and regulatory oversight. Moreover, the distance between individuals contributing data and systems outputs and benefits can be immense. However, signs of data ownership from LMIC are emerging; for example, a new network, critical of existing data-sharing approaches, is collating public health research data from health and demographic surveillance systems of over 3 million people in 48 populations [18]. Overcoming the analytic capacity challenges in LMIC may make it possible to leapfrog the nascent secondary use of health data in high-resource settings and embed secondary-use capacity in mHealth and eHealth projects in low-resource settings.

Further Challenges for Big Data in Low- and Middle-Income Countries

Large-scale implementation of big-data and secondary-use systems for health in LMIC faces many challenges. The collection of individual-level information—a prerequisite for big data—poses risks commensurate to the existing challenges of care delivery in low-resource settings. Opposing prospects for the future of big data in LMIC are outlined in box 15.2 and box 15.3, illustrating dystopian and utopian elements.

Box 15.2
Dystopian Big Data

In the worst-case scenario, big data becomes an expensive distraction driven by the global North, focused on disease-specific outcomes and unintelligible to those who most need data access. Siloed data that cannot be readily shared or compared could fragment an already fragile global health community. Breaches of data security could threaten personal safety, potentiating discrimination, violence, or genocide. The global health community could oversee spending of big money on big data with potentially little to show for the investment.

In brief, we could see:

1. diversion of focus and resources away from more-needed interventions.
2. poor data governance, with databases held by private companies, frequent leaks, and no recourse for citizens.
3. consent offloaded through poorly designed consent systems.
4. a lack of interoperability, with balkanized information systems that cannot be aggregated together.
5. poorly presented information and analysis considered not credible or illegible by patients, health care providers, entrepreneurs, and policy makers.

Box 15.3
Utopian Big Data

The era of big data may provide an opportunity for LMIC to leapfrog into robust secondary data use models. Decision makers in LMIC could develop a "demand side" platform to identify the information they need most. Partnerships formed with academia, industry, governments, international organizations, and the nonprofit sector could help innovate solutions. Although this idealized approach is optimistic, it is no less ambitious than the Sustainable Development Goals, eradicating polio, or controlling malaria. Indeed, achieving a "best case" model for deploying big data may be one of the keys to fulfilling these other promises.
  In brief, we could see:

1. individual data owned by patients.
2. robust governance processes developed to ensure respect of guiding values and principles in the use of data.
3. data automatically aggregated with little effort and decreasing cost.
4. interoperability standards required, with data seamlessly pooled and connected.
5. governments developing laws that allow the seamless sharing and pooling of data in real time while establishing adequate safeguards.
6. data presented in a usable format in a way that can be impactful to patients, health care providers, entrepreneurs, and policy makers.

Of universal concern is the threat to privacy posed by the digitization and centralization of personal health information. Although in practice, secondary use involves anonymized data, capacity to interpolate back to individuals may be intentionally or unintentionally retained. Sweeney claims that 87% of the US population can be uniquely identified simply using their date of birth, gender, and zip code [19]. For this reason, US health privacy regulation—HIPAA—stipulates that 18 specific identifiers must be removed before data is used for population health analysis [20].

Privacy concerns are further amplified when information is about individuals in vulnerable populations and communities. Even very basic health data—ethnicity, reproductive health history, sexually transmitted infections, diseases with a genetic basis, or risk exposures for disease—has the potential for misuse, discrimination, personal danger, or, in some cases, death [21]. Breaches to digital privacy in any setting are problematic, and there is concern the risk may be amplified by secondary use of health data. Certainly, the risk of accidental or intentional breaches of data security may be increased with limited literacy, high corruption, and rapid technological transitions [22]. Privacy management in high-resource settings is rapidly becoming counterproductive and outdated and is of little help to LMIC looking at ways to tackle these challenges. Traditionally, privacy laws have emphasized consent for data collection by an individual for a specific purpose. In direct opposition to this system, secondary use of health data is about linking and re-using data for a different purpose. Current approaches may involve long, cumbersome, and unwieldy consent forms that are meaningless to patients and leave individuals poorly protected, yet set up barriers to the beneficial use of data. In many LMIC settings, legislation supporting the privacy and security of information services is frequently underdeveloped and rarely enforced. These issues highlight the difficulties in data-sharing guidelines between LMIC stakeholders that not only hamper the benefits of big data for health but can also compromise those in play [21]. The solutions inevitably lie in moving from individual purpose-specific consent to emphasizing data access monitoring, ethical use of data, and data governance.

Increasingly, poorly designed privacy safeguards are having dangerous consequences in limiting the benefits of data. Data is accumulated in silos, but it is increasingly clear that linkages and secondary use can result in potentially lifesaving intervention at the level of care delivery and planning. Direct secondary data for health is grossly underutilized, and the neglect of indirect secondary data is likely to be even greater. One review found that many of the variables collected in epidemiological studies were never cleaned or coded—the primary researchers could not even use the data [23]. Pisani and AbouZahr articulate that "undervalued and underfunded, inadequate data management undermines the rest of the scientific enterprise" [24]. Indeed, it undermines population health.

By default, it is impossible to imagine all possible secondary uses of data at the time of collection. Consequently, purpose-specific consent processes at the time of collection need to be replaced with selective sharing capability and transparent, traceable data access. There is increasing need for an educated transparent process for data governance on behalf of patients and populations, rather than piecemeal and undecipherable consent protocols that provide little effective choice or protection. Such a process needs to translate societal values and concerns into best practices on complex issues balancing benefits and risks of data use. Concerns about consent and data sharing will persist, particularly around the power imbalance between high- and low-resource settings [25]. An open, transparent process of data governance is necessary as societal values and technological feasibility continue to rapidly evolve.

This vision is tempered by today's reality in low-resource settings: weak health systems and limited governance structures complicate the emergence of a coherent and safe health data strategy. Many countries in greatest need of health metrics struggle to collect vital, simple statistics on births and deaths, while epidemiological data of variable reliability come from small sentinel sites. Moreover, little information is reliably digitized. Health interventions—food, water, and sanitation—remain top priorities for over two billion people. Data alone cannot address development challenges [26]. However, as the cost of aggregating and coordinating resources and services electronically falls, big data stands to deliver disproportionately large benefits to LMIC. The more limited the resources for interventions, the more valuable targeting and focusing can be.

The application of big data to global health amplifies potential benefits, risks, and challenges. The persistent tension between vertical or disease-specific programs and horizontal or health system–focused approaches remains unresolved. Big data fits best with a horizontal approach—potentially improving data for all diseases in the spirit of the ambitious and valuable Global Burden of Disease project [27]. However, global health remains a relatively siloed undertaking driven by disease-specific interests. Disease-specific advocacy groups may well be at the forefront of applications for big data—risking further fragmentation of the enterprise. Ensuring universal standards that allow data linkage, inclusive data collection, and data dissemination and application is critical for maximizing big data's potential.

The Next Step in Secondary Use of Data for Health

Linkage of data sets for the improvement of health remains in its infancy in LMIC. It offers both unprecedented promises, but also great challenges. Informed, reflective, and resourced stewardship is critical to enable positive outcomes. However, the structures for global health governance are relatively fragile [28]. The United Nations established Global Pulse in 2009 as an initiative of its Executive Office. The division is charged with "fostering development of the analytical, technological and organizational capacities that decision makers need to access and utilize new digital data sources and real-time analytics" [29]. However, data protection standards for Global Pulse are grounded in a 1990 UN resolution named "guidelines for the regulation of computerized personal data files"—which remains an iconic example of how the division falls short of providing much-needed contemporary guidelines for governance [30].

Guidance efforts have been made in the World Economic Forum's Global Health Data Charter, framed around the vision for "better data for better health" [31]. Eight key data health challenges have been identified, and "enabling" activities highlighted. However, few practical steps are articulated. Given the scope, cost, and risks of big-data projects, far stronger governance is needed. Unfortunately, the global health community has a patchy record of cohesive governance and stewardship of technical developments [32]. Optimizing the application of big data is much more than establishing confidentiality safeguards and minimum standards. A broad effort to establish enforceable interoperability standards is imperative to creating linkages between datasets that can offer insight. Big data then needs a strategically driven approach to maximize benefits in the global health setting. Global health governance needs to move from a reactive model to a proactive, norm-forming approach.

Conclusion

An unprecedented number of datasets are created around the world for commercial, administrative, or humanitarian purposes. Together with eHealth, they could contribute to a new evolution from evidence-based medicine to results-based health care, enabling more targeted therapy for individuals to better the health of entire populations. Big data's mechanism of action is magnification, but sheer size makes both risks and benefits larger. This amplification is greater in low-resource settings, where data is most needed and most vulnerable to fragmentation and misuse. Conscious and committed leadership, analysis, and technical guidance are needed to minimize these risks. Complexities should not be underestimated; the growth of information may be exponential, but the shift from paper to petabytes in LMIC is seismic. Shepherding that transition provides another opportunity for global health institutions to demonstrate the powerful impact of positive global governance for health.

Questions for Discussion

- Discuss the risks and benefit of secondary data use. How does this differ between high-resourced and low- and middle-income settings?
- How can a rights-based approach to health data be reconciled with allowing for the benefits of secondary data use to be fulfilled?
- What do you think are the key elements to global governance of big data? Describe three principles you would include in a secondary-use data charter.
- As a recipient of health care, how would you want secondary health data to be used?

References

1. Safran C, Bloomrosen M, Hammond E, Labkoff S, Markel-Fox S, Tang P, et al. 2007. Towards a national framework for secondary use of health data: An American Medical Informatics Association white paper. *J Am Med Inform Assoc* 14(1): doi:10.1197/jamia.M2273.

2. Webster P. 2010. Electronic health records a "strong priority" for US government. *CMAJ* 182(2): E315–E6.

3. Wang SJ, Middleton B, Prosser LA, Bardon CG, Spurr CD, Carchidi PJ, et al. 2003. A cost-benefit analysis of electronic medical records in primary care. *Am J Med* 114(5): 397–403.

4. Menachemi N, Collum TH. 2011. Benefits and drawbacks of electronic health record systems. *Risk Manag Healthc Policy* 4: 46–55.

5. Hsiao C-J, Hing E. *Use and Characteristics of Electronic Health Record Systems Among Office-Based Physician Practices: United States, 2001–2013.* Hyattsville, MD: National Center for Health Statistics; 2014.

6. Marmot M, Allen J. 2014. Social determinants of health equity. *Am J Public Health* 104(S4): S517–S9.

7. Roth C, Foraker R, Payne P, Embi P. 2014. Community-level determinants of obesity: Harnessing the power of electronic health records for retrospective data analysis. *BMC Med Inform Decis Mak* 14: 36. doi:10.1186/1472-6947-14-36.

8. Miranda M, Ferranti J, Strauss B, Neelon B, Califf R. 2013. Geographic health information systems: A platform to support the "triple aim". *Health Aff* 32(9): 1608–1615.

9. Winickoff D. 2006. Genome and nation. Iceland's health sector database and its legacy. *Innovations* 1: 80–105.

10. Wesolowski A, Eagle N, Tatem AJ, Smith DL, Noor AM, Snow RW, et al. 2012. Quantifying the impact of human mobility on malaria. *Science* 338(6104): 267–270. doi:10.1126/science.1223467.

11. Talbot D. 2014. Cell-phone data might help predict Ebola's spread. *MIT Technology Review*, August 22. http://www.technologyreview.com/news/530296/cell-phone-data -might-help-predict-ebolas-spread/. Accessed November 10, 2014.

12. Gisore P, Shipala E, Otieno K, Rono B, Marete I, Tenge C, et al. 2012. Community based weighing of newborns and use of mobile phones by village elders in rural settings in Kenya: A decentralised approach to health care provision. *BMC Pregnancy Childbirth* 12(15): doi:10.1186/471-2393-12-15.

13. Aminpour F, Sadoughi F, Ahamdi M. 2014. Utilization of open source electronic health record around the world: A systematic review. *J Res Med Sci* 19(1): 57–64.

14. London School of Economics and Political Science. 2007. Electronic health privacy and security in developing countries and humanitarian operations. A report prepared by the Policy Engagement Network for the International Development Research Centre, The London School of Economics and Political Science.

15. Kumar K. 2013. Unique ID program introduces instant verification services [blog]. *New York Times*, May 24. http://india.blogs.nytimes.com/2013/05/24/aadhar-program -introduces-instant-verification-services/. Accessed July 20, 2013.

16. Kannan S. 2013. Apollo hospitals working on linking e-health records with Aadhaar. *The Hindu BusinessLine*, February 10. http://www.thehindubusinessline.com/companies/ apollo-hospitals-working-on-linking-ehealth-records-with-aadhaar/article4400591.ece. Accessed July 20, 2013.

17. Boyd C. 2012. RapidSMS: Saving a life in 160 characters. BBC, August 3. http://www .bbc.com/future/story/20120803-saving-a-life-in-160-characters. Accessed September 1, 2013.

18. Sankoh O, Herbst A, Juvekar S, Tollman S, Bayass P, Tanner M. 2013. INDEPTH launches a data repository and INDEPTHStats. *Lancet Glob Health* 1(2): E69.

19. Zetter K. 2009. Medical records: Stored in the cloud, sold on the open market. *Wired*. http://www.wired.com/2009/10/medicalrecords. Accessed November 3, 2014.

20. Klein C. Cloudy Confidentiality: Clinical and Legal Implications of Cloud Computing in Health Care. *J Am Acad Psychiatry Law* 39: 571–578.

21. Policy Engagement Network. 2010. *Electronic health privacy and security in developing countries and humanitarian operations.* London: Policy Engagement Network, London School of Economics and Policy Science.

22. Thomson Reuters Foundation, TrustLaw Connect. 2013. Patient privacy in a mobile world. A framework to address privacy laws in mobile health. http://www.mhealthknowledge.org/sites/default/files/10_trustlaw_connect_report.pdf.

23. Corti L, Wright M. *MRC Population Data Archiving and Access.* London: Medical Research Council; 2002.

24. Pisani E, AbouZahr C. 2010. Sharing health data: Good intentions are not enough. *Bull World Health Organ* 88: 462–466.

25. Tangcharoensathien V, Boonperm J, Jongudomsuk P. 2010. Sharing health data: Developing country perspectives. *Bull World Health Organ* 88: 468–469.

26. UN. *Big Data for Development: Challenges and Opportunities.* New York, NY: Global Pulse, United Nations 2012.

27. Institute for Health Metrics and Evaluation. *the Global Burden of Disease: Generating Evidence, Guiding Policy.* Seattle, WA: Institute for Health Metrics and Evaluation; 2013.

28. Ottersen O, Frenk J, Horton R. 2012. The Lancet University of Oslo Commission on Global Governance for Health, in collaboration with the Harvard Global Health Institute. *Lancet* 378(9803): 1612–1613.

29. UN Global Pulse. 2013. Strategy and roadmap. http://www.unglobalpulse.org/roadmap. Accessed September 9, 2013.

30. UN Global Pulse. Our privacy and data protection principles. 2013. http://www.unglobalpulse.org/privacy-and-data-protection. Accessed September 2, 2013.

31. World Economic Forum. 2011. Global Health Data Charter: World Economic Forum.

32. Gostin L, Mok E, Friedman E. 2011. Towards a radical transformation in global governance for health. *Michael.* 8: 228–239.

III IMPLEMENTING A HEALTH INFORMATICS PROJECT

The subsequent chapters delve into the practical process of implementing a health informatics project. While not a comprehensive manual or cookbook, the text presents particular challenges unique to developing a technology innovation in the global health setting.

We begin with an overview of the entire project life cycle and its many complicated participants and components, highlighting the cross-disciplinary nature of designing, developing, and deploying an informatics project. The next chapter then starts at the top of the project team, acknowledging the necessity of strong and knowledgeable leadership with uncommon abilities to communicate and coordinate across fields and experiences. This segues to bringing together the multidisciplinary team, calling for collaboration, co-creation, and capacity building. Once you have the team together, we continue onto the crucial design stage, where we expound on essential processes that facilitate connecting a technology innovation with quality improvements in health.

It is not until chapter 20 that we dive into specifics relating to software development. This chapter provides an introductory discussion on various software project-management approaches, and may seem rudimentary for experienced engineers; however, the text addresses particular methodologies that are necessary in the resource-limited global health setting. Usability and user experience retain their own chapter, since designing specifically to appropriate audiences will yield great influence on project adoption.

Finally, we close with three chapters on high-level topics that have strong influence on the implementation and sustainability of any innovation. Privacy and security have a growing influence on technology innovations, with the growing preponderance of generated health data and the overarching question of who owns that data. We then touch on the need to fund a project, glancing on the complicated financing options. Innovative business models are too often short-changed (and don't get enough emphasis here either), but will necessarily play an increasing role in resource-limited settings where direct beneficiaries often cannot pay. Finally, the section closes with critical material on monitoring and evaluating your informatics project, which are fundamental to ensuring that a project avoids simply being an inefficient tool for the sake of technology, and instead advances toward a sustainable innovation making a positive impact on lives and outcomes.

16 A Global Health Project Life Cycle

Cory Zue and Kenneth Paik

Take-Home Messages

- Key phases for a global health project include design, development, and deployment. These interdependent processes are flexible and adaptable to a variety of solutions, but have particular challenges unique to global health implementations.
- Technology is only a small part of any global health informatics project, since existing resources, workflows, regulatory environments, and so on are necessary to consider for the successful implementation of any technical solution.

Introduction

As the previous chapters of the book have established, there is a great potential for digital solutions to make a profound impact in the access and delivery of health care in the global context. In particular, rapidly evolving technology improvements in power, cost, and ubiquity afford the opportunity to overcome significant resource and infrastructure limitations. The prevailing questions: how can we ensure that technology is making a positive impact in health outcomes, and what are the steps we can take to build a sustainable solution?

Here we introduce a global health informatics project life cycle as a framework for developing a technology solution. This is not intended as a comprehensive, step-by-step guide, but rather to provide a high-level understanding of key considerations and practical insights toward a successful implementation. Incorporating technology into global health is complicated and requires a holistic approach to address unique challenges. An underlying theme throughout the process is to bring together many diverse perspectives to engage situational specificities and complex clinical scenarios.

Overview of the Project Life Cycle

While there are many ways to generalize and sequence a project life cycle, in this overview, we will be describing a conceptual three-phase system comprising design, development, and deployment (figure 16.1). While we present these stages as largely flowing in order, it is important to note that most projects do not move linearly forward and may have work going on in multiple stages at the same time, since there is substantial crossover and overlap across any phase. Furthermore, following a process of testing and validation within constantly changing environments, we often find that projects call for adaptation, so certain steps may need to be repeated or revised to adjust to changing requirements. We will describe each phase briefly in this chapter, then focus on certain specific segments for further detail in subsequent chapters.

Design

We begin with the design phase, which in many ways is the most fundamental, as it defines and frames the entire process and subsequent phases. The overarching objectives are to gain a better understanding of the problem being solved, defining what the product is trying to do, planning how the project may be built, and bringing together an appropriate team to accomplish these goals.

There are many different ways for a project to get started, perhaps driven by a governmental organization attempting to control an outbreak or escalating societal costs, an NGO targeting proposals within their mission purview, entrepreneurs trying to make a positive impact with their work, or driven by popular demand to solve a pressing need.

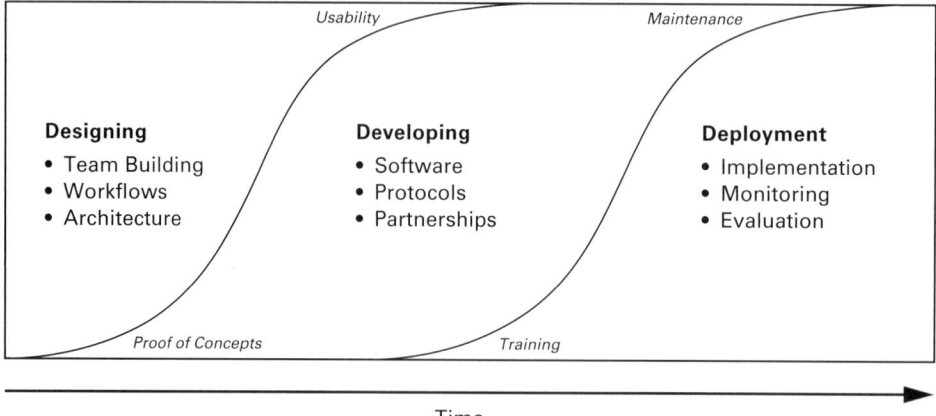

Figure 16.1
Diagram of the three steps, in process or summarized.

Thus, some steps may be predetermined or preempted, but every project needs to complete the design process to identify gaps and needs.

We are using the term "design" here as a catchall for many aspects of the planning process, but must emphasize the importance of these steps. Fundamentally, the design process determines requirements for development and the mechanisms for integrating a technology solution within existing environments. While this sometimes entails reproducing a technical solution that worked well in another setting, we also want to avoid replicating broken systems or attempting to force a solution into an environment merely because it uses the latest technologies. The design process hopefully leads to a deep understanding of the local environment, adapting its unique challenges and integrating with the unique workflows, leading to an effective and usable solution. The essential components of the design process include those described below.

Forming the Idea   Determining what problem to solve is almost as important as the actual solution. Targeting the wrong problem can lead to wasted time and avoidable revisions. For optimal impact, it is most crucial to generate ideas that will have a positive effect on health rather than simply being a solution using the latest technologies.

Bringing Together the Team   Team makeup is ultimately the most significant indicator for project success. Health care is inordinately complicated, involving many more sectors than just the practice of clinical medicine (operations, logistics, finance, and legal, to name a few). The best teams combine multidisciplinary perspectives, leading to holistic and effective solutions. It is paramount to either include in the process or consider deeply the perspectives of all stakeholders, as their compliance or engagement will be crucial to success.

Planning the Project   Any substantial project will require significant coordination and planning. With a technology project, this includes coordinating the disparate development teams through the design and development stages. Depending on the scope of the project, this may include clinical testing through a pilot or business-model validation. There should be early considerations for sustainability and how the project may continue to make an impact in the long term.

Architecting a Solution   An initial system architecture should be considered early in order to better inform other steps. Identifying key system components will identify necessary technical skillsets and expertise that will be required to include on the team. This will allow for early feasibility input and set reasonable expectations for what technology can accomplish. During the design stage, it is also important to identify the flow of data and information and how any technical solution integrates with existing workflows.

Subsequent chapters that dive deeper into the topics of the design process including collaborating and building teams (chapter 18), as well as approaching the design challenges of cultural and workflow uniqueness (chapter 19).

Development

The development phase can paradoxically be the most straightforward or the most frustrating, partly depending on how well the other phases are completed. Software development is an intensive process requiring highly skilled resources and experience, but, with sufficiently defined requirements and understanding, the construction of prototypes can be uncomplicated. The crucial component of that previous statement is "understanding." It is strongly discouraged to merely outsource development with basic requirements, as that will often lead to generic or fragmented products that have unintended consequences. Instead, we recommend a design thinking approach to development, with the development team engaged with stakeholders throughout the process for a deeper understanding of the problem and environment. This continuous engagement will also allow for quicker validation and iteration of designs.

Multidisciplinary Coordination   While in this textbook we focus on the software development process, for a global health project there will also usually be accompanying clinical and business development. Clinical development may entail defining clinical protocols or guidelines to implementation that may influence workflow and practices. Business development may include establishing partnerships and validating business models. All of these development aspects need to be coordinated, since there will often be interdependencies between them, such as clinical protocols needing to be established before the prototype interface can be finalized or partnerships established before being able to identify the target user base.

Resource Management   Early in the development process, you must consider available resources and technologies and adjust plans accordingly. This includes the development resources available (such as the number and skill of the engineers), but also what technologies and platforms are available within the local environment. Technology is not globally universal, and what is common in one region may be different from what is dominant in another. An overview of the essential health information technologies has been reviewed in Part 2.

In subsequent chapters, we will go into more depth regarding the software development process and alternatives therein (chapter 20) and usability testing (chapter 21) to ensure effective deployment.

Deployment

After the solution is developed, deployment entails implementation of the project, evaluation of its effectiveness and impact, and scaling the project. This again is often distinct across projects, but the general objectives are to refine the solution and progress toward a sustainable health impact. Deployment is particularly challenging in a global health project, since there are several daunting challenges for any solution. Technology is ultimately only a small part of the success of any health informatics project, as any solution needs to be closely integrated within existing workflows, engaging key stakeholders along the entire process.

Human Resources Essential human resources play a hugely significant role in a global health project, as the health care workforce requires abundant amounts of specialty training and unique skillsets. The potential workforce in the target implementation region that meets the criteria is often limited, leading to a "zero-sum game" by creating a competition between global health projects. This could potentially overburden the health care workforce or drastically increase implementation costs.

Another aspect that is often forgotten during implementation is ongoing training costs of the workforce. With any new guideline, protocol, or technology, the workforce will need to be adequately trained in order to ensure effective deployment. Usability (chapter 21) plays an important role in end-user adoption; developers must consider baseline technical competence, since not every individual is comfortable with using the latest computer or smartphone technologies.

Sustainable Quality Improvement Ultimately, as previously stated, the goal for a global health informatics project is sustainable impact in improving health outcomes. Ongoing evaluation and monitoring (chapter 24) measuring outcomes and health metrics is required to support clinical effectiveness. More importantly, technology solutions must consider methods to "close the loop," wherein specific interventions are connected to positive outcomes. Too often, projects merely collect data about a patient for research and publication purposes. For many complicated health conditions, in order to drive sustainable impact, the intervention needs to yield a specific benefit to the patients, which often involves follow-up care beyond a software application.

Maintenance and Scaling After implementation, maintenance typically entails minor enhancements, fixing defects, addressing scale or performance issues, and continually evaluating the product's performance. Incremental improvements and iterations, responsiveness to user feedback, and managing technical debt (chapter 20) lead to happier users and increased adoption. These processes require significant costs and resources and must be included in the plan for ongoing projects.

Beyond maintenance is scaling a project to the next step and expanding beyond the original project scope. This can increase the impact of the program by integrating with more services or expand to additional regions to reach a larger population. This necessitates careful considerations of sustainability and business models (chapter 23) for all projects, whether they are supported by grants or are intended to be commercial ventures.

Unique Regulatory Barriers The unique regulatory barriers to health technologies are a frequently encountered impediment. Even with clearly identified needs and benefits, politics can still get in the way. For example, most public health initiatives require buy-in from local governments, which are sometimes bureaucratic or have their own focused initiatives for limited resources. Another example is the regulatory environment for medical devices across differing regions: a product that was developed in one region may need to undergo extensive testing and evaluation from other local regulatory bodies.

The sensitive nature of health information and the need for patient privacy and security are an additional aspect to the regulatory environment (chapter 22). With the growing pervasiveness of electronic health data, there is growing concern over the vulnerabilities exposed by these expanding centralized data stores. Immense amounts of sensitive patient information can be exposed due to a software bug, security intrusion, or simple human error. Navigating these intricacies is important to consider throughout the project life cycle to avoid a violation and protect vulnerable populations.

Conclusion

The global health project life cycle described in this chapter is a simplified process highlighting the essential requirements for an effective solution. All three phases—design, development, and deployment—are interconnected and crucial to appropriately plan and manage the multidisciplinary aspects. These principles are applicable to all projects, though the process and order may need to be adapted to your specific project needs.

Questions for Discussion

- Why is design important when building a technical solution? What are some examples that come into play in each of the three phases of a project life cycle?

- At what stages of the project life cycle should you investigate and involve various stakeholders?

- What are some deployment challenges you might encounter when you are implementing a project?

17 Leadership Skills for Global Health Care Innovators

Laura J. Mintz and James K. Stoller

Take-Home Messages

- Leadership involves a set of skills that can be learned and implemented throughout organizations.
- Leadership can be distinguished from management by its aims, scale, and component parts.
- Collaboration is a critical component of leadership, and should be especially emphasized in settings where resources are scarce.
- 360-degree evaluation using well-validated tools and strategies is a critical element of effective leadership development.

Introduction

In order to successfully bring new technologies, modes of care delivery, and other innovations to under-resourced communities, effective leaders must manage the interests of multiple parties. Funders, government officials, existing health care structures, and the needs of the community must all play a role in successfully implementing new approaches and technologies. To achieve these goals, leaders and innovators must have the skills to address the needs of competing parties while they provide care that is accessible and has both high quality and low cost. Though these challenges apply to health care in all settings, they are amplified and especially daunting in resource-poor countries.

Overcoming these challenges in health care requires many critical success factors, arguably the most important of which is effective leadership. This chapter reviews the issue of leadership needs for innovating in global health. Specifically, we first discuss why leadership development is especially important for health care providers. Next, we review leadership competencies, both in general and in the specific context of health care. Finally, we review the leadership competencies that are most relevant to health care in resource-poor settings.

Why Is Leadership Development Needed for Innovation in Global Health?

Leadership skills are needed for innovators in global health to address the competing priorities and other challenges in this area. The need for leadership development is compounded by the fact that, at least in the case of physicians, the training experience cultivates behaviors that are antithetical to teamwork and collaboration [1]. Stoller has pointed out the four features of medical training that conspire against physicians' having teamwork behavior: (1) long and hierarchical training; (2) a heavy emphasis on individual performance throughout training; (3) the risk of "extrapolated authority;" and (4) deficit-based thinking. He suggests that "doctors are collaboratively challenged" [2]. A recent literature review suggests similar dynamics confound nursing education [3] and practice [4]. These insights are not new. Writing in 1978 regarding "why organizational development had not worked (so far) in medical centers," Weisbord pointed out that "science-based professional work differs markedly from product-based work. Health professionals learn rigorous scientific discipline as the 'content' of their training. The 'process' inculcates a value for autonomous decision making, personal achievement, and the importance of improving their *own* performance rather than that of any institution" [5]. Taken together, this divergence between the need for effective leadership and teamwork [6] in health care and the innate and trained behaviors of health care providers creates a paradox that must be addressed by developing leadership competencies among care providers.

In business sectors outside of health care, leadership skills are widely acknowledged to drive success, and leadership development programs have been widely implemented in a range of businesses (e.g., General Electric, IBM, Boeing, Federal Express, Toyota, Motorola, etc.). Requirements for a successful leadership development program have been studied and include [7]:

- having an influential champion
- having an institutional perspective that leadership is needed throughout the organization
- ensuring that the development program is tied to a current business imperative
- ensuring that programs are integrated as a process in an overarching strategy, not as standalone activities
- having dedicated facilities, with preference for an off-site location
- patience by organizational leadership.

For example, General Electric (GE) invests $1 billion a year in supporting the Jack Welsh Leadership Development Center in Crotonville, New York, which annually invites both junior and senior GE employees to engage in progressive learning about leadership competencies. Reflecting a longstanding commitment to developing leaders at GE, the center was established in 1956. In addition to similar commitments to developing leaders in other traditionally successful companies, leadership development programs also continue to be important in younger, emerging companies like Mozilla, developer of the Firefox browser [8–10].

Multinational companies also recognize the need for leadership competencies to ensure the success of global business endeavors. Terrell and Rosenbusch [11] examined the characteristics of successful global leaders and reported that they:

- develop through firsthand global leadership experience
- understand the importance of cultural sensitivity, relationships, and networks
- are driven by curiosity, openness, and a desire to learn.

The health care industry has generally lagged behind other business sectors in focusing on leadership development; indeed, in health care organizations (and particularly in academic medical centers), the selection of leaders has usually been based on traditional criteria of academic, clinical, or scientific prowess rather than on candidates' distinctive leadership competencies [12]. These traditional criteria overlook the fact that leadership competencies differ from scientific, clinical, or academic competencies and are not generally taught as part of traditional health care training. As such, attention to developing the leadership competencies of health care workers has been relatively sparse [13]. These competencies are discussed next.

Leadership Competencies for Health Care

Many models of leadership have been proposed and debated [14–16]; much of the debate has centered on the discussion of leadership as an innate "trait" (e.g., as something analogous to extraversion) versus an "ability," a set of skills that can be learned, practiced, and developed by individuals [17,18]. The latter models, in which leadership is characterized as a set of competencies that can be evaluated and cultivated, are especially relevant for health care providers.

In our experience, the leadership model proposed by Kouzes and Posner [19] offers a useful approach in health care, because the competencies can be both evaluated [14] and developed. The leadership assessment instrument for the Kouzes and Posner model, called the Leadership Practices Inventory (LPI), was developed by surveying leaders in the public and private sectors from a variety of countries; factor analysis was then performed to confirm the validity and reliability of the instrument.

In this model, Kouzes and Posner describe five components of leadership: (1) challenging the process; (2) inspiring a shared vision; (3) enabling others to act; (4) modeling the way; and (5) encouraging the heart. Each aspect of effective leadership is described below:

- "Challenging the process" describes the drive of leaders to grow, improve, take risks, and learn from mistakes.

- "Modeling the way" describes those leaders who describe and then act on high standards in all aspects of their work.

- "Inspiring a shared vision" describes those leaders who are able to inspire and appeal to all of their team members to create a vision together.

- "Enabling others to act" is the skill of cultivating leadership in the whole team.

- "Encouraging the heart" describes leaders who understand and recognize the critical contributions of each team member to the overall success of the team, and who celebrate those accomplishments regularly.

All five of these competencies have been consistently identified in great leaders and can be evaluated by an individual, by persons who are their supervisors, their peers, and by the individual who reports to them. In other words, these traits are amenable to analysis in a so-called "360-degree feedback analysis." Such a 360-degree evaluation is a key component of a successful leadership development program, since it provides leaders with others' feedback and with the self-awareness necessary to develop areas of relative weakness [20]. As an example of many such instruments, the LPI has 30 items, which are scored on a Likert scale, and the instrument can be used to identify areas of strength in individual leaders or to identify where leaders can improve on their already existing skills and practices. The inventory has been consistently useful in studies of persons in a wide variety of fields [14,21,22] and offers a concrete resource for measurement of leadership and targeting improvement. Many other examples of such feedback tools exist, including the Emotional Competence Inventory [23], the Global Leadership Life Inventory [24], books and reviews dedicated to the various tools [25–28], and several health care–specific tools, often used in evaluating physicians [29–32].

What Competencies Are Critical for Health Care Leadership?

In her scholarship on the competencies of exceptional leaders in a wide variety of settings, Goodall suggested that technical competency is necessary but not sufficient for great leadership. Boyatzis [33] agrees, and frames this notion as being composed of two different sorts of competencies. First, "threshold competencies" are the baseline skills necessary to be considered for a leadership position. In the case of health care workers, the threshold competencies for leadership are expertise and experience in one's field of clinical or scientific specialty and cognitive competencies such as memory and deductive reasoning. Examples of "threshold competencies" include what are traditionally considered as criteria for advancement to leadership positions in academic settings like grantsmanship, academic accomplishments, achievement of funding, clinical respectability, and so on. In contrast to these threshold competencies, so-called "differentiating competencies" may have little to do with traditional promotional criteria and are the traits that will determine one's leadership effectiveness. These differentiating competencies include more complex cognitive competencies like pattern recognition and systems thinking and, importantly, the four domains of emotional intelligence: self-awareness competencies, self-management competencies, social awareness competencies, and relationship management competencies. Emotional intelligence, defined as "the ability to perceive and express emotion, assimilate emotion in thought, understand and reason with emotion, and regulate emotion in the self and others" [34], describes a set of behaviors that are explicit and can be taught to and cultivated by leaders seeking to increase their skills. These models are often chosen by health care institutions that wish to develop leadership skills in their providers, with frequently favorable results [35–37]. For example, in a review of key competencies in programs devoted to physician leadership development, Stoller [38] proposed the following clusters as differentiating competencies in health care providers:

1. technical knowledge and skills (i.e., of operations, finance and accounting, information technology and systems, human resources [including diversity], strategic planning, legal issues in health care, and public policy)

2. knowledge of health care (i.e., of reimbursement strategies, legislation and regulation, quality assessment and management)

3. problem-solving prowess (i.e., around organizational strategy and project management)

4. emotional intelligence (i.e., the ability to evaluate self and others and to manage oneself in the context of a group)

5. communication (i.e., in leading change in groups and in individual encounters, such as in negotiation and conflict resolution)

6. commitment to lifelong learning.

Similarly, Davidson et al. [39] interviewed 21 senior leaders in health research organizations using the Health Leadership Competency Model [40] and found that the most critical skills needed for leadership included: talent development, collaboration, strategic orientation, and team leadership. They differentiated those priorities for senior members of leadership teams—financial skills and scientific achievement—from those needed by emerging leaders—scientific competence, information seeking, and a strong work ethic. In addition, in a study of nurses, residents, and physicians in an academic medical center, Dine et al. [41] found that four leadership concepts were important but lacking in training of leaders: management of the team (utilizing the skills of the persons on the team to maximum effect), establishing a vision (inspiring persons to push themselves for the sake of improved care), communication, and personal qualities such as being approachable and supportive. In a survey of chairs of departments of psychiatry, Keith et al. [42] found that 46% of respondents prioritized interpersonal communication skills in leaders and that 36% described altruism, perseverance, integrity, and honesty as critical features of successful academic chairs. Finally, Taylor et al. reported that critical differentiating competencies for established leaders in health care organizations included organizational altruism—the ability to subjugate one's personal advancement to the needs of the organization and of those being lead [43]. Others [44] have framed this via the concept of "servant leadership."

Leadership matters not only for navigating the financial and administrative components of health care, but because it can also directly impact patient outcomes. For example, Goodall [45] reported a significant association between physician leadership and hospital performance (e.g., in *US News and World Report* rankings); Bulmer Smith endorsed attention to emotional intelligence and patient outcomes in hiring and evaluating nurses [35]; and Stoller and Wheeler [6] summarized a large number of studies showing that teamwork, an important leadership competency, enhances patient outcomes in critical care medicine and in respiratory care. In addition, Baggs et al. [46] endorsed nurse-physician collaboration as a critical concept in enhancing outcomes in the critically ill [47]. Lobas [48] and Buckley et al. [49] advocated using an assessment of emotional intelligence in assessing candidates for leadership positions in academic medical centers, noting that great leadership was associated with greater organizational effectiveness. Importantly, effective leadership is associated with increased satisfaction from employees as well as patients.

Leadership must be distinguished from management. Both are complementary and are required for organizational success. Table 17.1 presents the distinction according to Kotter [50]. Management focuses on preserving order and structure, with activities like ensuring adequate staffing and budgeting. In contrast, leadership regards engaging and aligning people and effecting change to improve organizational performance. In the specific context of a field project, for example, management is required to ensure the budget is defended and that adequate staffing is available on all shifts, whereas leaders change the way services are delivered in order to enhance the project's effectiveness.

Table 17.1
Leadership versus Management

Managing	Leading
Aim: predictable, orderly results	Aim: to produce change
Involves planning and budgeting	Involves vision and setting direction
Involves organizing and staffing	Involves aligning people
Involves controlling and solving	Involves motivating and inspiring

From Kotter [50], with permission.

Leadership Competencies Especially Needed to Optimize Care in Resource-Poor Settings

In the context of specific leadership competencies for providing health care in resource-poor areas, the question arises: what are the leadership and management competencies needed to optimize health in underserved or under-resourced areas? To what extent, if any, do these competencies differ from the more generic health care leadership competencies discussed above? The issue has received some formal attention in the peer-reviewed, published literature and has also been the subject of active discussion in online forums.

Table 17.2 summarizes the literature on leadership skills required in global health. The overarching critical need for more research in this area has been emphasized by some authors [51–55]. For example, in reflecting on the elements of the global efforts that allowed the conquest of smallpox, Banta [56] noted, "smallpox was eradicated because of effective public health practice. ... There was effective health leadership, there was public involvement, and the campaign lent itself well to operation by objective. There had also been almost two centuries of research and development." Reflecting on the challenge of ensuring global vision health, Di Stefano [57] commented: "Global challenges demand global leadership."

A synthesis of the leadership competencies that are recommended suggests several common attributes that are, not surprisingly, also represented among the more general health care leadership competencies discussed above (table 17.2)—vision, a community and service orientation, systems awareness and thinking, innovation and a strong ability to improvise, altruism, change management expertise, and honesty. Still, the context of providing care in under-resourced areas lends specific nuances to these leadership competencies, as reflected in selected quotes from these reports below.

Both the challenge and paramount importance of vision were articulated by Banta [56]: "A major requirement of leadership is for the leader to know where he is going. ... How simplistic. How transparently obvious. Yet upon reflection, is it not the most difficult aspect of health leadership, i.e., defining which way to go?"

On the important issue of innovation and improvisation, Jain [54] commented: "This information and the process need to be mobilized to develop situation-appropriate solutions. This is a highly creative process and the quality of the outcome depends on the ability of the key actors to master the available information, the strength of their commitment to the projected goals of the health services as well as to the strategy to achieve these goals, and their perception of the gravity of the problems in hand. Critically important competencies include: system awareness, authority, exercise of power, peer relations, superior-subordinate relations, familial and ethnic obligations, use and value of systematic data, and scores of other socioeconomic concepts. Each culture seems to have marked preferences for certain types of behavior." Banta [56] concurred: "Any health worker who does not understand the world-view, the value system, the taboos, the dietary laws or the moral imperative of family customs, and attempts to establish a health programme

Table 17.2
Summary of Leadership Competencies Cited for Health Care in Under-Resourced Areas

Competency	Reference(s)
Focus on quality of care	Moss et al. [58]
	Bradley et al. [78]
	Sherman et al. [79]
	Yamey [80]
	Gantz et al. [61]
	Macphee and Suryaprakash [64]
	de Leon Siantz [81]
	Hughes [65]
	Epping-Jordan et al. [82]
	Knapp [83]
	Trofino [68]
	Wojtczak [8]
	Holt et al. [63]
Focus on measurement	Moss et al. [58]
	Swanson et al. [85]
	Yamey [80]
	Baker and Orton [86]
	Cowan et al. [60]
	Archaya [87]
	Epping-Jordan et al. [82]
	Knapp [83]
Change management expertise	Moss et al. [58]
	Conn et al. [88]
	Swanson et al. [85]
	Anazor [70]
	Yamey [80]
	Macphee and Suryaprakash [64]
	Haffeld [89]
	Douglas [90]
	Baker and Orton [86]
	Hughes [65]
	Fenderson and Fenderson [91]
	Porter-O'Grady [92]
	Trofino [68]
	Holt et al. [63]
Spirit of collaboration and teamwork	Moss et al. [58]
	Conn et al. [88]
	Bradley et al. [78]
	Anazor [70]
	Shaw and Meads [93]
	Gillespie et al. [62]
	Ackerman et al. [94]
	Gantz et al. [61]
	Haffeld [89]
	Douglas [90]
	Seedat et al. [95]
	Séguin et al. [96]
	Hardy et al. [97]
	de Leon Siantz [81]
	Gardner et al. [98]
	Hughes [65]
	Archaya [87]
	Fenderson and Fenderson [91]
	Nash and Gremmillion [55]
	Trofino [68]

Table 17.2 (continued)

Competency	Reference(s)
Systems perspective	Moss et al. [58] Jain [54] Banta [56] Palamountain et al. [99] Anazor [70] Sherman et al. [79] Yamey [80] Haffeld [89] Douglas [90] Gardner et al. [98] Archaya [87] Knapp [83] Porter-O'Grady [92] Battistella and Weil [52] Wojtczak [84] Holt et al. [83]
Commitment to quality improvement	Moss et al. [58] Anazor [70] Wilson et al. [71] Gantz et al. [61] Macphee and Suryaprakash [64] Baker and Orton [86] de Leon Siantz [81] Hughes [65] Porter-O'Grady [92] Trofino [68] Holt et al. [83]
Transparency	Moss et al. [58] Palamountain et al. [99] Ackerman et al. [94] Haffeld [89] Seedat et al. [95] Gardner et al. [98] Archaya [87] Wojtczak [84]
Honesty	Moss et al. [58] Bradley et al. [78] Shaw and Meads [93] Gardner et al. [98]
Service orientation and community engagement	Moss et al. [58] Palamountain et al. [99] Bradley et al. [78] Sherman et al. [79] Shaw and Meads [93] Gillespie et al. [62] Ackerman et al. [94] Yamey [80] Douglas [90] Séguin et al. [96] de Leon Siantz [81] Hughes [65] Addo [100] Holt et al. [83]

Table 17.2 (continued)

Competency	Reference(s)
Ability to manage in uncertainty	Moss et al. [58] Palamountain et al. [99] Sherman et al. [79] Douglas [90] de Leon Siantz [81 Hughes [65] Porter-O'Grady [92] Wojtczak [84]
Vision	Banta [56] Palamountain et al. [99] Ackerman et al. [94] Yamey [80] Gantz et al. [61] Baker and Orton [86] Seedat et al. [95] de Leon Siantz [81] Hughes [65] Fenderson and Fenderson [91] Knapp [83] Porter-O'Grady [92] Trofino [68] Wojtczak [84]
Innovativeness and ability to improvise	Jain [54] Bradley]et al. [78] Shaw and Meads [93] Gillespie et al. [62] Ackerman et al. [94] Wilson et al. [71] Gantz et al. [61] Macphee and Suryaprakash [64 Haffeld [89] Douglas [90] Baker and Orton [86] Knapp [83] Wojtczak [84] Holt et al. [83]
Leadership development at multiple levels of authority	Palamountain et al. [99] Bradley et al. [78] Shaw and Meads [93] Gillespie et al. [62] Ackerman et al. [94] Wilson et al. [71] Yamey [80] Gantz et al. [61] Macphee and Suryaprakash [64] Haffeld [89] Seedat et al. [95] Séguin et al. [96] de Leon Siantz [81] Hughes [65] Archaya [87] Fenderson and Fenderson [91] Knapp [83] Trofino [68] Lerer and Matzopolous [101] Holt et al. [83]

dependent upon some modification of human behavior is doomed to failure." Finally, commenting on the need for new leadership competencies to deliver care in under-resourced areas, Moss et al. [58] noted: "This has needed a style of leadership compared with a traditional controlling that manages projects through steering groups, emphasizes patience, enthusiasm, ability to manage in uncertainty, and has the courage to allow initiatives to evolve."

Our literature review especially emphasized the cultivation of leadership in nursing [59–69]. Several studies emphasized the current leadership in global health care by nurses [61,64,65,67], while others emphasized that mid-level nurse leadership is critical for successful implementation and effectiveness of health care interventions, and that nurses are and must remain at the forefront of global health innovation [68,70]. Regarding the current and ongoing importance of nurse involvement in global health care leadership, Wilson et al. [71] stated: "Nurses comprise the largest proportion … of the health workforce and are considered to be the front line staff across the health continuum in most health services and countries. In spite of the immense and significant role that nurses play in the healthcare system, they are seldom considered equal partners in multidisciplinary healthcare teams. As a result, the unique skills held by generalist and specialist nurses are often underutilized across the health continuum."

Complementing the relatively sparse published literature regarding leadership competencies for innovation in under-resourced areas, online forums regarding global health care delivery (e.g., GHDOnline) have featured conversations regarding the leadership and management competencies needed to optimize global health care delivery. Specifically, a September 2013 expert panel on "Managing Healthcare Delivery: Your Expertise" [72] attracted 183 respondents from 74 countries and 130 organizations, who responded to five focused questions:

1. What kind of management duties or responsibilities do you perform in health care delivery or see others perform?

2. How important is management of people, processes, and resources, compared to other issues or challenges in health care delivery? How do you prioritize this element of your work?

3. What core skills to those who manage delivery need to be effective? How did you or others gain the skills management training or capacity building opportunities available in your work?

4. What factors in health systems, organizations, or communities impacts the work of those who manage delivery? What are the main barriers to improving the efficacy of your management?

5. How can the global health delivery project address the challenges and barriers faced by those who manage delivery, especially at the front lines? What kinds of resources or programs would be most helpful to you in your work?

Expert panelists and respondents strongly endorsed the importance of leadership and management skills for global health care workers. For example, a Ugandan worker noted: "There is a feeling that the biggest problem affecting the health sector is poor management and leadership and not necessarily lack of resources." A a nurse-midwife working in northern India also noted: "The management/leadership of a facility is paramount to the success in making improvements. The leader can bring an expectation of quality and a respect for his/her staff, which changes all other functions within a facility. From my vantage point, that leadership—with clarity of vision, and respect for the staff—can create the space where improvement can occur."

In reviewing all the responses, a total of 101 pages of text were analyzed for themes regarding the specific leadership needs and competencies respondents reported were essential for optimal global health care delivery. Fifty three of the 183 respondents (29%) specifically addressed the leadership competencies needed for optimizing global health.

Conclusion

Business leaders around the world have long recognized the necessity for effective leadership, and many models exist to train individuals to be effective leaders. Providers have increasingly recognized that health care requires effective leadership but that these skills are not traditionally taught during training.

The generally lauded competencies in health care—clinical or scientific expertise and technical mastery—appear insufficient to bring innovations to under-resourced settings [39,73,74]. The innovative leaders who are especially needed for global health must navigate and negotiate the various interests involved in implementing new interventions. They must have a clear vision that is aligned with health care goals and must be champions of their own strategies, while working collaboratively with stakeholders to advance this vision.

Health care providers today generally have a dearth of resources or mentors to learn these skills. We must advocate for capacity building and training in leadership as a key component of success in global health. There are many benchmark models available from the business sector and some, though fewer, best practices in health care [75–77]. The literature suggests that many of the identified skills for effective leadership translate to under-resourced settings, particularly those of vision, collaboration, community orientation, systems thinking, and the ability to cultivate leadership at all levels of organizational authority.

As we continue to understand the role of leadership in helping to achieve accessible, high-quality, and low-cost health care, the nuances of the leadership skills needed for specific environments and communities will become even clearer. Overall, the leadership competencies needed for innovation in global health call upon generalizable leadership skills: clinical expertise; emotional intelligence; deep commitment to mission; and respect for patients, colleagues, and collaborators.

Questions for Discussion

- How might organizations go about identifying potential leaders and harnessing their talents in global health?
- How does my current organization support current leaders and identify new ones?
- How can large global health organizations cultivate the leadership skills inherent in local communities?
- How might large organizations collaborate meaningfully with smaller, community-based organizations?

References

1. Lee TH. 2010. Turning doctors into leaders. *Harv Bus Rev* 88(4): 50–58.

2. Stoller JK. 2004. Can physicians collaborate? A review of organizational development in healthcare. *OD Pract* 36: 19–24.

3. Pearson A, Laschinger H, Porritt K, Jordan Z, Tucker D, Long L. 2007. Comprehensive systematic review of evidence on developing and sustaining nursing leadership that fosters a healthy work environment in healthcare. *Int J Evid-Based Healthc* 5(2): 208–253. doi:10.1111/j.1479-6988.2007.00065.x.

4. Paliadelis P, Cruickshank M, Sheridan A. 2007. Caring for each other: How do nurse managers "manage" their role? *J Nurs Manag* 15(8): 830–837. doi:10.1111/j.1365-2934.2007.00754.x.

5. Weisbord MR. 1978. Why organization development hasn't worked (so far) in medical centers. *Organ Dev Public Adm Part 1 Organ Dev Prop Public Sect Featur* 5: 247.

6. Wheeler DT, Stoller JK. 2011. Teamwork, teambuilding and leadership in respiratory and health care. *Can J Respir Ther* 47(1): 6–11.

7. Day DV, Zaccaro SJ, Halpin SM. *Leader Development for Transforming Organizations: Growing Leaders for Tomorrow.* Psychology Press; 2004.

8. Bahrami H. 2013. People operations at Mozilla Corporation: Scaling a peer-to-peer global community. *Calif Manage Rev* 56(1): 67–88.

9. Avolio BJ, Sosik JJ, Kahai SS, Baker B. 2014. E-leadership: Re-examining transformations in leadership source and transmission. *Leadersh Q* 25(1): 105–131. doi:10.1016/j.leaqua.2013.11.003.

10. Thite M. National human resource development and firm performance: Lessons from emerging Indian multinationals. In Agrawal NM, Joman MG, Varkkey B,

Bannerjee C, eds. *Inclusiveness, Sustainability & Human Resource Development.* India: McGraw Hill Education; 2013: 109–114.

11. Terrell RS, Rosenbusch K. 2013. How global leaders develop. *J Manage Dev* 32(10): 1056–1079. doi:10.1108/JMD-01-2012-0008.

12. Garman A, Harris Lemak C. 2011. *Developing healthcare leaders: What have we learned, and what is next.* National Center For Healthcare Leadership: 12. http://www .nchl.org. Accessed March 3, 2014.

13. Stoller JK. 2009. Developing physician-leaders: A call to action. *J Gen Intern Med* 24(7): 876–878. doi:10.1007/s11606-009-1007-8.

14. Posner BZ, Kouzes JM. 1988. Development and validation of the leadership practices inventory. *Educ Psychol Meas* 48(2): 483–496.

15. Bar-On R. 2006. The Bar-On model of emotional-social intelligence (ESI). *Psicothema* 18(Suppl): 13–25.

16. Heifetz RA. *Leadership Without Easy Answers.* Harvard University Press; 1994.

17. Dulewicz V, Higgs M. 2000. Emotional intelligence—A review and evaluation study. *J Manag Psychol* 15(4): 341–372. doi:10.1108/02683940010330993.

18. Conte JM. 2005. A review and critique of emotional intelligence measures. *J Organ Behav* 26(4): 433–440.

19. Kouzes JM, Posner BZ. *The Five Practices of Exemplary Leadership: Healthcare— General.* John Wiley and Sons; 2011.

20. Boyatzis RE. 2008. Leadership development from a complexity perspective. *Consult Psychol J Pract Res* 60(4): 298–313. doi:10.1037/1065-9293.60.4.298.

21. Zagorsek H, Jaklic M, Stough SJ. 2004. Comparing leadership practices between the United States, Nigeria, and Slovenia: Does culture matter? *Cross Cult Manag Int J.* 11(2): 16–34. doi:10.1108/13527600410797774.

22. Tourangeau A, McGilton K. 2004. Measuring leadership practices of nurses using the Leadership Practices Inventory. *Nurs Res* 53(3): 182–189.

23. Boyatzis RE, Sala F. 2004. The emotional competence inventory (ECI). http://doi. apa.org/psycinfo/2004-19636-007. Accessed April 8, 2014.

24. Kets de Vries MFR, Vrignaud P, Florent-Treacy E. 2004. The Global Leadership Life Inventory: Development and psychometric properties of a 360-degree feedback instrument. *Int J Hum Resour Manage* 15(3): 475–492. doi:10.1080/0958519042000181214.

25. Lepsinger R, Lucia AD. *The Art and Science of 360 Degree Feedback.* John Wiley & Sons; 2009.

26. Brutus S, Fleenor JW, London M. 1998. Does 360-degree feedback work in different industries?: A between-industry comparison of the reliability and validity of

multi-source performance ratings. *J Manage Dev* 17(3): 177–190. doi:10.1108/EUM0000000004487.

27. Ghorpade J. 2000. Managing five paradoxes of 360-degree feedback. *Acad Manage Exec* 14(1): 140–150. doi:10.5465/AME.2000.2909846.

28. Wood L, Hassell A, Whitehouse A, Bullock A, Wall D. 2006. A literature review of multi-source feedback systems within and without health services, leading to 10 tips for their successful design. *Med Teach* 28(7): E185–e191.

29. Lockyer J. 2003. Multisource feedback in the assessment of physician competencies. *J Contin Educ Health Prof* 23(1): 4–12.

30. Higgins RSD, Bridges J, Burke JM, O'Donnell MA, Cohen NM, Wilkes SB. 2004. Implementing the ACGME general competencies in a cardiothoracic surgery residency program using 360-degree feedback. *Ann Thorac Surg* 77(1): 12–17.

31. Lelliott P, Williams R, Mears A, Andiappan M, Owen H, Reading P, et al. 2008. Questionnaires for 360-degree assessment of consultant psychiatrists: Development and psychometric properties. *Br J Psychiatry* 193(2): 156–160. doi:10.1192/bjp.bp.107.041681.

32. Rodgers KG, Manifold C. 2002. 360-degree feedback: Possibilities for assessment of the ACGME core competencies for emergency medicine residents. *Acad Emerg Med* 9(11): 1300–1304. doi:10.1197/aemj.9.11.1300.

33. Boyatzis RE. 2009. Competencies as a behavioral approach to emotional intelligence. *J Manage Dev* 28(9): 749–770. doi:10.1108/02621710910987647.

34. Sternberg RJ, Kaufman SB. *The Cambridge Handbook of Intelligence.* Cambridge University Press; 2011.

35. Bulmer Smith K, Profetto-McGrath J, Cummings GG. 2009. Emotional intelligence and nursing: An integrative literature review. *Int J Nurs Stud* 46(12): 1624–1636. doi:10.1016/j.ijnurstu.2009.05.024.

36. Arora S, Ashrafian H, Davis R, Athanasiou T, Darzi A, Sevdalis N. 2010. Emotional intelligence in medicine: A systematic review through the context of the ACGME competencies. *Med Educ* 44(8): 749–764. doi:10.1111/j.1365-2923.2010.03709.x.

37. Sahafi E, Danaee H, Sarlak M. 2011. The impact of emotional intelligence on citizenship behavior of physicians (with emphasis on infertility specialists). *J Family Reprod Health* 5(4): 109–115.

38. Stoller JK. 2008. Developing physician-leaders: Key competencies and available programs. *J Health Adm Educ* 25(4): 307–328.

39. Davidson PL, Azziz R, Morrison J, Rocha J, Braun J. 2012. Identifying and developing leadership competencies in health research organizations: A pilot study. *J Health Adm Educ* 29(2): 135–154.

40. Calhoun JG, Dollett L, Sinioris ME, Wainio JA, Butler PW, Griffith JR, et al. 2008. Development of an interprofessional competency model for healthcare leadership. *J Healthc Manag* 53(6): 375–390.

41. Dine CJ, Kahn JM, Abella BS, Asch DA, Shea JA. 2011. Key elements of clinical physician leadership at an academic medical center. *J Grad Med Educ* 3(1): 31–36.

42. Mintz LJ, Stoller JK. 2014. A systematic review of physician leadership and emotional intelligence. *J Grad Med Educ* 6(1): 21–31. doi:10.4300/JGME-D-13-00012.1.

43. Taylor CA, Taylor JC, Stoller JK. 2008. Exploring leadership competencies in established and aspiring physician leaders: An interview-based study. *J Gen Intern Med* 23(6): 748–754. doi:10.1007/s11606-008-0565-5.

44. Greenleaf RK. *Servant Leadership: A Journey Into the Nature of Legitimate Power and Greatness.* Paulist Press; 2002.

45. Goodall AH. 2011. Physician-leaders and hospital performance: Is there an association? *Soc Sci Med* 73(4): 535–539. doi:10.1016/j.socscimed.2011.06.025.

46. Baggs J, Schmitt M, Mushlin A, Mitchell PH, Eldredge DH, Oakes D, et al. 1999. Association between nurse-physician collaboration and patient outcomes in three intensive care units. *Crit Care Med* 27(9): 1991–1998.

47. Baggs J, Schmitt M, Mushlin A, Mitchell PH, Eldredge DH, Oakes D, et al. 1999. Association between nurse-physician collaboration and patient outcomes in three intensive care units. *Crit Care Med* 27(9): 1991–1998.

48. Lobas JG. 2006. Leadership in academic medicine: Capabilities and conditions for organizational success. *Am J Med* 119(7): 617–621. doi:10.1016/j.amjmed.2006.04.005.

49. Buckley PF, Rayburn WF. 2010. The care and feeding of chairs of departments of psychiatry. *Am J Psychiatry* 167(4): 376–378. doi:10.1176/appi.ajp.2009.09070949.

50. Kotter JP. *Leading Change.* Boston, MA: Harvard Business Review Press; 2012.

51. Alon I, Higgins JM. 2005. Global leadership success through emotional and cultural intelligences. *Bus Horiz* 48(6): 501–512. doi:10.1016/j.bushor.2005.04.003.

52. Battistella RM, Weil TP. 1996. The new management competencies: A global perspective. *Physician Exec* 22(7): 18–23.

53. Buse K, Tanaka S. 2011. Global public-private health partnerships: Lessons learned from ten years of experience and evaluation. *Int Dent J* 61: 2–10. doi:10.1111/j.1875-595X.2011.00034.x.

54. Jain SC. 1992. Improving health manpower: A global perspective. *J Health Hum Resour Adm* 14(4): 373–401.

55. Nash MG, Gremillion C. 2004. Globalization impacts the healthcare organization of the 21st century. Demanding new ways to market product lines successfully. *Nurs Adm Q* 28(2): 86–91.

56. Banta JE. 1987. Leadership in health for all in developing countries: Quo vadis? *Asia Pac J Public Health* 1(3): 6–10. doi:10.1177/101053958700100302.

57. Di Stefano A. 2002. World optometry: The challenges of leadership for the new millennium. *Optometry* 73(6): 339–350.

58. Moss F, Palmberg M, Plsek P, Schellekens W. 2000. Quality improvement around the world: How much we can learn from each other. *Qual Health Care QHC* 9(1): 63–66. doi:10.1136/qhc.9.1.63.

59. Barrow M, McKimm J, Gasquoine S. 2010. The policy and the practice: Early-career doctors and nurses as leaders and followers in the delivery of health care. *Adv Health Sci Educ* 16(1): 17–29. doi:10.1007/s10459-010-9239-2.

60. Cowan DT, Jenifer Wilson-Barnett D, Norman IJ, Murrells T. 2008. Measuring nursing competence: Development of a self-assessment tool for general nurses across Europe. *Int J Nurs Stud* 45(6): 902–913. doi:10.1016/j.ijnurstu.2007.03.004.

61. Gantz NR, Sherman R, Jasper M, Choo CG, Herrin-Griffith D, Harris K. 2012. Global nurse leader perspectives on health systems and workforce challenges. *J Nurs Manag* 20(4): 433–443. doi:10.1111/j.1365-2834.2012.01393.x.

62. Gillespie BM, Chaboyer W, Lingard S, Ball S. 2012. Perioperative nurses' perceptions of competence: Implications for migration. *ORNAC J* 30(3): 17–18, 20–22, 24 passim.

63. Holt J, Barrett C, Clarke D, Monks R. 2000. The globalization of nursing knowledge. *Nurse Educ Today* 20(6): 426–431. doi:10.1054/nedt.2000.0497.

64. Macphee M, Suryaprakash N. 2012. First-line nurse leaders' health-care change management initiatives. *J Nurs Manag* 20(2): 249–259. doi:10.1111/j.1365-2834.2011.01338.x.

65. Hughes F. 2006. Nurses at the forefront of innovation. *Int Nurs Rev* 53(2): 94–101. doi:10.1111/j.1466-7657.2006.00463.x.

66. Mannahan CA. 2010. Different worlds: A cultural perspective on nurse-physician communication. *Nurs Clin North Am* 45(1): 71–79. doi:10.1016/j.cnur.2009.10.005.

67. Mcsherry R, Douglas M. 2011. Innovation in nursing practice: A means to tackling the global challenges facing nurses, midwives and nurse leaders and managers in the future. *J Nurs Manag* 19(2): 165–169. doi:10.1111/j.1365-2834.2011.01241.x.

68. Trofino J. 2003. Power sharing. A transformational strategy for nurse retention, effectiveness, and extra effort. *Nurs Leadersh Forum* 8(2): 64–71.

69. Willcocks SG. 2012. Exploring leadership effectiveness: Nurses as clinical leaders in the NHS. *Leadersh Health Serv* 25(1): 8–19. doi:10.1108/17511871211198034.

70. Anazor C. 2012. Preparing nurse leaders for global health reforms. *Nurs Manag* 19(4): 26–28. doi:10.7748/nm2012.07.19.4.26.c9167.

71. Wilson A, Whitaker N, Whitford D. 2012. Rising to the challenge of health care reform with entrepreneurial and intrapreneurial nursing initiatives. *Online J Issues Nurs* 17(2): 5.

72. Global Health Delivery Project. 2013. Managing health care delivery: Your expertise [expert online panel]. http://www.ghdonline.org/managing-health-care-delivery/ discussion/managing-health-care-delivery-your-expertise/. Global Health Delivery Project, Harvard University. Accessed March 15, 2014.

73. Snell AJ, Dickson G. 2011. Optimizing health care employees' newly learned leadership behaviors. *Leadersh Health Serv* 24(3): 183–195.

74. Snell AJ, Briscoe D, Dickson G. 2011. From the inside out: The engagement of physicians as leaders in health care settings. *Qual Health Res* 21(7): 952–967. doi:10.1177/1049732311399780.

75. Schwartz RW, Pogge CR, Gillis SA, Holsinger JW. 2000. Programs for the development of physician leaders: A curricular process in its infancy. *Acad Med* 75(2): 133–140.

76. Viggiano TR, Pawlina W, Lindor KD, Olsen KD, Cortese DA. 2007. Putting the needs of the patient first: Mayo Clinic's core value, institutional culture, and professionalism covenant. *Acad Med* 82(11): 1089–1093. doi:10.1097/ACM.0b013e3181575dcd.

77. Hopkins MM, O'Neill D, FitzSimmons K, Bailin PL, Stoller JK. 2011. Leadership and organization development in health care: Lessons from the Cleveland Clinic. *Adv Health Care Manag* 10: 151–165. doi:10.1108/S1474-8231(2011)0000010015.

78. Bradley EH, Curry LA, Taylor LA, Pallas SW, Talbert-Slagle K, Yuan C, et al. 2012. A model for scale up of family health innovations in low-income and middle-income settings: A mixed methods study. *BMJ Open* 2(4). doi:10.1136/bmjopen-2012-000987.

79. Sherman R, Dyess S, Hannah E, Prestia A. 2013. Succession planning for the future through an academic-practice partnership: A nursing administration master's program for emerging nurse leaders. *Nurs Adm Q* 37(1): 18–27. doi:10.1097/NAQ .0b013e31827514ba.

80. Yamey G. 2012. What are the barriers to scaling up health interventions in low and middle income countries? A qualitative study of academic leaders in implementation science. *Global Health* 8: 11. doi:10.1186/1744-8603-8-11.

81. De Leon Siantz ML. 2008. Leading change in diversity and cultural competence. *J Prof Nurs Off J Am Assoc Coll Nurs* 24(3): 167–171. doi:10.1016/j.profnurs .2008.01.005.

82. Epping-Jordan JE, Pruitt SD, Bengoa R, Wagner EH. 2004. Improving the quality of health care for chronic conditions. *Qual Saf Health Care* 13(4): 299–305. doi:10.1136/ qhc.13.4.299.

83. Knapp ML. 1997. Finishing big by starting small. Continuous improvement is the key to enhancing community health. *Health Prog St Louis Mo*. 78(5): 22–25, 33.

84. Wojtczak A. 2003. Leadership development: Prerequisite for successful public-private partnership. *World Hosp Health Serv Off J Int Hosp Fed* 39(1): 27–29, 31, 33.

85. Swanson RC, Cattaneo A, Bradley E, Chunharas S, Atun R, Abbas KM, et al. 2012. Rethinking health systems strengthening: Key systems thinking tools and strategies for transformational change. *Health Policy Plan* 27(Suppl 4): Iv54–iv61. doi:10.1093/heapol/czs090.

86. Baker EL, Orton SN. 2010. Practicing management and leadership: Vision, strategy, operations, and tactics. *J Public Health Manag Pract* 16(5): 470–471. doi:10.1097/PHH.0b013e3181f5164b.

87. Acharya T, Rab MA, Singer PA, Daar AS. 2005. Harnessing genomics to improve health in the Eastern Mediterranean region—an executive course in genomics policy. *Health Res Policy Syst BioMed Cent* 3(1): 1. doi:10.1186/1478-4505-3-1.

88. Conn CP, Jenkins P, Touray SO. 1996. Strengthening health management: Experience of district teams in the Gambia. *Health Policy Plan* 11(1): 64–71. doi:10.1093/heapol/11.1.64.

89. Haffeld J. 2012. Facilitative governance: Transforming global health through complexity theory. *Glob Public Health* 7(5): 452–464. doi:10.1080/17441692.2011.649486.

90. Douglas MR. 2011. Opportunities and challenges facing the future global nursing and midwifery workforce. *J Nurs Manag* 19(6): 695–699. doi:10.1111/j.1365-2834.2011.01302.x.

91. Fenderson BA, Fenderson DA. 2004. Balancing traditional values in academic medicine with advances in science and technology. *Croat Med J* 45(3): 259–263.

92. Porter-O'Grady T. 1996. Into the new paradigm: Writing the script for the future of health care. *Collegian* 3(4): 5–10.

93. Shaw SE, Meads G. 2012. Extending primary care: Potential learning from Italy. *Prim Health Care Res Dev* 13(4): 289–293. doi:10.1017/S1463423612000011.

94. Ackerman Gulaid L, Kiragu K. 2012. Lessons learnt from promising practices in community engagement for the elimination of new HIV infections in children by 2015 and keeping their mothers alive: Summary of a desk review. *J Int AIDS Soc* 15(Suppl 2): 17390.

95. Seedat M, Van Niekerk A, Jewkes R, Suffla S, Ratele K. 2009. Violence and injuries in South Africa: Prioritising an agenda for prevention. *Lancet* 374(9694): 1011–1022. doi:10.1016/S0140-6736(09)60948-X.

96. Séguin B, Hardy B-J, Singer PA, Daar AS. 2008. Universal health care, genomic medicine and Thailand: Investing in today and tomorrow. *Nat Rev Genet* 9(Suppl 1): S14–S19. doi:10.1038/nrg2443.

97. Hardy B-J, Séguin B, Ramesar R, Singer PA, Daar AS. 2008. South Africa: From species cradle to genomic applications. *Nat Rev Genet* 9(Suppl 1): S19–S23. doi:10.1038/nrg2441.

98. Gardner CA, Acharya T, Yach D. 2007. Technological and social innovation: A unifying new paradigm for global health. *Health Aff (Millwood)* 26(4): 1052–1061. doi:10.1377/hlthaff.26.4.1052.

99. Palamountain KM, Stewart KA, Krauss A, Kelso D, Diermeier D. 2010. University leadership for innovation in global health and HIV/AIDS diagnostics. *Glob Public Health* 5(2): 189–196. doi:10.1080/17441690903456274.

100. Addo D. 1996. So far and yet so near? *Bull Med Libr Assoc* 84(1): 100–104.

101. Lerer L, Matzopoulos R. 2001. "The worst of both worlds": The management reform of the World Health Organization. *Int J Health Serv Plan Adm Eval* 31(2): 415–438.

18 Building a Global Health Team

Andrea Ippolito and Jacqueline DePasse

Take-Home Messages

- We propose the mantra of "collaboration, co-creation, and capacity building" for individuals, teams, and organizations interested in participating in innovations in global health settings.
- Collaboration is promoting multidisciplinary teams to tackle complicated problems for the challenge of health care improvement.
- Co-creation focuses on creating teams that leverage local clinicians and experts, to better understand each unique environment and culture.
- Capacity building focuses on long-term sustainability, to ensure that future innovation can be locally derived and maintained.

Introduction

In recent years, there has been a surge of interest from students and professionals in innovation in global health settings. For example, the involvement of medical graduates from the United States in global health innovation and care-redesign efforts has increased 10-fold in the past 35 years [1], with similar trends observed in other countries [2,3]. Likewise, engineering and computer science students have shown increased desire to work with communities abroad, motivated to make a social impact with their work. As a result, university degree programs focused on global health and development for both clinicians and nonmedical professionals have emerged. Transformation in information technology has significantly contributed to this intellectual focus on global health by enabling faster and more seamless communication across the globe. Travel and virtual work in global health settings has never been easier due to technological leaps forward that have been called "the most transformative single event in development work of our generation" [4].

The Fragmented System

Although the convergence of interest and improved communication has led to increased attention and action surrounding innovation in global health settings, there are several flaws with the current approach. First, too often "global health work" consists of teams from high-income countries traveling to low- and middle-income countries (LMIC) for short periods of time, leading to inconsistent and lackluster results. These teams, while well intentioned, attempt to roll out new technology or provide care without developing sustainable models for moving forward with innovations and, worse, often without understanding the true urgent needs of the local communities. A recent article by Jane Cockerell highlighted that "at least 40% of medical equipment in developing countries is out of service (some studies cite 50–80%) and that doesn't account for what equipment should be present and isn't. By comparison, less than 1% of medical equipment is out of service in high-income countries" [5–7]. In cases of novel technology, the ground-level stakeholders often do not know how to resolve issues when the new equipment malfunctions or requires a replacement part. This leads to "graveyards of technology" taking up space or left to age without providing value in these resource-constrained settings. Additionally, the sporadic status quo efforts often fail to understand the unique cultural, societal, and political needs of the local settings, with a spectrum of consequences. As stated by Howitt et al., "technologies from high-income countries are often deployed in these [low- and middle-income country] settings without enough thought of the consequences, and such technologies might rapidly become useless … donations can place a burden on recipients; oxygen concentrators donated to a Gambian tertiary hospital required a voltage incompatible with the electricity supply in that country" [7]. Users are inadequately trained, or there is insufficient infrastructure to support the often-sensitive medical equipment. At best, this approach wastes or displaces needed time and resources; at worst, it may create what Peter Buffett has (controversially) labeled "philanthropic colonialism," [8] leaving negative impressions to disincentivize potential future efforts.

Secondly, innovations utilizing mobile health, or "mHealth," have often failed to integrate into the existing social, cultural, and organizational fabric and infrastructure in global health settings. They have stayed as isolated projects outside of traditional care pathways, with limited incorporation to the existing system or current improvement efforts. Mobile health innovations are often attractive to teams or individuals with entrepreneurial mindsets because they present lower barriers to initially deploy these technologies. However, many of these initiatives suffer from "pilot-itis" where they do not move forward into integration with existing systems. Often, the end result of these pilots may be a published paper, at best, without focusing on sustainability beyond the research phase. Furthermore, negative results are rarely reported, so many pilots are reinventing broken wheels that are doomed to failure. The speakers at the 2012 Groupe Speciale Mobile Association mHealth Summit in South Africa "bemoaned that 'pilot-itis'—the inability to break out of pilot stage—is holding back mobile health in developing countries" [9]. The failure to get out of the pilot stage can take away resources and supplies in already constrained settings, leading to fragmentation and little improvement in health outcomes. In many cases, these efforts remain isolated, insignificant projects taking away valuable time from local stakeholders.

Thirdly, this wave of interest in global health settings has attracted diverse groups of stakeholders, including involvement from engineers, public health workers, medical professionals, and computer scientists. However, the formation of projects from various disciplines in parallel has often led to fragmented and redundant work in global health settings. With little coordination taking placing across these stakeholder groups, segregated fiefdoms are formed, negatively impacting health outcomes. For instance, an mHealth program for obstetric care, diabetes care, HIV care, or another specialized disease process that does not integrate into the existing public health and governmental infrastructure will ultimately create fragmentation and redundancy [10].

A New Mantra for Innovation

One of the central themes highlighted above is the failure of programs in global health settings to develop sustainable plans and models to ensure they both fit into the existing system of care and are maintainable and adaptable to meet local needs. To address these challenges, we propose a mantra of "collaboration, co-creation, and capacity building" [11].

Collaboration

Medicine and health systems are immensely complicated, as discussed in earlier chapters of this textbook. With so many interacting fields along the entire health care vertical, it is a given that no group can solely control quality outcomes; even front-line clinicians directly treating patients are impacted by government regulations, medical supplies, and market forces. This is why this principle calls for collaboration across fields, purposefully pulling together multidisciplinary teams. Innovators need to pursue new modes of collaboration in global health settings.

While skills often overlap across fields for any individual, the following generalizes some simplified stereotypes for illustration. Clinicians should remain abreast of the latest developments in medical practice via continuous medical education, but generally are only aware of the latest well-marketed technology development. Therefore, clinicians should collaborate with the technologists who are aware of the limitations and constraints for what is feasible on a platform. Conversely, for the engineers who think their technology can solve every problem, they are usually unaware of the complexities and complications of delivering medical care, especially when focused on quality improvement. Only when clinicians and engineers work together can a team implement an intelligently designed and effective innovation.

By definition, entrepreneurs are risk takers and often drive toward the path of least resistance. They are incentivized to build barriers around their intellectual property to protect themselves against competitors and ensure that their venture is a profitable, sustainable entity. However, when engaging in global health settings, taking time up front to involve local stakeholders to build entrepreneurial teams results in superior outcomes [12]. Although engaging community members early in an innovation effort may initially feel like an "obstruction," it will ultimately lead to more productive, collaborative efforts and in the long run will create a more sustainable innovation. Interdisciplinary teams create a learning environment in which stakeholders are free to share ideas to develop best practices surrounding the newly proposed innovations.

Co-Creation

Co-creation in the context of global health innovation is making sure to partner with collaborators from the local environment. For foreign innovators, it is crucial to develop a cultural sensitivity to what makes the locale unique. This includes knowing which problems are most urgent for the local community, accounting for wide differences in disease prevalence across borders and socioeconomic status. Co-creation is also required, since what works in one locale won't necessary translate to a global location. Often there are local resource limitations, such as poor roads, limited power infrastructure, or lack of Internet access. More difficult to navigate are often-undocumented cultural differences, such as understanding who the primary decision maker is for a family. In the United States, it is biased toward the individual or spouse, but in many cultures outside the United States, there is a much more extended familial influence, in which parents or other relatives have a significant influence over the medical decisions of even other adults. Rather than having design driven by researchers from high-income countries applying their tools and processes to familiar problems, it is crucial to have core members of the team who are integrated with the target community and familiar with the specific local characteristics.

Capacity Building

The overarching goal for any innovation should be a long-term sustainable impact. However, many global health projects currently are supported by governmental and nongovernmental organization and foundations. These are wonderful initiatives and lead to incredible work and progress in the public health; however, they are often time-limited and have restricted funding. This is one of the strongest culprits for "pilot-itis," as many projects simply end once the grant period is over. In order for a project to be more sustainable, development resources and even the innovation itself should be at least partially derived locally, so that team members will retain a long-term view and commitment to maintain a sustained impact for their local community. To achieve this lofty goal, organizations will need to focus on local capacity building to build necessary skills and train the next generation of digital health innovators.

Recommendations in Practice

For individuals, teams, and organizations interested in participating in innovations in global health settings, we have proposed this mantra of "collaboration, co-creation, and capacity building" using the lessons learned from the organizations of Sana; the Consortium for Affordable Medical Technology Co-Creation laboratories; MIT's Hacking Medicine; and GHDonline. These organizations have all pursued successful strategies in global health settings by practicing and upholding this mantra, and we recommend several strategies to achieve these goals in LMIC settings.

Under the guise of this mantra, we first recommend initiating innovation projects by responding to a clinical need affecting care delivery in the local setting. One example of this is Sana, a volunteer organization hosted by the Computer Science and Artificial Intelligence Laboratory at the Massachusetts Institute of Technology, which begins each project, program, or venture with this approach. Over time, Sana has developed an open-source mobile telehealth platform that allows for capture, transmission, and archiving of complex medical data such as ECG and EEG waveforms, in addition to patient demographic and clinical information to help meet needs in LMIC settings [13]. Sana begins each of its efforts with a thorough discussion and identification of clinical needs by the interdisciplinary team, which includes international NGOs, universities, governments, and private ventures, with strong emphasis on local stakeholders. Local organizations approach Sana with specific problems or "pain points" to solve, and Sana utilizes their core, enabling mobile telehealth platform to address the specific local needs. The team moves ahead only when buy-in is established from clinical providers, informaticians, and engineering and public health experts at the local level who will be pushing the project forward themselves. Having local clinicians on the team is essential, as they have the connections and influence. Sometimes the local culture—often sequestered by paternalistic medical traditions—might not be ready for quality improvement movements, so ministries of health or medical associations may resist cooperating. These local clinicians serve as barometers by which the team can determine if the innovation may be successful.

Secondly, we recommend building the capacity of the local community using a co-creation pathway. Because resources are often constrained in LMIC settings, it is critical to amplify the existing resources using co-creation, further supported by enabling technological infrastructure. The Co-Creation Laboratories, administratively housed at Massachusetts General Hospital in partnership with a consortium of partners in Uganda and

India [12], emphasize this iterative design process. Starting with the health needs identified by LMIC, the Co-Creation Laboratories work closely with local partners to tailor technologies through rapid prototyping and iterative creation. Utilizing Steve Blank's "lean start-up" [14] and Bill Aulet's "disciplined entrepreneurship" principles [15], they emphasize creating a "minimum value product," or MVP, needed to test out a potential solution to meet the clinical need. This initial prototype is tested and validated in the local context and setting. In a process they term "role flexing," the end user becomes "a designer, a physician, a policy advisory and anthropologist, and an engineer" [12]. These quick, iterative developmental cycles allow for the innovation team to obtain feedback in real time to propel the development of a solution that meets the unique needs of the community.

Another example of building capacity through co-creation is through the concept of "hackathons." Hackathons are focused, 48-hour innovation sessions that have created a number of successful companies and technological solutions [16]. At the time of writing, MIT's Hacking Medicine group has organized 47 hackathons across four continents that bring together engineers, scientists, designers, entrepreneurs, and front-line providers (including nurses and medical staff) to address painpoints identified during routine clinical practice. Traditionally, hackathons were developed as a forum for computer programmers to rapidly develop solutions in a short period of time (24–48 hours). Health care–focused hackathons provide new opportunities for providers to collaborate with engineers and quickly make an impact by offering the clinical perspective required to pose meaningful questions and to explain the context in which medical data is collected. Similarly, hackathons present a great forum for engineers and data scientists to gain access to real problems impacting medicine and to engage with stakeholders who have expert domain knowledge. By entrenching engineers and data scientists with clinicians, hackathons in LMIC settings provide a rare opportunity to impact care by bringing together diverse stakeholders in a shortened timeframe to prototype and iterate on ideas and solutions. For instance, one example of a sustainable project developed out of the hackathon model is the Augmented Infant Resuscitator [16]. The initial "pain point" was presented by Dr. Data Santorino, a pediatrician at the Mbarara University of Science and Technology in Uganda. He discussed the gaps in newborn resuscitation skills and training in LMIC despite the need for effective care, with over 6 million infants requiring basic resuscitation [17]. After pitching this problem, Dr. Santorino attracted a team composed of an MIT engineer, a business entrepreneur, and an MGH clinician who joined him to develop a new approach to this problem. During the hackathon event, they generated multiple ideas and prototypes and ended the event by presenting a working prototype of the resuscitator. This working prototype consisted of a microprocessor embedded in a bag-valve mask sized for infants. They continued to work together after the weekend to refine the prototype and business model. Currently, they are deploying their technology in the field in Uganda and have attracted the interest of investors and partners.

The third and last recommendation emphasizes multidisciplinary collaboration. There are great untapped opportunities to further accelerate innovation in global health settings through crowdsourcing innovation directly from the users and embedding it in user-driven communities. Eric von Hippel speaks extensively about the concept of the "democratization of innovation" [18]. This is a paradigm that allows front-line users to "develop exactly what they want, rather than relying on manufacturers to act as their (often very imperfect) agents. Moreover, individual users do not have to develop everything they need on their own: They can benefit from innovations developed and freely shared by others" [18]. Embedding these user-driven innovations in communities (both online and in-person) can create connections that "short-circuit" the innovation process and increase the speed and effectiveness of disseminating new evidence.

This concept has been well documented in other industries. For instance, the Defense Advanced Research Projects Agency developed ARPAnet to create a network of researchers and defense contractors to accelerate the exchange of software and data, while Linus Torvalds developed LINUX in 1991 as free and open-source operating system that enabled anyone to contribute to its development. Global health brings a unique set of challenges, and a more democratized approach is needed.

GHDonline is one example of a democratized platform that enables the formation of cross-disciplinary partnerships to help build the capacity and extend the skills of local community workers with a global network of experts. The platform brings together clinicians (including community health workers), researchers, public health experts, engineers, policy makers, social scientists, and students with an interest in global health [19]. Members of GHDonline can post questions or propose discussion topics to engage and obtain feedback from this virtual community in a diverse range of topics, from global surgery and anesthesia to health information technology. This online forum enables participants to access experts and promotes best practice sharing. It removes geographic, cultural, and socioeconomic boundaries to increase the pace and availability of collaborative efforts. GHDonline creates a horizontal network of partnerships across global health settings, removing any bureaucratic or top-down cultural barriers.

Conclusion

Our recommendation is to accelerate the development of sustainable solutions to solve the diverse and expansive problems facing stakeholders across global health settings by applying the mantra and recommendations discussed above. Several challenges still remain to pursue innovative activities in LMIC. First, despite the impressive gains and improvements in information and communication technologies across the globe, it is still quite difficult to coordinate teams of diverse stakeholders across geographic locations. This model requires patience from team members, along with rigorous project management to ensure efforts are propelled forward in an appropriate manner. In addition, it is important to avoid individualistic approaches often pursued by members of the entrepreneurial community and to embrace different paradigms practiced across the vast number of contexts across the globe. Finally, it is critical to obtain buy-in of political leadership in both organizations and LMIC to encourage them to develop policies, processes, funding mechanisms, infrastructure, and organizations to support innovations. Nevertheless, we believe that those who are able to follow the mantra, "collaboration, co-creation and capacity building" stand a far better chance of producing real and lasting improvements in global health.

Questions for Discussion

- What are some unique aspects of your local culture that benefit or hinder innovation in health care?
- How would you go about building local capacity to train and support the next generation of digital health innovators?

Acknowledgments

We would like to acknowledge Kris Olson and the Consortium for Affordable Medical Technologies (CAMTech) for their contribution to this article.

References

1. Drain PK, Primack A, Hunt DD, Fawzi WW, Holmes KK, Gardner P. 2007. Global health in medical education: A call for more training and opportunities. *Acad Med* 9: 226–230.

2. Coltart CE, Black ME, Easterbrook PJ. 2011. Global health in the UK government and university sector. *Infect Dis Clin North Am* 25: 555–574.

3. Izadnegahdar R, Correia S, Ohata B, Kittler A, ter Kuile S, Vaillancourt S, et al. 2008. Global health in Canadian medical education: Current practices and opportunities. *Acad Med* 83: 192–198.

4. Jeffrey S. Information technology and the revolution in health care. Unite for Sight Conference, 14 April 2013.

5. Cockerell J. Making donations of medical equipment work. The Lancet, 20 January 2014. http://globalhealth.thelancet.com/2014/01/20/making-donations-medical-equipment-work. Accessed 15 February 2015.

6. Perry L, Malkin R. 2011. Effectiveness of medical equipment donations to improve health systems: How much medical equipment is broken in the developing world? *Med Biol Eng Comput* 49(7): 719–722.

7. Howitt P, Darzi A, Yang GZ, Ashrafian H, Atun R, Barlow J, et al. 2012. Technologies for global health. *Lancet* 380(9840): 507–535.

8. Buffett P. 2013. The charitable-industrial complex. *New York Times*, 26 July. http://www.nytimes.com/2013/07/27/opinion/the-charitable-industrial-complex.html. Accessed July 28, 2013.

9. Chamberlain S. 2012. Pilot-itis: What's the cure? BBC Media Action, June 20. http://www.bbc.co.uk/blogs/bbcmediaaction/entries/e00fc35a-0c0f-3e35-8280-38d048c34487. Accessed February 15, 2015.

10. Byrnes N. 2014. Mobile health's growing pains. *MIT Tech Review* 117(5): 7–8.

11. DePasse J, Celi LA. 2013. Collaboration, capacity building and co-creation as a new mantra in global health. *Int J Qual Health Care* 30(3): 260–264. doi:10.1093/intqhc/mzt077.

12. Caldwell A, Young A, Gomez-Marquez J, Olson KR. 2011. Global health technology 2.0. *IEEE Pulse* 2: 63–67.

13. Sana. http://sana.mit.edu. Accessed July 27, 2013.

14. Blank S. 2013. Why the lean start-up changes everything. *Harv Bus Rev* 91(5): 63–72.

15. Aulet B. *Disciplined Entrepreneurship: 24 Steps to a Successful Startup.* John Wiley & Sons; 2013.

16. DePasse JW, Carroll R, Ippolito A, Yost A, Santorino D, Chu Z, et al. 2014. Less noise, more hacking: How to deploy principles from MIT's hacking medicine to accelerate health care. *Int J Technol Assess Health Care* 30(3): 1–5.

17. Wall SN, Lee AC, Niermeyer S, English M, Keenan WJ, Carlo W, et al. 2009. Neonatal resuscitation in low resource settings: What, who, and how to overcome challenges to scaleup? *Int J Gynaecol Obstet* 107(Suppl 1): S47–S62, S63–S64.

18. Von Hippel E. 2005. *Democratizing Innovation.* Cambridge, MA: MIT Press.

19. GHDonline. www.ghdonline.org. Accessed July 28, 2013.

19   The Health Informatics Design Process

Kenneth Paik, Biyeun Buczyk, and Cory Zue

Take-Home Messages

- The health informatics design process requires close multidisciplinary collaboration along clinical, technical, funding, and policy lines.
- Stakeholder analysis involves individuals and organizations beyond just the eventual end users, critically including payers, providers, and policy makers.
- Workflow integration involves linking technical innovation with clinical outcomes, plus reducing barriers to adoption, such as added work.
- Test, validate, and learn early during the design and development process in order to adjust and adapt the solution for improved outcomes.

Introduction

Design has often been misconstrued as merely pertaining to aesthetic or graphic design, but in the context of this book, it more holistically constitutes the robust planning and functional specifications for the entire project. Analogous to architectural plans detailing what materials to use and how everything fits together, the health informatics design process requires an understanding of the technical components as well as the setting in which it will be implemented. The primary challenge is integrating an innovation with the established environment to yield a beneficial impact without disrupting effective processes.

There are many factors that could potentially lead to the failure of a health informatics project; however, a common breakdown from the outset is the design of the project. One common mistake is presumptively applying the blueprints from a previous project to a new situation. Unfortunately, what works in one area does not necessarily translate to another, particularly when entering a different cultural or socioeconomic environment. Maintaining a social awareness of the characteristic patients and health workers is crucial to implementing a usable application, while understanding and navigating the political and regulatory habitat is pivotal to avoiding insurmountable barriers.

Other failures derive from errors in process, without appropriately considering dependencies. Projects can be too compartmentalized, segregating the clinical design from the technology development. Too often, principal investigators simply hand off design specifications to developers to produce the software. This amplifies errors on both ends, as the clinical investigators fall into traps of feasibility and the engineers make flawed assumptions of implementation, resulting in buggy software nobody wants to use.

A crucial aspect emphasized throughout this textbook is the frequent disconnect between technical innovation and quality improvement. Engineers often get caught thinking a solution will succeed because it is the latest and greatest, deploying "technology for technology's sake." However, blindly designing solutions based on the newest advances ignores the crucial user base and potential clinical impact. A new technology without the accompanying commitment to improving health care will inevitably lead to failed, unsustainable pilots, since clinicians won't want to use it and there would be no monetary cost benefit. Returning to the architectural analogy, we want to design a solution where "form follows function," so that the design of the technology innovation is based primarily on an intended positive clinical impact rather than designing around a core technology.

Essential Recommendations

Before any technology development begins, we must first determine the required components through an intensive design process. This chapter is not a detailed process manual to be followed step by step, nor is it an explicit implementation of the various "design thinking," "human centered design," or "integrative thinking" processes, which are excellent models to follow. Instead, we present here the crucial elements to consider when integrating an informatics solution in a global health environment. The primary focus on quality improvement brings attention to capturing and communicating the right information, while also connecting to the workflow loop for appropriate clinical intervention. Equally important, we must focus on making applications easy to use in order to encourage adoption and sustainability. In order to accomplish these challenging, often conflicting goals, we recommend incorporating the following mechanisms into your design process.

Stakeholder Analysis

Understanding the key players involved with an intervention is central to deploying a usable and effective solution. This goes beyond just end users to include anyone that is involved in the health care delivery process for your intervention.

Many mHealth solutions are intended to interface with multiple users, such as clinicians, health workers, or patients. It is important to consider how each group will actually use the application and their aptitude for adapting to a new interface, and to allow for individual variance. This is a challenging step for engineers, since they are steeped in the latest technologies and tend to want to deploy the latest advances in user interfaces. The engineers are often trapped building complicated interfaces with which they are familiar, but that can seem like a foreign language to others. To overcome this, it is important to bring an advocate for the end user into the design process to better understand their adeptness and preferences. One illustrative example from our project work at Sana is our postsurgical project in Haiti, where the end users are local community health workers. While designing the user interface, we had to reconcile that most of the workers were farmers or worked extensively in manual labor, leading to predominantly calloused hands that sometimes struggled with small dexterity-requiring touch interfaces. To adapt to this user base, we adjusted with larger buttons and hotspots for easier input. Further information about usability and usability testing is available in chapter 21.

When considering other stakeholders to design for, it is important to be comprehensive in considering who else is in the process. This means not just individual end users of the technology but any individual or organization involved in the process, directly or indirectly, since they can have a significant influence on the design of the solution. It is helpful to consider any group that can influence the funding, implementation, or public policy around an intervention. Common stakeholders to recognize include providers who deliver care, payers who reimburse for procedures or care delivery, funders who may fund the overall pilot program, or governmental organizations that establish public policy or drive health initiatives. Each of these groups can have a significant impact on the sustainable success of an intervention, while not considering any single one can obstruct project progress regardless of the success of other aspects. For example, even with a successful clinical pilot and evidence of quality improvement, if the local government does not provide supportive public policies or instantiates prohibitive policies in regard to data or treatment regulations, an intervention cannot be scaled up.

Workflow Integration

Any technical innovation needs to be thoughtfully integrated within the clinical workflow. Rather than designing around a novel technology, it's often constructive to begin with the clinical intervention and analyze where technology can play a role and improve processes. At the outset, it is helpful to investigate any significant barriers to implementation, such as preexisting systems, user hesitance, immutable processes, or insufficient human resources.

An aspect of workflow integration is a strong emphasis on workflow efficiency. Clinicians are notoriously overworked, with limited time and significant amounts spent on documentation already. As much as possible, any innovation needs to avoid adding work or the solution won't be adopted by the clinician user base, nearly regardless of the potential benefit. Therefore, it is imperative to design efficient clinical interfaces that minimize the amount of additional work, with improving efficiency an ideal objective. An important caveat comes from including the previous recommendation of end-user analysis, where the clinician users will likely have different biases toward what interface improves efficiency from the implementing engineers, so it is prudent to include clinicians in the design process.

Most importantly, for any mHealth solution to yield a lasting impact, it must be directly tied to quality improvement. This requires "closing the loop" with a clinical intervention, so it is strongly recommended that a holistically designed intervention connect the informatics innovation with the clinical process. This is a challenging proposition, and it requires clinicians to collaborate closely with technologists to push the envelope of combining what is technically feasible with what can make a clinical impact.

Prototype Validation and Rapid Iteration

The final recommendation is to learn during the design process and adapt and adjust accordingly throughout development in order to facilitate the best outcomes. This can be built into the process through prototype validation and rapid iteration. For prototype validation, this might include planned "proofs of concept," which are small prototypes that attempt to answer any significant questions from the design stage. These can be as varied as a questionnaire to determine target users' needs or acceptance of a new technology, to a technical prototype validating an exchange protocol. Another possibility includes mockups or screenshots to test usability for a target audience. These prototypes should test and validate or disprove questions so you can adjust your plan early rather than be caught delivering an ineffective project.

Even after the design stage, if possible it is recommended to implement a process of rapid iteration during the development phase. This entails getting feedback quickly from stakeholders in order to quickly adjust the solution. This entails not locking into what is in the technical specifications and keeping an open mind to what the feedback is telling you. The quicker the development team learns what will actually work, the less significant the impact on the ultimate development timeline or cost is likely to be. The potential utility of various project management methods will be covered in chapter 20.

Conclusion

The health informatics design process is a pivotal balancing of stakeholders and outcomes, requiring close multidisciplinary collaboration. It is beneficial to maintain a wide perspective and pursue stakeholder input to reduce barriers and promote adoption.

Implementing these processes will encourage the connection of quality improvement and sustainable program impact to your technology innovation.

Questions for Discussion

- Considering a potential innovation. Who are some of the crucial stakeholders that might have an impact on its implementation?
- What are significant barriers to adoption for a potential mHealth innovation?
- What are some "proofs of concept" that might test the previously identified barriers?

20 Software Project Management

Daniel Myung and Cory Zue

Take-Home Messages

- Delivering technology is not a singular event; it is a process and a learned skill to manage expectations and deliver on time.
- Methods and tools—be it Agile or Waterfall—depend on the engagement model you and your customer agree upon.
- Building software is an iterative process that should involve frequent testing and validation of ideas and collecting feedback from different stakeholders at every stage.
- It is crucial to understand the different stages of the process, what to focus on in each stage, and how the requirements and process changes at each stage.
- Software development processes in the information and communication technologies for development, or ICT4D, space are not so different from any other, except that sometimes understanding your target users or markets can be more challenging.

Introduction

Implementing a project to advance the health informatics capabilities in an organization is a multidisciplinary endeavor. It is far more than installing some new appliance or using some new software. Many strong technology approaches applied to important challenges have failed to solve the problem at scale because of challenges in executing the product development life cycle. This points to the heavy reliance on coordinated project management, particularly when integrating new technologies into complicated systems such as global health.

There are numerous books, lectures, and philosophies surrounding the art and science of effective project management, and we encourage you to find and utilize the practice that matches well with your organization. This chapter on fundamentals will seek to provide some basic background on project management specifically for projects developing information and communication technologies. There will be a particular emphasis on the essentials a technical implementer needs to consider when deploying a global health project in a global resource-limited setting.

When coordinating a cross-disciplinary team in a complicated setting such as global health, the biggest hurdles are coordinating diverse members and tasks while ensuring each of the stakeholders' views are accounted for. There is an essential tension in balancing the dual goals of deploying a new and innovative technology with the necessary focus on clinical quality improvement. Therefore, it is paramount that the engineering process closely harmonizes with the clinical design process, ensuring an effective and usable solution. Given this set of needs, can you, the implementer, shepherd resources appropriately to meet these needs in a timely manner?

Common Software Project Management Methodologies

Over the decades, the software industry has employed many different frameworks to manage development projects. Broadly speaking, these software-development life-cycle guidelines provide good parameters for implementers to follow. As technologies, regulatory requirements, human resources, and business requirements have changed, so too has the development process. We will highlight two common practices currently employed with divergent philosophies of management: Waterfall and Agile.

Waterfall Development

Waterfall project management seeks to follow a sequential order of events building up to the finished product (figure 20.1). Its core methodology is attributed to Winston W. Royce [1]. Each stage of the project's life cycle must be completed before the next stage of the project is to begin.

At face value, the sequential stages of a project's life make intuitive sense. For projects large and small where a clear vision and plan are known, Waterfall is widely used and promoted. Due to its sequential nature, there is a strong emphasis on clear requirements and documentation. This makes it easy for both stakeholders and implementers to understand a project's progress.

Waterfall Advantages:
• The project has a clear overarching plan and objective at the outset
• Each stage is clear in its outcome

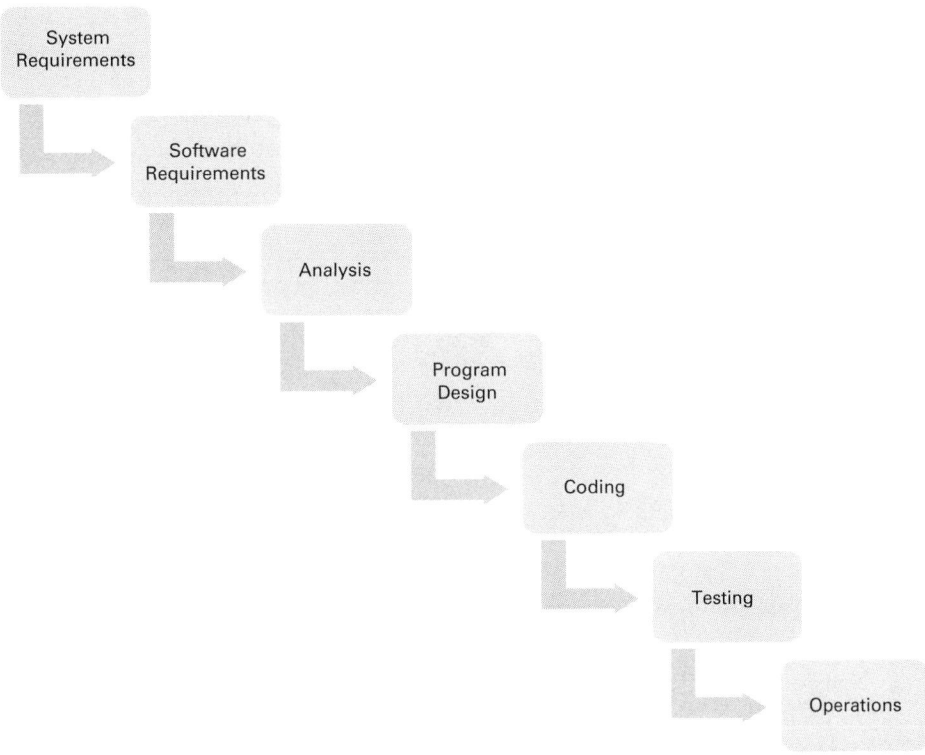

Figure 20.1
Stages of the Waterfall development life cycle.

- Up-front customer engagement
- Contractual nature of milestones and deliverables

Waterfall Disadvantages:
- Significant up-front planning and design may diverge from actual reality quickly
- Rigidity of stages makes change management difficult
- Incorporating feedback from stakeholders in later stages is complicated

Agile Development

Agile project management came about in 2001 from a group of software developers seeking to simplify the software-development process as a reaction to what were seen as drawbacks to "traditional" Waterfall development [2]. While the original manifesto itself is a series of statements emphasizing a more lightweight means to producing quality software, in practice there have been various iterations of running Agile projects. Its variants include SCRUM (the most widely used; see figure 20.2), Extreme Programming, Lean, Kanban, and others [3].

At its core, Agile focuses on frequent short-cycle iterations of gathering requirements, development, and deployment of a unit of work or feature within the project. Rather than bundling up a large release of features for a major release, Agile focuses on frequent iteration with customers throughout the life cycle of the project.

A typical Scrum sprint is shown above. They are typically triaged and placed on a backlog list for the product. In every sprint, which can be 2–4 weeks in length, a subset of the most important items project management thinks can be completed during the constraints of the sprint are prioritized. These items are then specified "just in time," developed, tested, and deployed during the sprint. At the end of the sprint, the features deployed are validated by the customer as completed, and the process repeats.

Agile Advantages
- Just-in-time requirements for a given feature
- Frequent customer feedback throughout life cycle of project
- Expects and handles changes to project scope well

Agile Disadvantages
- Potentially high workload on customer for iteration and approval through project life cycle

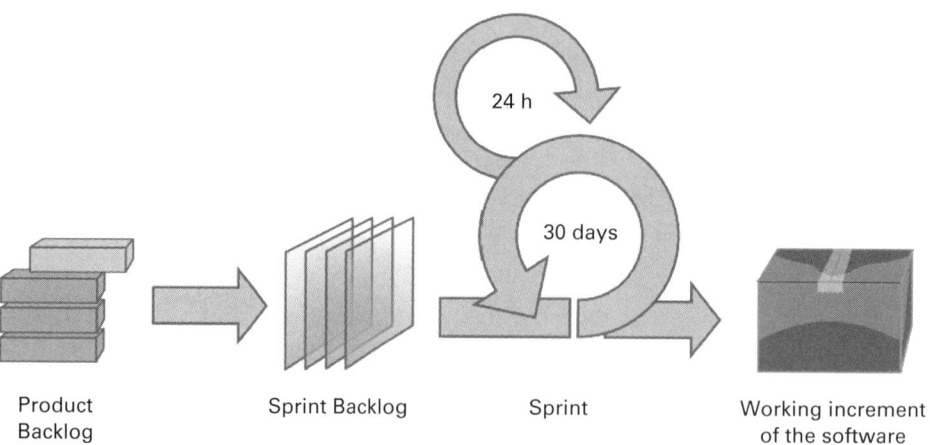

Product   Sprint Backlog   Sprint   Working increment
Backlog   of the software

Figure 20.2
A typical Scrum sprint [4].

- Need expectation management and buy-in of customer for process
- Staff will need to be highly skilled with both the process as well as technical needs; customer engagement and domain knowledge are helpful as well
- Planning for fixed deliverables difficult due to iterative nature of delivery

Agile or Waterfall?

Is one philosophy inherently better than the other? Not necessarily. While Agile sought to address some deficiencies in the Waterfall model specific to software development, it still has its drawbacks and burdens on staff and customer. Depending on the size and scope of the project, one may be more advantageous than the other. This is also dependent on the makeup of your stakeholders as well as the makeup of your team.

In general, if your customer is committed to being available to give continuous feedback and iteration, then Agile may be the more appropriate choice. If developing and deploying new technology is a new and unknown endeavor, then with the right partnership, the project should be a process, which Agile can provide. However, if up-front requirements can be known and evolving iteration is not necessary or practical, then a Waterfall approach is advisable.

Life of an Example Project

The following is largely built upon the collective experiences of Dimagi (http://www.dimagi.com/), a company spun out of the Massachusetts Institute of Technology that designs and implements open and innovative software to help care for underserved communities in low- and middle-income countries (LMIC). The team assembled its practices from its peers in NGO spheres and combined them with the lean and agile methods from modern software-development firms. In practice, information and communication technology (ICT) projects in LMIC generally lend themselves well to a hybrid Agile and Waterfall approach. With the large scope of an ICT intervention, a significant amount of effort is devoted up front to prepare the overarching mission and vision with the partners on the ground. This up-front effort generally has fallen under a Waterfall approach for defining scope and initial requirements. However, once a project is under way and the software is actively developed, an Agile approach with iterative, continuous feedback has been the norm.

This chapter will not cover the financial aspect of negotiating rates and bills for projects such as these. We will stay high-level here on methods of management. Specific details of IT implementation strategies are a complex topic on their own and vary greatly depending on the type of project being executed, especially in LMIC. As such, day-to-day project-specific actions will not be covered in this chapter.

Project Inception

Figure 20.3 depicts the stages of software development. As with any health informatics IT project, it is important to establish a clear and compelling set of reasons and requirements for why an intervention is necessary. Whether it is done at the management level or government ministry level, or by a person more intimately involved with front-line workers' (FLWs) needs, these questions generally follow a familiar pattern of assessing the perceived benefit:

• What pain points does this project seek to solve?

• What are the benefits you will gain?

• How will the quality and delivery of service by your FLWs improve?

• How will the organization improve its management of FLWs?

• How will monitoring and evaluation and reporting become more effective, efficient, and transparent?

It is recommended that for a project to be undertaken, these high-level questions be answered. They will establish the initial boundaries of need and expectation. Project approval is a mutual agreement by you, the implementer, agreeing to the scope of desire, and the customer accepting the costs for what is promised.

Whether managing a project in Agile or Waterfall, this crafting of a vision for the project is important for a stakeholder. For an Agile practitioner, this up-front declaration of a project may seem to front-load expectations on a project; however, for ICT projects, especially in health ministry or government-related fields, we have found it to be necessary to be "Waterfall first" in this stage of the project. In more formal software life-cycle deployments [5], these planning phases are necessary before formal Agile iteration can begin.

Project Approved—Kicking it Off

Once a project has been approved, it is a good idea to organize a plenary meeting of users, beneficiaries, and stakeholders of the project. It typically serves as a way to get all

Stages of Software Development

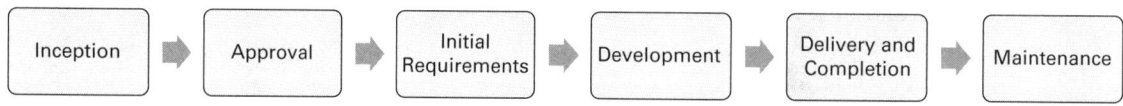

Figure 20.3
Stages of software development.

actors in one place to understand the dependencies and workflow needs for the project. The key here is that the actual users and beneficiaries of the system being developed should have a seat at the table early on. It is also important to get these parties to understand the roles they play in the system and to build ownership across all levels of the project.

This ownership building is important for all users of the system. Often, health ministries or larger NGOs may impose new projects and interventions with little feedback or input from their FLWs. A project's success depends on execution and motivation from actual workers using the system, so it is important to provide an environment where their feedback and participation is heard and utilized.

This initial meeting should also provide familiarity with users to help lower the barrier to easy communication. This will prove key for getting timely and frequent user/stakeholder feedback in the necessary iterations of the product's development.

Following the kickoff meeting, limit the size and frequency of meetings to those stakeholders and users most directly impacted or needed for the project or task at hand.

Roles and Responsibilities

Typically, a project team's structure should follow the makeup shown in figure 20.4.

The Project Team

Your ICT implementation project should have a *project team* in place to execute and shepherd the project to completion. At its core, it should consist of a *product owner* representing the interests of the customer or stakeholder. The owner will be the primary

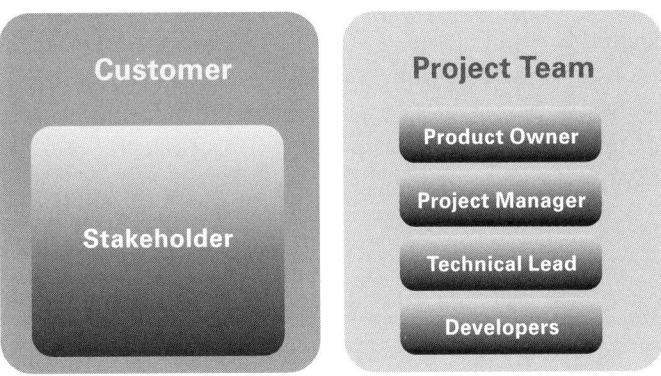

Figure 20.4
Typical project team structure.

person your customer will interact with. It is their conversations that will establish the particular requirements for the project, and they will be the primary conduit through which feedback will be gathered. They should have an exceptional ability to empathize and identify with the customer's needs. Note that while the product owner represents the customer's interests, they are still employed by you, the implementer.

On the technical side, a *project manager* and *technical lead* will represent the technical team's interests. These people must work alongside each other to prioritize and agree upon customer features and desires feasible for the project.

Depending on the particular management and execution philosophy, the titles, roles, and number of these people may differ. The key for all these roles and responsibility structures is ensuring that effective communication channels remain open from the customer/stakeholder's perspective to the technical team.

From the Customer

We cannot stress enough the need for a primary *champion* or *customer advocate* of the project. This individual, or small group of people, should be wholly employed to represent the customer's interests. In fact, we recommend the customer advocate be the one who requested the project in the first place. This individual will be the primary point of contact for the product owner. It is vital that a vocal and invested party be present to work alongside the product owner and that they have the time and initiative to oversee the project along its many phases, instead of being a distant executive present only at the beginning and end of the project. As important as it is for the technical team to have a competent project manager, there needs to be an equal counterpart to the technical project manager advocating for the end users to drive the project forward at every important milestone.

We feel that this customer advocate must be local to the eventual deployment and be in close or direct contact with the end users. If the customer advocate is, for example, a central manager too far removed from the day-to-day operations of the FLWs, in particular, it may produce a mismatch of expectations and ownership of issues and problems. It is important that the customer advocate has direct incentives for the project's success.

Gather Initial Requirements

Central to any project actually executing is the distillation of the core needs of the users and consumers of the system to base units of functionality. These core needs must then be digestible by the technical team to implement. In traditional "Waterfall" project management styles, the requirements-gathering phase may be a major, one-time event. Once collected, these requirements would then be executed by the technical team and delivered at a certain point in time. In contrast, the Agile methodology of continuous customer feedback has made this process an iterative, incremental process. Depending on the scope and scale of the ICT project, this first requirements-gathering phase may be a significant amount of work, regardless of the management methodology used.

User Stories

One popular technique for requirements gathering and distilling functionality for the engineers is the creation of *user stories*. User stories are succinct statements that capture a clear unit of work, with all the actors and outcomes. It helps bridge the communication between end user and engineer and keeps core needs focused within the particular tasks. Multiple user stories can describe a process within the project, and many more can eventually capture the entirety of the project at hand. Typically, a product owner will work with the customer or stakeholder in crafting these statements.

A typical user story starts out as a statement needing parts filled, such as:

"As a <user>, I want to be able to do <blank action> so that I can do <additional action>:"

An example user story in telemedicine could be filled out like this:

"As a nurse, I want to be able to upload a photo taken by my smartphone so that I can ask for a referral from a doctor."

What is key is that these user-story statements must originate from the customer and be expressed in terms that a customer would want as a particular feature of the product. It should not, and likely will not, be sufficient in detail for the technical team to actually implement, because elaborating a user story with specific technical details such as SQL statements or programming languages will only confuse both users and developers.

The statement should be sufficient to get the technical team to get started on the project. In Agile projects, this is where specification and design happen "just in time" for development. When the user-story feature is accepted for the project sprint, the product team should allocate resources for specifying the implementation. These just-in-time requirements and specifications at the time of development are key both to getting the essence of the user-story request as close to implementation as possible, and to getting customer acceptance quickly, both in the specification and design phase and in implementation and acceptance of completion.

From this entry statement, further functionality and operational background can be elaborated. If using a centralized issue- and task-management system, these could all be added as background information.

Additional information on the background of the story could include the current state of the system and highlighting the difficulty of the existing process to reveal additional operational and workflow benefits that the feature will unlock.

Use succinct and specific language for the functionality that matches the user experience. There are various resources to consider for training in user stories and general Agile management of projects.

A project with a well-defined list of user stories can now paint a narrative of all the features being implemented. Furthermore, tasks and accomplishments can be tracked by the user stories being completed by the implementation team, so they provide a clear indicator for both the client and implementer of the progress of a project.

For the technical team, the user story may be too high-level. In the prior example, it makes rather large assumptions that there is a smartphone platform that can be developed upon as well as other infrastructure needed for referrals. For engineers, it is common practice to break down a larger task into subtasks based upon the technical task needed. End users and customers may not need to see the particular implementation details, but it will help engineers focus on particular functionalities with broken-up tasks. To go back to the example story, the smartphone application could hypothetically be broken down into two to three tasks—one for the smartphone application, one for image capture, and one for upload capabilities. Furthermore, the referral functionality could be broken down into one task for image capture and processing, and a second task for referral alerting and tracking.

Breaking down a primary user story into smaller subtasks for implementers to use makes to easier to assign time and labor costs to the particular tasks. With these estimates on labor and degree of difficulty, it is possible to triage implementation of features and communicate to the customer timelines, costs, and sequence of deliverables.

Development

The above sections highlighted some of the typical up-front work needed to get a project going. The actual course of development and delivery of features moving forward from the initial phases is where the need for choosing a particular management philosophy happens. It is here where Agile or Waterfall methodology should be chosen and ultimately followed.

For Agile development, close customer contact is needed for the specification of the particular features being developed, but also for confirmation and sign-off of the particular set of features at the conclusion of a sprint. For geographically distributed teams, this consistent contact and communication may be difficult to obtain. It is this need for clarity of communication that has led to the proliferation of a variety of collaboration tools and techniques to help project teams and customers stay synchronized regardless of their location. Whether it is using the Scrum method and utilizing an online tool, or using a marker board with sticky notepaper and maintaining a Kanban board by hand, some sort of tracking system needs to be employed to help track the progress of development.

These tools and methodologies are important in order to measure and document the completion of work, record issues, and communicate and retain knowledge throughout the project. With each task in your backlog completed, you are able to take on new tasks and be one step closer to completion.

The burn-down chart [6] is a graphical representation of the completed versus remaining tasks for a given iteration or sprint within a project (see figure 20.5). Over the course of multiple iterations, the remaining backlog of committed tasks should eventually go to zero as you complete your tasks.

Delivery and Completion

As the project's features are delivered, it is important to communicate early and often with the stakeholder on the general state of the project and provide estimates of timelines for completion.

Arriving at agreement for completion and measuring success can be challenging. Did the customer fully understand their needs when requirements were agreed upon? Do their stakeholders agree on the features you delivered being complete? Features have been delivered according to the specifications set by the initial requirements as well as signed off at respective sprints—is that sufficient? What if the stakeholders and users are unhappy?

It is the role of the project manager to set expectations with the customer on establishing timetables, deadlines, and limits to the feature backlog and when to consider the

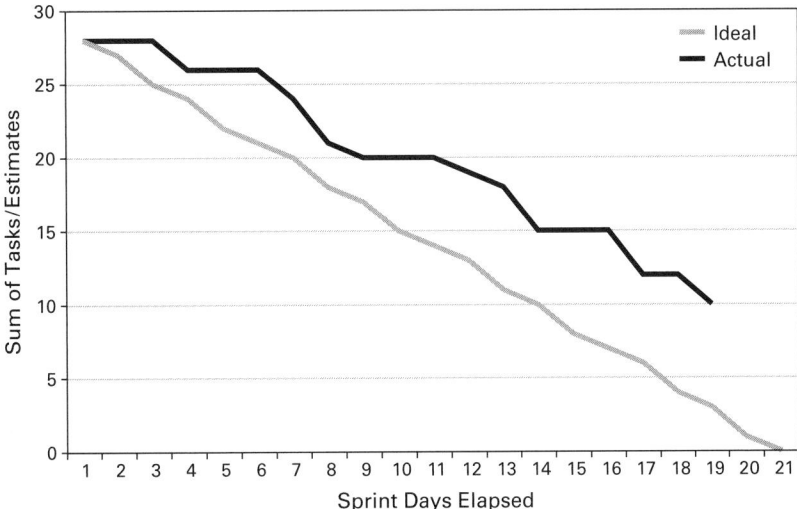

Figure 20.5
Example burn-down chart.

project complete. Some projects may be time-boxed for a fixed delivery date, so not all features may be implemented and a best-effort implementation may be needed. Other projects may be completely groundbreaking in terms of what is being delivered, so completeness criteria may not be known ahead of time. These projects may need to be constrained by time, material, and budget after an agreed-upon level of functionality and satisfaction is established.

Finally, delivery of a system hinges upon the successful handoff of responsibility to both the customer's end users as well as their administrators. Are the trainers and eventual administers properly equipped to champion the product on their own? Can their IT staff troubleshoot and repair issues without your direct intervention? Can they install, configure, and extend your solution without needing to call and e-mail you at every moment? In addition to feature delivery, there is also a crucial knowledge-transfer and training component needed for closing out a project.

Maintenance

ICT systems will eventually develop problems. Whether it is the fault of the technology or other factors, skilled assistance will be needed to troubleshoot and remedy inevitable problems.

As mentioned above, delivery and completeness of a project is dependent upon sufficient knowledge transfer and training of the customer and its users. But just as no system is error-free, there will be inevitable knowledge gaps. Providing customers an official channel in which to engage with you post-project completion is an important step to take. It ensures that your customer is operating the product well, but also helps maintain your reputation. It is important to set an appropriate time and labor constraint on the amount of maintenance and support. There are various models throughout the ICT industry to follow for how to maintain contracts after an actual project or product is delivered.

How and when to give support and maintenance on your end is entirely determined by the scope of the project and the capabilities you built into the system and your team to provide such support. If the customer has a support team in-house, it may be more appropriate to provide deep training for technical issues to their staff and reserve your staff only for higher levels of support. In other circumstances, your customer may have zero capacity to self-manage your system, so you may need to incur additional overhead to support this customer.

Understanding and Measuring Usage

After releasing a product to the world, it is extremely important to understand how that product is being used. There are important subjective and objective ways to accomplish this.

On the subjective side, it's important to continually engage with and observe your users. Ensuring that there is a mechanism for users to provide input on the product and feel like their voices are being heard is an incredibly useful way to get suggestions on how to improve the product, and if users can see their input being rolled out as changes to the product, they will feel more connected to the product and be more likely to keep using it (and recommend it to others). This can be more challenging in the information and communication technologies for development (ICT4D) space when it is logistically harder to reach out to, and engage with, end users of the system. In scenarios where users are very difficult to reach through normal channels, we recommend having intermediaries who talk with users and collect their feedback and bring that back to the product team.

Oftentimes, it can be easier to understand usage via objective measurement using tools like logging or web analytics. These can be incredibly powerful ways to see how frequently features are being used, and also can facilitate A/B testing for usability enhancements. There are many products to help execute A/B testing and references that cover this topic in more depth.

Project Considerations in LMIC

The previous sections addressed project management in general guidelines. In practice for ICT in LMIC, traditional project management methodologies for stakeholder interaction and customer feedback need contextual awareness to the prevailing industry standards. The following addresses some suggestions for structuring projects in LMIC.

Incorporating Feedback for Projects in LMIC

The kickoff meeting, while an important milestone and overview of the particular needs of a project, only touches upon the particular needs and issues at a high level. The information gathered from that meeting will invariably be insufficient for the particular needs for the varying users in the system. With requirements gathering and user validation of features being developed, it is important that the feedback mechanisms for your project are robust and accessible. In LMIC, however, getting the right feedback, in particular from your eventual end users, can prove challenging.

Direct Feedback   Descriptions workflows for FLWs or management can differ widely from original specification once they are field tested by actual users. Especially for community health workers, cultural norms may complicate getting direct, substantive feedback, even for glaringly obvious issues.

In communicating directly, it is important to be as clear as possible when probing and unpacking issues that will arise in the testing of the system. If the customer encounters a bug that causes an error or other unexpected behavior, be sure they are trained to communicate in a way the implementer can understand. Conversely, ensure that the product manager, or other customer-facing personnel, are able to ask the right probing questions to understand the exact situation in a way that can be understandable by your technical staff. Whether this is done via face-to-face communication or electronically, the key is to capture as much information as possible to minimize back-and-forth communication (which could span days if across multiple time zones). Note this is not to minimize communication in general, but to minimize miscommunication. The end goal should be that your technical team should feel confident that they have enough information from the user to reproduce whatever issue they encountered. The end user and customer should feel confident that their issue has been received and understood.

Indirect Feedback   Opportunities to monitor the actual issues from afar are critical. If users have a safe place where they feel they can give honest feedback, especially regarding bugs, it will facilitate more candid responses. It may not be direct criticism, but rather observations and interactions of your system completely outside your expectations.

Asking "do you like it" will likely yield positive feedback, but will not be substantive. Instead we recommend giving tasks or observing actual FLW work with minimal prompting. The key here is to understand user behavior.

As you observe the user behaviors and implement features according to the agreed-upon user stories, use the tracking system to incorporate the feedbacks and changes to how the actual solution is implemented. As the story gets refined, it must be reflected as more knowledge is gained. This in turn will help the implementers change course if necessary or improve upon initial designs. It is this continuous feedback and refinement that makes the process successful.

The end goal with the features being implemented is that these particular user stories can be marked as completed from the issue list initially agreed upon. Validating the story's desired outcome with the customer confirming success helps finalize each agreed-upon component of the system.

Getting the Right Feedback

Be aware of the context in which a project is being implemented in the organization or ministry. High-level ownership and the hierarchy in which a project is imposed could profoundly affect the quality and quantity of feedback necessary to improve the system. Power dynamics will greatly differ between the high-level stakeholder (the funder, or signer of contracts), the implementer (you and the project) and the ultimate end user (FLWs).

Typically, in other large IT projects, the end user may have more power and agency to dictate feedback. In a resource-constrained setting, the IT implementer may be coming in as a more powerful entity with the perception that it is immune or not beholden to stakeholder feedback—especially FLWs. This perception could be developed due to projects being imposed from high organizational decrees instead from grassroots-level needs. Alternatively, FLWs may never be given the opportunity to give feedback to levels above them.

The unfortunate result of organizational structures mentioned above is that feedback from the ultimate and most important users of the system—the FLWs—will be difficult to receive.

Perceptions of this new system could also intimidate your users as well. A system being brought in could be seen as perfect or complete, without fault. If the IT implementation is going to be the first implementation of such technology and techniques, then it could magnify the assumptions of perfection.

However, the opposite may be true. Being the first implementation of IT also magnifies the need for early, frequent, and effective feedback. If FLWs are not familiar with IT, then any particular error or issue they run into could be interpreted as user error or unfamiliarity with IT instead of a particular defect or usability flaw in the system. Discerning the distinctions among user error, user unfamiliarity, and design flaws is difficult and time-consuming for projects in these situations. Be aware of cultural or organizational norms as well. For example, negative feedback for new processes or systems may not be vocalized in an official capacity.

With these challenges in getting direct feedback, take extra effort to build into the project's roadmap specific mechanisms for receiving it. During usability assessments, if developers and designers are present, they cannot guide or prompt the users evaluating the system. Try to create situations where supervisors, administrators, or people with power over the users are not visible or present to intimidate or otherwise influence the feedback of the users. Consider having a trained peer or similar person present to observe and receive feedback and workarounds that the target user might recommend.

Staffing needs for getting effective front-line feedback should consider a full-time presence alongside the actual FLWs. This individual or group should report to the product manager. Depending on the size of the project, it could in fact also be the product manager, too.

Feedback and Testing by Monitoring

Proactive outreach to customers and users is one dimension of getting the appropriate feedback for iteratively improving your project. This proactive effort can communicate enthusiasm and care to customers. It is, however, time-consuming and could introduce behavior alteration that may not reveal true behavior. So while the planned feedback sessions are important, we also would stress having an effective monitoring strategy that allows for passive data collection around your system. In ICT projects utilizing web technology or mobile technology such as phones, there are various methods and frameworks to collect usage data from your users. As with any monitoring and tracking technology, ensure that your stakeholders and users consent to such technologies and be clear that this is for feedback and customer improvement.

These monitoring techniques can allow you to monitor behavior and observe how a user would navigate through your website or mobile phone application. It could highlight design flaws or workflow deficiencies you otherwise might not notice.

In additional, errors or bugs user may encounter can be set to send an alert your technical team immediately. Users may never report some issues they encounter. The reasons could range from the FLWs thinking it is their own error causing the issue, or error fatigue. By receiving these issues directly, it allows you to notify the customer that you are proactive in finding and remedying issues. That builds additional trust and enthusiasm from your customers.

This monitoring framework also aids the maintenance of the system. Should issues crop up, an automated error and monitoring system will greatly reduce the times between issue reports and diagnosis to actual resolution. Whether maintained by the customer staff, or by you the implementer, real data and information recorded from the point of a problem removes guesswork and communication breakdowns.

Practical Takeaways

Centralized Task Management

Employ a centralized issue-management system to track tasks, defects, and store knowledge. The feedback system should be the go-to place all members of the development team can refer to and use to update work on issues, be it new development or troubleshooting and solving an issue observed in the field.

For multinational teams spread across multiple time zones, it is important to use a centrally accessible online system so that correspondences can be shared and viewed by all. This will greatly facilitate communication and resolution of issues. If the deployed region reports an issue, but is halfway across the world from another team, the central management system can make the resolution process more efficient. The customer can leave questions on the issue tracker and greatly reduce miscommunication. Instead of waiting for phone calls or long e-mail conversations spread out over many days, the central tracker can act as the sole and trusted source for all knowledge around an issue.

If the region of deployment is in a place of poor Internet connectivity, systems like these become even more important. We recommend prioritizing Internet airtime to the project's budget to enable use of such a system. The project's members at all levels should commit to a culture of using such a system as well. So if there is a challenge for reliable bandwidth to such a site, reiterate the importance to use the site despite the network challenges. These services vary in how efficient they are at using bandwidth, so we recommend trying them out in your locales to see which is the right fit from a management perspective as well as technical perspective. The savings gained in time and institutional knowledge creation from using these systems we believe far outweighs the usage costs they may incur.

Feedback Monitoring and Collection Systems

Your system should utilize active and passive data-collection systems agreed upon with the customer for getting detailed information about the active system. This active and passive collection of information can be in the form of user behavior, error reports, or other feedback, and should be only utilized for the improvement of the system.

Dealing with Setbacks

In any project of significance, there will always be setbacks that could cause delays. Implementing health informatics is difficult for a variety of reasons. The technology is new and complex; the logistics of people, training, and materials could be out of your control. Regulatory or bureaucratic hurdles could add unanticipated additional overhead. Mistakes from your designs and assumptions could lead to mismatched expectations, requiring new, unexpected work.

Whatever the setbacks may be, it is important to communicate early and often on the need to shift deadlines or pivot priorities. Hopefully, with proper tracking of tasks completed via the centralized tracking system and clear documentation of communication around user stories, these can be both minimized, and anticipated.

Conclusion

As with any project that seeks to inject IT into a situation where IT did not exist before, it is important to set limits and constraints to what is possible to accomplish given the budget and time constraints you may have. It highlights the need to agree with the customer on the scope and language spelled out in your user stories. Keeping stories realistic and grounded in the realities of what is available in that region is important for both *feature creep*—the continual incremental accumulation of features—and for preventing never-ending projects due to open-ended user stories. It is important in agreeing on the user stories that both sides concur on what is feasible within the timeframe of the project as well as how a particular feature of set of features can be evaluated as completed.

We have only scratched the surface of what effective project management can entail. We mainly focused on the management from an IT and informatics project perspective. As you embark on your projects, we encourage you to find the strategy that makes the most sense. Build a sensible structure for how to negotiate the features of the project, monitor your execution, and get appropriate feedback. The bottom line is that this need not result in an onerous set of rules and regulations for every task your project must complete, but provide enough structure to make these guidelines natural and enable you and your team to work effectively.

Questions for Discussion

- Why is handling change such an important selling point for Agile over Waterfall?
- What are some reasons to choose one method, Agile or Waterfall, over the other?
- How closely do you think the software-development life cycle in information and communication technologies for development, or ICT4D, mirrors that of normal software companies? What are key things to consider specifically in the ICT4D space?
- Which of the different phases of development is most important? Why?

Additional Resources

Agile Project Management Tools

A sample of web-based tools for online task management collaboration:

- Fogcreek's Fogbugz: http://www.fogcreek.com/Fogbugz/
- Trello: https://trello.com/
- Atlassian's Jira: https://www.atlassian.com/software/jira
- Pivotal Tracker: http://www.pivotaltracker.com/
- Asana: https://asana.com/
- Basecamp: https://basecamp.com/.

Further Reading on Agile Project Management

- Agile retrospectives: http://shop.oreilly.com/product/9780977616640.do
- The art of agile development: http://shop.oreilly.com/product/9780596527679.do
- Essential Scrum: http://www.safaribooksonline.com/library/view/essential-scrum-a/9780321700407/app04.html

References

1. Royce WW. 1970. Managing the development of large software systems. *Proc IEEE WESCON* 26(8): 1–9.

2. See http://agilemanifesto.org/history.html.

3. See http://www.versionone.com/pdf/2013-state-of-agile-survey.pdf.

4. Lakeworks. 2009. Scrum process (own work). Licensed under GNU Free Documentation License via Wikimedia Commons. http://commons.wikimedia.org/wiki/File:Scrum_process.svg#/media/File:Scrum_process.svg.

5. Ambler SW. 2005. The agile system development life cycle (SDLC). Ambysoft. http://www.ambysoft.com/essays/agileLifecycle.html. Accessed May 24, 2010.

6. I8abug. 2011. Burn down chart (own work). http://commons.wikimedia.org/wiki/File:Burn_down_chart.png#/media/File:Burn_down_chart.png.

21 Usability and User Experience

Biyeun Buczyk and Clayton Sims

Take-Home Messages

- Usability plays a crucial role in the success and adoption of any technology innovation.
- The global health informatics design process requires close interaction and engagement with the eventual users through considerable user testing, evaluation, and engagement.

Introduction

Careful and thoughtful design plays a role in the success of any technology, and is essential in information and communication technologies for development (ICT4D) settings. Designers creating interfaces for developing regions face unique challenges in engaging users, who can present major barriers to adoption or scale and are often identified too late in a project's lifecycle to be properly addressed. In this chapter, we will discuss four major areas for consideration in the design of systems specifically in the global health space, both at the user-interface level and in building the overall structure of user experience.

Design Thinking

A principal challenge when thinking about the design of systems in a global health intervention is that users may have an entirely different foundation of skillsets, experience, and knowledge compared to the baseline user. Consequently, many of the ideas covered in other design courses, while still applicable and useful in the global setting, may be prioritized differently from what is commonly expected. Therefore, a rigid approach to design based on standard conventions is not advised. Assumptions that are otherwise considered established in a baseline setting—levels of user literacy, technological familiarity, and shared mental models—are now given immediate attention due to increased variability. Meanwhile, minute details—typography, use of white space and screen real estate, colors, and other design-centric considerations—typically marked with the highest priority, while still relevant and valid, no longer become primary areas of focus.

In a typical ICT4D project setting, the likelihood of encountering lower rates of literacy among users is far greater than what is typically considered in higher-resource settings. Focus should first be placed on content organization and flow of information, rather than specific attention to typographic detail and layout. Visual consistency ultimately takes precedence over aesthetics, as any slight variation in interface may signal a new mode of action to the user. As these changes cannot be readily explained with text, the user must rely entirely on previous experience with familiar colors, shapes, and arrangement of components when deciding how to proceed. If a change is too jarring, the user may prematurely close the application or place the tool aside due to fears of losing progress or data.

Alongside visual consistency is regularity in the number of actions or mental modeling required at a single point or screen. Imagine an application where nearly every screen requires one level of interaction from the user to proceed—for instance, entering text then pressing a button to move to the next view. A second screen is now presented that first requires text entry in the form of a search box and then displays a filtered list below the search box. While staying within the same visual context, the user is now required to select a result to proceed to the next screen. This second screen introduces a new mental model and a feedback mechanism that establishes the possibility of two different interactions within the same context, rather than one. While subtle, this change may startle a new user encountering this workflow for the first time, especially if he or she is new to the technology encapsulating this solution—whether a mobile phone, tablet, or computer—and is unfamiliar with its established user-interaction paradigms. Rather than introducing a new mental model, a simpler approach would be to first present a screen with the search box and then move to a new screen for item selection after text to the search box was submitted. Of course, depending on the application, this may disrupt the forward linear progression of interactions, as the user may need to move backward to change the text in the search box. Regardless, this change of model is something to be aware of when designing solutions. It's generally best to select the simplest workflow and, if necessary, only branch out to workflows most commonly used by other solutions utilizing the same core technology.

However, familiarity with the core technology in general may vary greatly with culture, regardless of similarities in age or socioeconomic background. For instance, users from villages in rural India have had access and availability to mobile phones and smartphones for a greater period of time compared to users of similar economic, gender, and educational backgrounds in rural Africa. Consequently, these users are likely to be more comfortable with a greater variety of mental models required for interacting with core technologies supporting various ICT4D solutions, and may adapt more easily to changes in mental modeling states or utilizations of established workflow patterns.

Audience Identification

The most important step when approaching any topic related to user experience is to first consider and identify the audience (or audiences) using the tool. Answers regarding the question "who is my audience?" will increase proportionally with a rising degree of complexity and outcomes of the tool in question. In cases where the tool is capable of solving a wide variety of problems, the grouping of audiences will likely funnel into three workflows: basic, intermediate, and advanced. From these workflows, commonalities of expectations can then be established among users in each category.

Establishing the profile of a solution's primary-level user is central to later identifying whether certain workflows are easily discoverable or intuitive. Typical characteristics of primary-level users might include some degree of unfamiliarity with technology in general, as well as a lack of awareness, desire, or ability to read any available documentation. Interactions targeting such users should rely more on visual cues rather than textual explanations of the interface. Additionally, primary-level users might typically be engaging with technology as a supplement or aid to their core work. The technology is not their main focus, and these users are interested in completing tasks in the fastest way possible.

With this in mind, primary-level workflows should be as directed as possible, with few to zero options available to the user that may alter the direction or outcome of a particular task. Options should be broken into smaller, less complex workflows that are presented as separate tasks from the beginning, rather than adding complexity during the middle of a workflow. Additionally, whenever options are present, the most commonly used option should be provided as the default choice.

When considering the design of primary workflows, it's also advisable to draw inspiration from common experiences across all basic-level users. With access to technology becoming more prevalent even in the most remote regions, it is safer to assume that certain experiences—social media and applications like Facebook or search applications like Google—are shared among the majority of primary-level users. Once these shared experiences are identified, they can be used as an excellent basis for visual components, computer-human interactions, and information display that can be utilized as elements in ICT4D solutions. The more universal a workflow or design can be, the more it will be readily understood by a wider range of users, requiring less time spent learning the interface and more time accomplishing the core task at hand.

Once the primary-level user is identified, the characteristics of intermediate and advanced users can be established. Intermediate users are less likely to be completely comfortable with technology than their advanced counterparts, but perhaps are more willing and able to read documentation relevant to accomplishing higher-level tasks. Advanced-level users have a higher probability of having technology be central to their work and are very comfortable seeking out documentation to achieve complex tasks.

Options that may fall under the advanced category may include advanced search string formatting or use of APIs, and can rely exclusively on documentation to be discoverable. For the most part, advanced workflows should be last on the list of considerations when thinking about the user experience of ICT4D solutions. However, this does not mean that intermediate workflows should be ignored altogether.

Intermediate options should still remain relatively discoverable by users, but may require the aid of help text, simple documentation, or tutorials. These tasks might add complexity by allowing the user to choose from several nondefault options midway through their workflow. While it's easy to compound tasks together and create levels of complexity, it's important to make sure that intermediate workflows still remain fairly directed. The less documentation a user must reference to complete a particular task, the faster they will be able to achieve the end goal.

Holistic Design

Designing systems for use in global health can often involve introducing an entire technology stack in order to support a specific intervention. An algorithm to screen for malnutrition in rural areas requires the introduction of a platform to run that algorithm, carrying with it an entire chain of logistics and training associated with the platform. In contrast with a more isolated software design, in which a designer may be responsible only for the user interface presented for their product, everything from the keyboard used to type to the way that electricity is provided to project sites may require careful consideration as a component of a tool being introduced. Being mindful of this full end-to-end experience of a user's interaction with technology is a key differentiator for successful adoption and sustainability of ICT4D projects.

Balancing Best Practices and Innovation

One of the challenges facing designers creating health systems in developing regions is balancing the extent to which they rely on existing "host" platforms (operating systems, devices, etc.) that are commercially available with the specific needs of their users. User-interface designers are generally accustomed to isolating their responsibilities while working within a platform. Operating system manufacturers, for instance, provide software developers with guidelines to follow in their products. Successful software more often than not will conform to these common design guidelines, because it allows users to interact with the software in a familiar and intuitive way that leverages and reinforces their prior experience.

For a project whose target user population has sub-60% literacy and speaks a language that is not translated in an operating system's distribution, however, it is unlikely that users will be able to benefit from a tool following the same patterns as the other software products on that operating system. Software that focuses on platform standards while ignoring the needs of its specific users faces steep training costs and poor consistency.

The techniques for meeting the needs of users who are not well served by existing platforms can be broken down into a balance between three rough domains:

- platform targeting
- sandboxing
- training.

Platform Targeting

Platform targeting involves identifying what common technology platforms are common to a project's target user base and determining whether they are an appropriate foundation. Some of the essential and often overlooked aspects of this targeting involve not just how familiar that platform is to users, but the overhead introduced by its maintenance. Projects that rely on a data connection require that connection to be configured and kept up to date. A project that utilizes a wireless device will require the training not merely to use the device, but also to establish and troubleshoot its connection to the host.

Take, for example, a project whose goal is to deliver regularly updated information to rural and disconnected communities with very limited training capacity. Utilizing a smartphone or laptop requires consistent charging, which introduces new problems. A feature phone application often requires a significant amount of training to be used reliably. An IVR (interactive voice response) or USSD (unstructured supplementary service data) approach, however, depending on the availability and experience of the users, could eliminate the majority of training needs associated with maintaining the host platform while still providing the needed complexity, but requires either a high level of familiarity and literacy for USSD, or a significant cost to utilize IVR.

Sandboxing

Sandboxing techniques assimilate functionality from the host platform in an attempt to tailor them directly to target users. This allows a tool to adopt the advantages of a host platform (cost, accessibility, capabilities) while minimizing its limitations. Sandboxing techniques can range from simple (using built-in menu customization on a platform to make it easier to launch a tool) to complex (creating a custom Linux distribution that is tailored only to provide the interface needed to use a tool), depending on a project's needs.

The most significant advantage of sandboxing is that it allows a designer to shift the costs associated with complexity from recurring events (more expensive device platforms or regular and widespread training) down to one-time costs by incurring that complexity when designing and creating a tool. Sandboxing is an important aspect of a user-centered design practice when implementing interfaces in ICT4D settings as a way to minimize training and improve the degree to which a tool can meet the needs of unique user bases.

Despite the overall value of the technique, over-reliance on sandboxing can introduce hidden costs and risks for global health projects. Modern technology platforms are expected to evolve and grow to better meet their users' needs over time, as is the case with all operating systems and most mobile phone platforms. Tools relying on existing best practices and platform functionality can expect to receive these advantages over time, while tools which have re-implemented those behaviors must eschew the new benefits or themselves adapt over time. A best practice is to utilize user testing and to identify critical events that could present barriers to adoption of a tool and focus sandboxing efforts on the minimal set of functionality necessary to ensure its usability.

User Testing and Evaluation

User testing is one of the cornerstones of successful interface design, and its value is demonstrated clearly when designing for global health applications. The usability mantra of "You are not the user" is particularly true across cultural and international boundaries, requiring frequent inclusion of user testing into successful iterative design. In practice, however, this need is threatened by significant challenges. Limited access to users, language or cultural barriers, and imperfect testing situations all raise the level of difficulty for achieving successful testing. While there are no universal solutions to these problems, some strategies can be employed to maximize the value of user testing and overcome limitations.

Planned User Testing

Working around limitations is at the core of user testing in ICT4D applications, and understanding the target user population and the available testing facilities as much as possible will assist in that process. If testing will need to be performed in an outdoor setting, creating a binder full of small pieces of paper for an interactive paper prototyping testing session will likely lead to frustration and limited value. Designers should be mindful that some common usability techniques like "Wizard-of-Oz" testing may not be culturally appropriate or possible with their sample users, and users who have limited exposure to computing can have major difficulties interacting with abstract low-fidelity paper prototypes.

The advantages of low-fidelity prototyping (low cost, low barrier to change, etc.) remain valid in global health settings, but testers should be aware that their testing may require significant time to explain the abstractions, work around language issues, and appropriately convey scenarios. Designers should plan tests around those limitations and consider the balance of introducing higher-fidelity fixtures for ease of experience. Since user attention in testing sessions is always limited, planning low-fidelity tests may require more users than expected to cover all scenarios intended.

User-Story Formats

When performing user-testing sessions in ICT4D settings, designers should expect to be as flexible as possible. A myriad of potential complications can arise to derail a complex testing process, such as limited participation, the need for or success of a facilitator or translator at driving the session, and unexpected divergences from profiled users or the testing facilities. For instance, a user-story session could be planned for 15 doctors from local facilities, but in practice 15 nurses or practitioners with different backgrounds could arrive from those facilities instead. Alternatively, eight hours of testing could be scheduled, but interruptions or delays could result in a smaller testing window being available.

The key to effective testing in these contexts is flexibility and preparation. It is helpful to break testing down into separate pieces and prioritize which elements should be completed first. Having a significant number of different experiments prepared for testing will ensure that time with users can be optimized, even if not all of the experiments can be completed. A similar approach is helpful for breaking down the process of experiments. It is ideal to be able to perform a paper prototyping test with rigid discipline (no coaching, individual users, etc.), but in practice that may not work effectively with users who are unwilling to explore. Having backup plans prepared, like paired exploration between multiple users to make the situation more comfortable, will help ensure that testing sessions produce useful outputs. Allowing users to share roles and responsibilities in testing, either as a pair or including users as a part of the prompting processes, can generally allow for much freer feedback and participation.

Testing Process and Outputs

For projects involving a mix of language skills, user-testing sessions for global health projects will often require a translator or facilitator to drive the overall process. Getting feedback directly from users during testing can present difficulties due to language barriers (for verbal feedback) or literacy issues (for issuing questionnaires or surveys). It is tempting for testers and designers to ease their testing sessions to include users who speak common languages or don't have literacy issues, but doing so can significantly bias the process and results of user testing and should be avoided when possible.

Clear, scenario-driven prompting and observation can be the most powerful tools during testing sessions. If users are presented with unambiguous goals and prompts during user testing, a significant number of issues can be determined directly from user interaction with the scenarios and direct feedback can be elicited more uniformly. When performing mid- to high-fidelity testing, in particular, such as user acceptance testing of actual interfaces or software, answering essential usability questions of uptake, learnability, and discoverability will be significantly more reliable when testing includes users picked for their representation of the target group rather than ease of communication.

User Engagement

Due to the global nature of many ICT4D solutions, it is important to consider not only the ease with which a user can understand and learn a workflow, but how well it caters to his or her culture or experience on a personal level. A more engaged user will be more likely to complete tasks thoroughly and with purpose, leading to greater accuracy and better results. Central to increasing the feelings of personalization and engagement of users is use of multimedia and language localization. With this in mind, an application can feel less like an intervention from an outside world with no cultural context, and more like a tool necessary to accomplish the task at hand.

Due to the varying levels of literacy that may be encountered by ICT4D solutions, it is important to reduce the amount of text presented to the user whenever possible and rely more on other forms of multimedia to disseminate information. Such forms of multimedia may include audio, images, or video. Audio is particularly useful in cases where the literacy of the user, beneficiary, or both may be low and the information presented is particularly complex. It is often useful to include both text and audio reading information displayed. In cases where a particular idea is more simply conveyed visually rather that textually—for instance, the proper way to hold a newborn—images or video should be included alongside or in place of text. When using imagery, it's also important to consider whether to use photographs or drawings. Due to the visual complexity that photographs can provide, it is often more effective to utilize drawings or cartoons instead, since specific control can be placed on what visual details to highlight. Additionally, certain scenarios may be easier to draw or symbolize rather than photograph. In particular, abstract ideas are more effectively communicated with drawings instead of photographs; for example, a warning sign or skull and bones can be used to indicate danger.

While multimedia should be preferred over text, any written language included by ICT4D solutions should always be localized to the user's native language. This not only improves the accuracy of information delivery, but improves the level of personalization and satisfaction from the user. In addition to providing local translations for text, it is equally as important to localize any audio present in multimedia files. Cultural features of people from the user's home region should also be considered when creating drawings and cartoons of humans for the application—even changes as subtle as type of clothing can have a profound effect on the reception of visual multimedia.

Conclusion

User preferences and abilities play a crucial role in how widely a technical solution is adopted and succeeds. End users or advocates should have a persistent voice during the multidisciplinary design stage, and any development plan should include extensive user testing and evaluation to ensure an optimal user experience.

Questions for Discussion

- What are some ways your target audience for your global health innovation is unique or different?
- What considerations for this audience do you think you would need to include during the design process, and how would you go about testing and evaluating these enhancements?

22 Privacy and Security: Privacy of Personal eHealth Data in Low- and Middle-Income Countries

William C. Philbrick

Take-Home Messages

- Principles of security and confidentiality of personal data are well recognized internationally but applied in a very variable fashion in low- and middle-income countries (LMIC).

- The rapid progression of technology is allowing increasing sharing of data between electronic health records and other health information systems, national registers of vital events, consumer data, and other sources, creating new risks and challenges for patient privacy.

- Privacy of personal data is covered by a range of different, laws, regulations, and conventions, with some regions such as the European Community applying omnibus data-protection regulation; others, for example the United States, having specific regulations for health data (such as HIPAA); and many LMIC having none.

- Differing attitudes toward privacy between many Western developed nations and LMIC create challenges in developing harmonized global privacy standards. For example, cultural barriers to health data privacy for women and girls in some communities can discourage them from seeking care.

Introduction

The roles that privacy and confidentiality play in eHealth (which includes "mHealth," described below, and is also referred to as "digital health") are inherently linked with hardware and software security.[1] Laws, policies, public health interests, and societal attitudes regarding the expectation of privacy over individual health data dictate how technology addresses security solutions to protect personal data. Often, however, business interests drive how technology addresses data security. These business interests do not necessarily reflect prevailing laws, policies, public health standards, and social attitudes regarding privacy. One of the greatest challenges in the evolution of eHealth is generating a unified approach to privacy so that laws, policies, and public health standards keep pace with the dizzying evolution of technology, while at the same time respecting individual attitudes toward the expectation and "right" of privacy.

The media is increasingly reporting instances of breaches in the security of large amounts of electronically stored personal data. These breaches, most notably the breach into Anthem, one of the largest health insurers in the United States, have included the unauthorized access to millions of records of personal health identification data [1]. As eHealth systems move toward handling larger and larger amounts of different kinds of data, a phenomenon known as "big data," addressing both security and privacy issues takes on a heightened urgency. Public dismay caused by security breaches is fueling intensified scrutiny of how the privacy of health information is protected by eHealth information systems. However, such scrutiny seems to focus on the role of technology security, and not so much on unpacking what the concepts of "privacy" and "confidentiality" mean in regard to personal health records.

This chapter will explore and provide an overview of the concept of privacy in the context of eHealth. It will present interpretations of what eHealth privacy means; identify some of the driving forces warranting examination of how privacy is protected under eHealth systems; and present the current state of how the global community acknowledges and protects privacy in an increasingly digital world.

What Does Privacy Mean and How Does it Link to Security?

"Privacy" with respect to eHealth can be viewed broadly to apply to an individual person, while "confidentiality" applies to data. Privacy generally refers to patients having substantial control over the extent, timing, and circumstances of sharing oneself and information about oneself with others [16]. Confidentiality refers to the treatment of identifiable information that has been disclosed to others in a relationship of trust and with the expectation that it will not be divulged to others except in ways that have been previously agreed upon [16]. For purposes of this chapter, the term *privacy* encompasses the concept of confidentiality.

Understanding all the implications connected with privacy, including what society's reasonable expectations to privacy of personal information ought to be in the rapidly growing world of eHealth, is vital to developing a secure eHealth system. Protecting the privacy of personal health data is particularly critical with sensitive issues such as HIV, sexual preference, and conditions relating to sexual and reproductive health. Safeguarding the privacy of personal health data is also critical when dealing with victims/survivors of sexual violence accessing health services to tend to their injuries. Victims/survivors of sexual violence might not seek help or appropriate health care if they feared personal information connected with the assault would not be kept confidential, exposing them to possible retribution from perpetrators and stigmatization within their communities [6].

There are many eHealth stakeholders with vested interests in eHealth data. An ideal eHealth information system should incorporate the interests of all these stakeholders:

- health care professionals who use the data to make decisions regarding the best possible care for their patients
- local, regional, national, and international health authorities responsible for ensuring public health, who use the data for making policy decisions and resource allocations to most efficiently protect the public health
- individual patients with a *right* to protecting the privacy of their personal health data so they can receive unfettered access to the best possible health care without judgment, stigma, or discrimination.

Driving Forces for Examining eHealth Privacy in LMIC

Proliferation of Mobile Phone Usage for Health

While much discourse around eHealth privacy has been occurring in the context of Western, developed economies, there are driving forces and considerations that warrant examining privacy implications for eHealth in the context of LMIC. In particular, an increasingly number of front-line health workers in even the poorest, most remote areas of the world are using mobile phones for health-related activities ("mHealth"), including the collection and management of patient-level health data [3,11,40,44]. Emerging electronic health information systems in LMIC, such as DHIS2 and OpenMRS, that leverage mobile phones and other information and communication technologies (ICT) for the collection of patient-level health data further contribute to the eHealth phenomenon.[2] Using mobile phone applications to collect critical, sensitive, private medical information, and eHealth information management systems to store and manage that data, warrant a special focus on security and privacy features to avoid the potentially harmful consequences that are associated with breaches of privacy [8,19,22].

Data for Decision Making: Demand for More Complete, Timely, Accurate, and Reliable Data

A global groundswell of demand in LMIC for better and more health, demographic, and other types of data is driving much of the push toward eHealth information systems [2]. Referred to as "data for decision making," the public health community views electronic data collection, particularly mobile phones, as a means to obtain more complete, timely, accurate, and reliable health data to better inform appropriate health interventions, prioritizations of activities, and the efficient allocation of resources [41]. While evidence exists that using mobile phones and ICT devices enables front-line health workers to collect more complete, timely, and accurate information, there is also evidence that using mobile phones in particular for collecting and analyzing data in LMIC is not failsafe and leads to accuracy errors comparable to using other traditional data-collection methods [4,28]. Yet, with an arguably mixed evidence base supporting the accuracy advantages of using mobile phones as the ICT entry point for collecting electronic health data, the trend for using mobile phones and SMS for health data collection moves forward.

Global health stakeholders, including the World Health Organization, are actively promoting eHealth and mHealth solutions for developing harmonized reproductive health registries [12]. Public health experts assert that population-based health registries are essential for monitoring progress in global health and development, particularly Millennium Goals 4 and 5 (reducing child mortality and improving maternal health) [42]. Electronically collecting population-based aggregated health data for health registries often starts at the level of the individual patient. Front-line health care workers use mobile phones and ICT (e.g., web-based technology) to collect and record individual health data when they meet with patients at hospitals, local clinics, and patients' homes. Even though the data will ultimately be aggregated, without failsafe protection that guards against transmitting and misappropriating personally identifiable patient information, electronically collecting data that starts with the entry of patient-level health information potentially exposes that data to vulnerability to breaches of privacy. Chapter 9 discusses registries in detail.

Data Sharing and the Interoperability of eHealth Information Systems

Connected with the drive to electronically collect more health data is the drive toward data sharing and the interoperability between and among information management systems [24]. Electronic health data can be increasingly shared between and among multiple systems, stakeholders, and environments, presenting new and unexplored challenges to individual privacy [32]. eHealth interoperability permits more data sharing between caregiver and patient; caregiver and caregiver; caregiver and administrative entity; administrative entity and national registry or information management system; and national health information management systems and international surveillance bodies. "Interoperability," for the purposes of this chapter, refers to connecting independent technological systems so they communicate, exchange data, and use the information that has been exchanged (see also chapter 11).

The issues of data sharing and eHealth system interoperability arise in numerous health-related contexts. The biological research community has been working toward establishing a framework for responsible sharing of genomic and health-related data [20,21]. Communities of patients with common health conditions such as cancer have benefited from online sharing of information [13]. In general, there is a growth of health information exchange, leading to more individual patient records shared across multiple health care settings separate from an individual's original point of care [5].

Global focus on supporting the expanding digitalization of national civil registration and vital statistics (CRVS) systems raises significant privacy concerns over personal health data. A CRVS system captures data and statistics on vital events such as births, deaths, marriages, divorces, and fetal deaths. One of the key functions of a CRVS system is to secure all citizens with a legal identity through the issuance of birth certificates, ensuring the right to access public services and social protection [45].

Many within the global health community assert that vital registries, as part of CRVS systems, are "global public goods" [25]. Electronic registries facilitate the collection, storage, retrieval, and analysis of accurate population and demographic data to inform national policy makers, who use the data for policy planning and efficient resource allocation. The international community also uses the data for monitoring progress against global health and development indicators under the Millennium Development Goals [25]. Promoters for electronically modernizing CRVS systems, which could include linking with mobile data-collection platforms, note the growth of mHealth within LMIC, enabling front-line health workers to use SMS messaging to enter data that will be used by registries [25].

The interoperability of eHealth information systems with CRVS systems that store personally identifiable data, notwithstanding any security precautions that may be in place, potentially heightens the risk of inadvertent sharing of personal health data (figure 22.1).

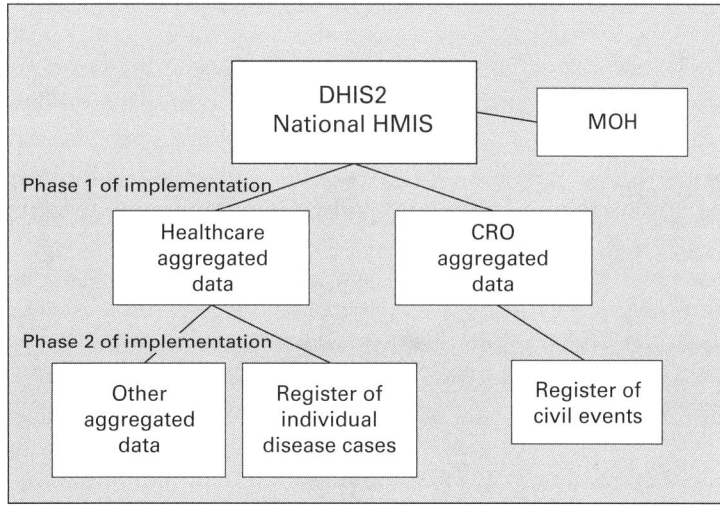

Figure 22.1
Vision for DHIS2: Linking of health and CRVS information management systems [45]. (DHIS2 is described in detail in chapter 42, found in the online supplementary section.)

The State of Privacy Protection in eHealth

Protecting the privacy of health and other personal information is dependent upon how privacy is conceptualized and defined. One cannot protect privacy without knowing exactly what privacy is and what sorts of information are deemed private. Accordingly, protecting privacy requires identifying standards that define with specificity the categories of health and personal data warranting privacy protection. Ideally, privacy standards also define the circumstances and conditions under which different kinds of health and personal data can be shared, and with whom. The word "ideally" is used because the challenges in identifying those standards are comparable to the search for the Holy Grail. Subjectivity and context play a large part in ascertaining standards regarding privacy. Different stakeholders have widely varying perspectives on the sorts of information that merit protection from disclosure, the limiting circumstances under which private data may be shared, and with which stakeholders that data can be shared.

Numerous initiatives acknowledge and underscore the importance of addressing privacy and security in eHealth and CRVS systems in LMIC [30,37]. The World Health Organization has reported that governments cite issues related to data privacy and security and the protection of individual health information as two of the top barriers to the expansion of mHealth [43]. A number of jurisdictions are drafting and considering eHealth Action Plans that specifically address data protection and personal privacy [9,46]. Privacy and data-protection frameworks should be foundational components of the architecture of national eHealth systems [47] (figure 22.2).

Organizations and initiatives including the International Organization for Standards; Health Level 7 International; Integrating the Health Care Enterprise; the World Health Organization; and the International Telecommunications Union are all playing roles and driving an agenda toward establishing interoperability standards (which would include addressing privacy and security) [29]. Their efforts include focusing on how to accom-

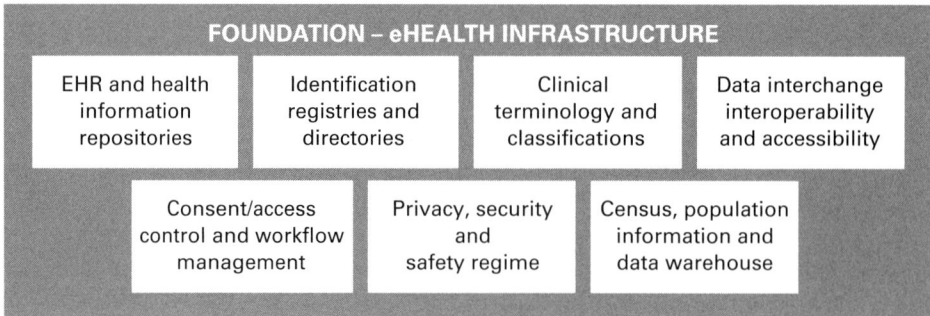

Figure 22.2
ISO National eHealth Architecture: Foundation of eHealth infrastructure [29].

modate LMIC needs [29]. While progress is being made, there is still no global consensus on a set of specific, harmonized standards regarding interoperability and protecting the privacy of personal health data [10,29].

With respect to electronic CRVS information systems (which, when interoperable with eHealth systems and registries, have implications for the privacy of personal health data), some global standards do exist [35,36]. However, many of those standards are buried in dense, highly technical documents that were written over 15 years ago when the technology, systems, and program contexts were different from those of today.

Laws and Policies

In the absence of an international consensus and a convention enshrining standards specifically addressing eHealth privacy in LMIC contexts, national laws, regulations, and policies generally dictate how eHealth systems handle privacy. Most legal approaches toward protecting privacy are grounded in the recognition of the individual right to privacy. Notwithstanding enshrining the legal right to privacy, those laws, policies, and regulations that have been enacted:

- are generally ad hoc
- vary significantly from one nation to another
- do not always explicitly address the electronic collection, management, and transmission of health data; and/or
- are vague and ambiguous.

International law, most notably the Universal Declaration of Human Rights, recognizes the individual right to privacy [38]. Numerous other international and multinational agreements and conventions, such as the International Covenant on Civil and Political Rights and the European Convention on Human Rights and Fundamental Freedoms [7], also acknowledge the individual right to privacy [14]. Most countries recognize the right to privacy in their constitutions, and when not explicitly recognized constitutionally, many courts have promulgated the right to privacy in their decrees, as they have done in the United States, Ireland, and India [14].

A 2013 comprehensive landscaping global review and analysis of current privacy laws and regulations revealed that privacy laws falls into one of three categories: (1) omnibus data-protection regulation in the style of European laws, which regulate all personal information equally; (2) United States–style sectoral privacy laws that address specific privacy issues arising in certain industries and business sectors, so that only certain types of personal information are regulated; and (3) the constitutional approach, whereby certain types of personal information are considered private and inviolate from a basic human rights perspective, but no specific privacy regulation is otherwise in place [34].

Europe and certain Latin American and Asian countries have enacted and implemented omnibus data-privacy laws [34]. The United States has enacted broad protection over health and medical data, notably through the Health Insurance Portability and Accountability Act, commonly known as HIPAA [18]. Comparatively, most African countries have undeveloped data-privacy legal regulatory frameworks with the exception of a handful of countries, including South Africa, Kenya, Mauritius, and Morocco [34].

The individual right to privacy is not universally recognized in many LMIC. For example, the African Charter on Human and People's Rights (Banjul) Charter, which has been adopted by more than 50 countries, fails to articulate the personal right to privacy [17,34]. A number African countries have, however, addressed privacy by conferring constitutional and other legal obligations, supplemented by ethical codes of practice, upon medical workers and others who typically come into contact with certain kinds of information, such as data relating to HIV/AIDS, DNA, and genetic information [34,39].

The recognition of the right to privacy specifically regarding patient information is found in the World Health Organization's 1994 Declaration on the Promotion of Patients' Rights in Europe and in the European Commission's Data Protection Directive 95/46/EC [34]. The 1994 World Health Organization Declaration, however, like many international declarations and conventions, is voluntary and does not have the force of law unless adopted by member states. Extending the right to privacy specifically to personal health data that is electronically collected and stored is gaining momentum, but is not universal, nor harmonized between jurisdictions.

Culture and Social Norms

Obligations conferred by constitutions, legislation, or ethical codes of practice for practitioners do not guarantee against breaches of confidentiality by health care workers in many LMIC where privacy concepts of informed consent are not culturally embraced [26,34]. Culture and social norms connected with living in communal societies in many LMIC, particularly in Africa, account for the relative absence of formal legislative and regulatory provisions recognizing and protecting the right to privacy over personal health data. The notion of personal privacy rights, including the expectation of confidentiality over personal health data, tends to conflict with traditional African society's sense of duty to help all who are sick within a community [26]. It is common practice for patients to be accompanied by family or other community members when visiting traditional medicine practitioners. Often a head of the family and other community members will consult among themselves to decide the appropriate course of action for a sick member of the community, with many having access to information regarding the condition of the patient [26].

Gender norms in many cultures that subordinate the rights of women and girls significantly undermine a woman's expectation to privacy over her personal information, particularly regarding sexual and reproductive health. Women in some cultures are reluctant to use health services because gender-insensitive health workers do not ensure privacy and confidentiality regarding treatments [31].

Emerging Challenges in Addressing Privacy

With the burgeoning growth of eHealth comes the breaking down of country borders. Devices that electronically collect data and the servers that electronically store the data frequently sit in different countries. Cross-border electronic transfers of health information implicate key issues of ownership and access to eHealth data. A key gap in most nations' legislative approaches toward privacy is how to address cross-border transfers of personal information [34]. Questions about ownership and control rights of national governments, the organizations managing servers, local administrative health authorities, and individual patients over patient-level eHealth data are yet to be resolved by global consensus [33]. However, some governments restrict the transfer of personal data of any citizens, other than aggregate data, outside their borders [23,48].

As the issues of eHealth privacy are sorted and frameworks for protecting the privacy of personal health data are developed and implemented, questions arise as to who enforces privacy standards and who is accountable for breaches. These questions include: who is accountable as duty bearers for breaches of privacy, and under what circumstances? Will front-line health care workers at rural health clinics be held accountable, and if so, under what circumstances? Will technology companies be held accountable for not putting in place effective security mechanisms into the hardware devices (mobile phones) and software applications? Are district and national health authorities accountable for eHealth information systems that do not possess failsafe security features and lead to inadvertent disclosures of private health information? When a breach of privacy does occur, will a patient living in a rural village in Africa have any realistic recourse to seek redress?

The evolution of "big data" and cloud computing, along with the never-ending introduction of new technologies, create privacy challenges that are yet to be completely identified [27]. The speed of new and emerging technologies and their ecosystems will indubitably outpace eHealth privacy frameworks and standards, making them anachronistic almost as soon as they are developed.

Conclusion

This chapter only scrapes the surface in exploring how privacy of personal health data is conceptualized and protected in an LMIC eHealth environment. The concept of privacy is multifaceted and complex, influenced by many factors. Laws, policies, culture, social norms, and technology all play roles in contributing to standards that impact privacy protection, including the duty to keep personal health data confidential. These factors are often intertwined with social norms regarding expectations of personal privacy influencing laws and policies, or laws and policies impacting how software developers design security features for ensuring the protection of personal health data. Sometimes these factors are incongruous, such as when, for example, laws and policies do not reflect the prevailing social and cultural norms regarding what sorts of personal health information should be afforded privacy protection. Differing attitudes toward privacy between many Western developed nations and LMIC create challenges in developing globally harmonized privacy standards.

The dizzying pace of development of new eHealth technologies creates constant challenges for addressing eHealth privacy. The framers of privacy laws, policies, and standards cannot always anticipate new innovations in technology that would impact the ability to electronically protect personal health data. The exuberance toward rolling out electronic health information systems and data sharing requires a tempered approach that reflects and addresses the individual right to privacy of personal health information.

Questions for Discussion

- What are some of the biggest risks to patients in low- and middle-income countries of the unauthorized sharing of personal data? What are the key technical and organizational actions an organization can take in implementing a new eHealth system to mitigate these risks?

- Countries such as Rwanda have enacted regulations to prevent personal medical data of citizens being transferred abroad. What are the pros and cons of this policy in terms of support for health care and clinical research?

- How might the design of health information systems help to mitigate the risks of inappropriate data sharing, including in settings where data is shared between systems and where legal frameworks may be weak?

Notes

1. For a more detailed overview of security, see chapter 13.

2. OpenMRS is an open-source electronic health record system now found in over 40 countries in Africa, Asia, Europe, and South and North America. DHIS2 is a health management information system used in 47 countries across four continents.

References

1. Abelson R, Creswell J. 2015. Data breach at Anthem may lead to others. *New York Times*, February 6. http://www.nytimes.com/2015/02/07/business/data-breach-at-anthem-may-lead-to-others.html.

2. Baldwin W, Diers J. 2009. Poverty, gender, and youth: Demographic data for development in sub-Saharan Africa. Working paper No. 13. Population Council. http://www.popcouncil.org/uploads/pdfs/wp/pgy/013.pdf.

3. Betjeman, TJ., Sogoian SE, and Foran MP. 2013. *mHealth in Sub-Saharan Africa. Int J Telemed Appl* 482324. http://dx.doi.org/ 10.1155/2013/482324.

4. Birnbaum B, DeRenzi B, Flaxman AD, Lesh N. 2012. Automated quality control for mobile data collection. Proceedings of the 2nd ACM Symposium on Computing for Development. http://dl.acm.org/citation.cfm?doid=2160601.2160603.

5. Caine K, Hanania R. 2013. Patients want granular privacy control over health information in electronic medical records. *JAMIA* 20(1): 7–15 http://www.pubmedcentral.nih.gov/articlerender.fcgi?artid=3555326&tool=pmcentrez&rendertype=abstract.

6. Monitoring CP, and the Evaluation Working Group. 2012. Ethical principles, dilemmas and risks in collecting data on violence against children: A review of available literature. New York: UNICEF. http://data.unicef.org/corecode/uploads/document6/uploaded_pdfs/corecode/EPDRCLitReview_193.pdf.

7. Council of Europe. 1950. European Convention on Human Rights and Fundamental Freedoms, amended by Protocols No. 11 and No. 14. Art. 8. November 4. http://conventions.coe.int/treaty/en/treaties/html/005.htm.

8. Dehling T, Gao F, Schneider S, Sunyaev A. 2015. Exploring the far side of mobile health: Information security and privacy of mobile health apps on iOS and Android. *JMIR Mhealth Uhealth* 1: 5. http://mhealth.jmir.org/2015/1/e8/.

9. European Data Protection Supervisor. 2013. Opinion of the European data protection supervisor on the communication from the Commission on eHealth Action Plan 2012–2020: Innovative healthcare for the 21st century. March 27. https://secure.edps.europa.eu/EDPSWEB/webdav/shared/Documents/Consultation/Opinions/2013/13-03-27_eHealth_Action_EN.pdf.

10. Fernández-Alemán JL, Señor IC, Lozoya PÁ, Toval A. 2013. Security and privacy in electronic health records: A systematic literature review. *J Biomed Inform* 46(3): 541–562. doi:10.1016/j.jbi.2012.12.003.

11. Fraser HSF, Blaya J. 2010. Implementing medical information systems in developing countries: What works and what doesn't. *AMIA Annu Symp Proc* (2010): 232–236. http://www.ncbi.nlm.nih.gov/pmc/articles/PMC3041413/.

12. Frøen F. 2013. An Initiative for harmonized Reproductive Health Registries … for Better Reproductive Health Data for Women and Children. hRHR Consultations Workshop Hanoi 2013. http://www.fhi.no/dokumenter/1aee010e3e.pdf.

13. Frost J, Vermeulen IE, Beekers N. 2014. Anonymity versus privacy: Selective information sharing in online cancer communities. *J Med Internet Res* 16(5): E126 http://www.ncbi.nlm.nih.gov/pmc/articles/PMC4051744/.

14. Global Internet Liberty Campaign. Privacy and human rights: An international survey of privacy laws and practice. http://gilc.org/privacy/survey/intro.html.

15. The Global Summit on Civil Registration and Vital Statistics. 2013. Civil registration and vital statistics. http://www.globalsummitoncrvs.org/crvs.html. Accessed February 11, 2015.

16. Gostin L, Hodge JG, Valentine NB, Nygren-Krug H. 2003. The domains of health responsiveness: A human rights analysis. World Health Organization. http://www.who.int/healthinfo/paper53.pdf.

17. Hansungule M. African courts and the African Commission on Human and People's Rights. In Bosi A, Diescho J, eds. *Human Rights in Africa: Legal Perspectives on Their Protection and Promotion*. Windhoek, Namibia: Macmillan Education; 2009: 233–271. http://www.kas.de/upload/auslandshomepages/namibia/Human_Rights_in_Africa/8_Hansungule.pdf.

18. 104th US Congress. 1996. Health Insurance Portability and Accountability Act. Public Law 104–191. US Statut Large 110: 1936–2103.

19. Helm AM, Georgatos D. 2014. Privacy and mHealth: How mobile health apps fit into a privacy framework not limited to HIPAA. *Syracuse Law Rev* 64: 131–150.

20. Knoppers BA. 2014. Does policy grow on trees? *BMC Med Ethics* 15: 21 http://bmcmedethics.biomedcentral.com/articles/10.1186/1472-6939-15-87/.

21. Kosseim P, Dove ES, Baggaley C, Meslin EM, Cate FH, Kaye J, Harris JR, Knoppers BM. 2014. Building a data sharing model for global genomic research. *Genome Biol* 15: 430 http://genomebiology.com/2014/15/8/430.

22. Martínez-Pérez B, de la Torre-Díez I, López-Coronado M. 2014. Privacy and security in mobile health apps: A review and recommendations. *J Med Syst* 39: 181.

23. Fulbright NR. 2014. Global data privacy directory. http://www.nortonrosefulbright.com/files/global-data-privacy-directory-52687.pdf.

24. Nuffield Council on Bioethics. 2015. The collection, linking and use of data in biomedical research and health care: Ethical issues. Nuffield Council on Bioethics. http://nuffieldbioethics.org/wp-content/uploads/Biological_and_health_data_web.pdf.

25. Oomman N, Mehl G, Berg M, Silverman R. 2013. Modernizing vital registration systems: Why now? *The Lancet* 381(9875): 1336–1337. http://www.thelancet.com/pdfs/journals/lancet/PIIS0140-6736(13)60847-8.pdf.

26. Osuji PI. *African Traditional Medicine: Autonomy and Informed Consent*. Switzerland: Springer; 2014: 1–4.

27. Pasquale F, Ragone TA. 2014. Protecting health privacy in an era of big data processing and cloud computing. *Stanf Technol Law Rev* 17: 595–694 https://journals.law.stanford.edu/sites/default/files/stanford-technology-law-review/online/protecting healthprivacy.pdf.

28. Patnaik S, Brunskill E, Thies W. 2009. Evaluating the accuracy of data collection on mobile phones: A study of forms, SMS, and voice. 2009 International Conference on Information and Communication Technologies and Development. ICTD 2009 Proceedings, 74–84.

29. Payne JD. 2013. The state of standards and interoperability for mHealth among low- and middle-income countries. mHealth Alliance. http://www.mhealthknowledge.org/resources/state-standards-and-interoperability-mhealth-among-low-and-middle-income-countries.

30. Principles for Digital Development. 2015. Principles for digital development. http://ict4dprinciples.org/wp-content/uploads/2014/06/Green_Tree_v5.pdf.

31. Sen G, Östlin P, George A. 2007. Unequal, unfair, ineffective and inefficient–gender inequity in health: Why it exists and how we can change it. Final report to the WHO commission on social determinants of health. Women and Gender Equity Knowledge Network. http://www.who.int/social_determinants/resources/csdh_media/wgekn_final_report_07.pdf.

32. Seppälä A, Nykänen P, Ruotsalainen P. 2014. Privacy-related context information for ubiquitous health. *JMIR Mhealth Uhealth* 2(1): e12. http://www.ncbi.nlm.nih.gov/pmc/articles/PMC4114417/.

33. Trotter F. 2012. Who owns patient data? O'Reilly Radar. June 6. http://radar.oreilly.com/2012/06/patient-data-ownership-access.html.

34. Connect T. 2013. Patient privacy in a mobile world: A framework to address privacy law issues in mobile health. http://www.trust.org/spotlight/Patient-Privacy-in-a-Mobile-World.

35. United Nations Department of Economic and Social Affairs. 1998. Handbook on civil registration and vital statistics systems: Computerization. http://unstats.un.org/unsd/publication/SeriesF/SeriesF_73E.pdf.

36. United Nations Department of Economic and Social Affairs. 1998. Handbook on civil registration and vital statistics systems: Policies and protocols for the release and archiving of individual records. http://unstats.un.org/unsd/publication/SeriesF/SeriesF_70E.pdf.

37. United Nations Statistics Division. 2013. Principles and Recommendations for a Vital Statistics System, Revision 3, Final Draft. http://unstats.un.org/UNSD/Demographic/standmeth/principles/unedited_M19Rev3en.pdf.

38. Universal Declaration of Human Rights. 1949. Article 12. http://www.un.org/en/documents/udhr/.

39. Veatch RM. 2000. *African Ethical Theory and the Four Principles: Cross-Cultural Perspectives in Medical Ethics*, 2d ed. London, UK; Jones and Bartlett Publishers: 252–53.

40. Weeks RV. 2014. The implementation of an electronic patient healthcare record system: A South African case study. *Management* 11: 101–119 http://repository.up.ac.za/bitstream/handle/2263/40963/Weeks_Implementation_2014.pdf?sequence=1.

41. Wilkins K, Nsubuga P, Mendlein J, Mercer D, Pappaioanou M. 2008. The data for decision making project: Assessment of surveillance systems in developing countries to improve access to public health information. *Public Health* 122(9): 914–922.

42. Wojcieszek A, Flenady V, Nankabira V, Middleton P, Crowther C, Lewis J, et al. 2014. Harmonised reproductive health registries: Developing indicators and minimum datasets to improve uptake of the WHO essential interventions in reproductive, child and maternal health. 18th Congress of the Perinatal Society of Australia and New Zealand, Crown Perth, Australia, Vol. 50. http://www.fhi.no/dokumenter/1d23cd1b4e.pdf.

43. World Health Organization. 2011. mHealth: New horizons for health through mobile technologies. http://www.who.int/goe/publications/goe_mhealth_web.pdf.

44. World Health Organization. 2012. Management of patient Information: Trends and challenges in member states. Global observatory of eHealth series, Vol. 6. Geneva, Switzerland: World Health Organization. http://apps.who.int/iris/bitstream/10665/76794/1/9789241504645_eng.pdf.

45. World Health Organization. 2013. Systematic review of eCRVS and mCRVS interventions in low and middle income countries. http://www.who.int/healthinfo/civil_registration/crvs_report_ecrvs_mcrvs_2013.pdf.

46. World Health Organization. 2012. Legal frameworks for eHealth. Global observatory of eHealth series, Vol. 5. Geneva, Switzerland: World Health Organization. http://whqlibdoc.who.int/publications/2012/9789241503143_eng.pdf.

47. World Health Organization and International Telecommunications Union. 2012. National eHealth Strategy Toolkit.

48. Wugmeister M, Retzer K, and Rich C. 2007. Global solutions for cross-border data transfers: Making the case of corporate privacy rules. *Georgetown J Int Law* 38: 449–498; see 464.

23 Financing and Commercialization

Jocelyn Ling, Abeezer Tapia, Rose Shuman, Biju Mohandes, F. Mita Paramita, and Sunil Nair

Take-Home Message

- Raising capital for enterprise is as much an art as science. The key is to use common sense and sound business judgment to choose the relevant form of capital from the appropriate source at the right time.

Introduction

Even in the second decade of the twenty-first century, the unmet health needs of emerging markets remain tremendous. Complementary to efforts to improve health worker competencies and health systems capacities, medical technology can result in an improved standard of care for poorer populations across a host of developing world diseases.

Unfortunately, the typical means of introducing medical technology to the developing world is to take developed-world technology, strip the "bells and whistles, " and provide a cheaper, less feature-rich solution for the emerging market. We argue this approach is mistaken. Patient needs and cultural paradigms of medical care are different in emerging markets—from location and accessibility of health services, to health worker–patient interactions, expectations of patients, and price points that patients and their families can afford. Technology designed for the hospital or clinic may be of little use on rural roads and distant homesteads.

We suggest a more effective approach is to conduct localized development, where a medical service or device is designed from scratch *in situ* with the express purpose of addressing the needs of the local population, who may indeed contribute to the financing and delivery of the technology. Vital to success are effective organization and financing of the enterprise (particularly the social enterprise model, though these recommendations apply to for-profit ventures too), as well as successful commercialization of the medical technology. These topics are covered in detail below.

Defining an Organizational Approach

Successful technologic launches are driven by effective organizations—though an organization will grow and evolve over time to adapt to changing conditions or internal stakeholders, a clear mission and vision for success at the outset will give the new venture a platform from which to base all its future efforts. Social business models vary greatly, and careful consideration should be given to which model to pursue. One should choose the social enterprise route (which will be the focus of this section) *only* after conducting an analysis of the available options and determining a best fit alignment with one's motivation, commitment, and definition of a satisfactory outcome. Simply put, founding a social enterprise may or may not be the most expeditious way to achieve the desired goal. Alternative models include:

- starting a profitable business entity, selling either a health care product or service, which serve both a social and financial purpose
- innovating a new open-source digital tool or hardware product, making the technology free to the global public to use and build from
- conducting research to validate a new concept and sharing the learning among health practitioners and researchers
- developing a methodology or product, and then merging this new innovation into the operations of an existing entity
- starting a grant-receiving nonprofit organization.

Each model carries a different balance of founder commitment; need for external validation and buy-in; funding requirements; administrative burdens; timelines for creation, and for return on investment (however defined); and control over outcomes. Successful products and projects have been launched out of all these models. Taking the time to establish the right fit will preserve motivation and conserve resources down the road for all involved.

The Social Enterprise Model

Henceforth, we proceed with the assumption that one's interest is in pursuing a social business model, although this content is relevant for other organizational structures as well. When starting a new social enterprise, it is important to evaluate three main factors, described below.

Commitment

Committing to an open-ended, complex health care product requires reflection. The great majority of developing-world health product companies require years of commitment prior to reaching financial sustainability. At early stages, grant funding often provides financial backbone for the organization, even for the social business. Obtaining such funding and further investments can be frustrating, and requires both determination and perseverance.

This reality requires a more flexible definition of success than just the balance sheet, particularly in the early years of the enterprise. It requires a clear sense of motivations, as the stresses of creating a social enterprise are commensurate to founding a traditional for-profit firm, but without promise of large payouts. Evaluate regularly: is the potential for saving lives and health system resources sufficient to take this project on? Both vision and measured outcomes must sustain the motivation to continue the longer journey.

Time commitment is crucial. The timeline to achieve reasonable success in a developing world–focused health care start-up often stretches to many years. International health initiatives generally require relocation or frequent overseas travel for the life of one's involvement in the project. Finally, a very competitive capital-raising environment and low returns in this sector lead to a slower scaling rate, and hence require longer commitments from both founders and investors before seeing return on investment.

Is founding a social enterprise a commitment one wishes to make? Assess whether this is a side project or a full-time pursuit. How many years and what percentage of time can the entire team commit up front?

Viability

Once the team is committed for the foreseeable future, evaluate whether this product is viable as a sustainable business. A complete analysis should include the following.

Product   Is this product capable of being built within the specifications needed for deployment locally? If the product involves hardware, what is the supply chain? If it is a digital product, is it appropriate given the communications and technology infrastructures as well as human capacity available at intended deployment sites?

Market   Field research up front increases the odds of successfully entering a new market with a new product. It is crucial to have a good grasp of customer purchasing and use behaviors, as well as the requirements to make a service or product market-ready.

In the medical sector, there are significant hurdles: business and medical industry regulations; customs importation; and entrenched health care systems that vary regionally. How does this new product enhance or threaten established stakeholders? Who are the natural allies of the product? Seek strong evidence for the marketability of your good or service, including similar examples of successful enterprises in the same field and market.

When possible, it is best to hone concepts over multiple pilots before building a company around promising ideas. That learning will yield significant insights regarding viability of the product, potential for impact, routes to market, and team composition and commitment.

Business Plan   Raising any form of capital is highly competitive and requires a strong business plan. Often, founding teams are unfamiliar at the outset with the challenges of doing business in emerging and developing-world market environments.

Building a business plan based on remote assumptions and developed-country business templates may secure initial funding. However, doing the field research up front to assess the true viability of the business provides a more accurate picture. Research on the ground at targeted pilot sites, as well as reviewing relevant case studies, better justifies the financial projections and capital-raising decisions, and aligns all partners' expectations for impact, scaling, and return on investment.

Team   Developing a product is but one of the many business challenges involved in starting a new enterprise. The same enthusiasm for research and development (R&D) problem solving must carry over to all facets of running the company. Does the team have the executive, administrative, legal, financial, operations, marketing, sales, and related skills and passions required to create a complete business? Success will depend on team strength all around.

Teams also grow and change over a company's life cycle. It is healthy to discuss with cofounders from the outset long-term goals for management transition. Transitions are often triggered by financial needs—both personal and organizational, as well as by investor requirements for a more professional management team. If the company sells a physical product, how will it transition from small-batch manufacture to a larger scale or outsourced suppliers?

Financing and Sustainability

Once convinced of the team commitment to move forward and that the intended venture is viable in the market, it is time to evaluate how to finance the company.

Projects and companies require funding at all stages of a life cycle, as will be covered in more detail below. Potential social enterprise founders should be aware that funding for social enterprises typically comes from a mix of sources, including grants. Also, once committed to founding an enterprise, fundraising commences immediately, never ends, and is rarely sufficient. The work of raising capital generally falls on the shoulders of the founders and requires balancing the work of building the company with the engagement needed to recruit and retain investors over the duration.

Funding and scaling look different for a medical hardware versus an eHealth service or software business. When building business models and projections, ensure that they are based on case studies. Building and distributing physical items is more expensive, more complex, and runs into more regulatory frameworks than launching digital products. In both scenarios, human and infrastructural constraints will come into play.

As a founder, one must consider the organizational structure carefully. Impact must be the core driver and should be quantifiable. Compared to a traditional for-profit company, the magnitude of financial gain for founders or investors is generally not competitive with opportunities in the traditional private sector. Raising capital is affected by the lower profit profile. Medical-social enterprises attract a specialized set of social impact investors willing to trade outcomes for return.

As a final note: when raising capital, founders typically start with their own resources as well as those loaned or gifted by friends and family. All start-ups, including social enterprises, have very high rates of failure. It is strongly recommended to raise no more than those investing are prepared to lose. The value of long-term personal relationships, as well as one's own financial security, often does not merit the risk of soliciting funds for uncertain gains. We recommend that founders be comfortable soliciting funds from the outset of their venture from a variety of sources, as this will remain a central activity throughout the life of the enterprise.

Still ready to go? Then let's delve into the details of raising capital!

Financing

The successful development of any medical technology requires money; that is to say, financial capital. Capital is the fuel that propels every business. Innovative eHealth and mHealth start-ups need to understand if, when, and how to raise capital, regardless of the venture's developmental stage. The capital needs of a venture can essentially be framed around three questions:

1. Do I need capital, and what types of capital are there?
2. How much capital do I need, and when?
3. Where can I find capital?

What Types of Capital Are There?

Finance in the developing world is no longer the privy of international aid agencies and nongovernmental organizations. There are now multiple types of capital available to the private entrepreneur, each with their own characteristics, terms, and conditions. It is important to understand how each type of capital fits into your venture's stage of growth and future profit goals. To understand the spectrum of choices available, table 23.1 defines various types of capital and describes their major characteristics.

Table 23.1

Types of Capital

Type	Definition	Characteristics
Grant capital	• Raised from donors, foundations, governments, and sometimes friends and family	• This is the cheapest form of capital in that the company does not need to pay it back and hence comes with enormous flexibility, especially during the blueprint and validation stage of a company's growth • The sums involved are often small, though, and donors only so generous! Companies will often need to proceed quickly to other forms of capital raising, as described above.
Equity	• Raised from investors by issuing common shares, which represent ownership in a company. The ownership entailed by sale of these shares is determined by the valuation of the company at that stage. For instance, if a company raises $100 by issuing shares for that amount to an investor at a pre money company valuation of $100, the investor will own 50% of the company • These shares are called common shares because, unlike preferred equity, they typically do not come with any special rights or privileges	• This type of capital does not require any collaterals, guarantees, or preferred returns and allows flexibility to the company as it navigates the ups and downs of the business cycle • The key risk inherent in the issue of common shares is the dilution of the entrepreneurs' ownership of the business and her share in the profit the business might generate. The key to raising capital through common equity is to time it well. It is recommended that any equity issuance be delayed to the extent possible, and come at stages in the company's growth when the entrepreneur is able to command a good valuation for her company as well as use the equity to drastically increase that value, so that even with dilution her ownership value continues to increase
Preferred shares	• Raised from venture capital and private equity investors by issuing preferred shares in the company • These are called preferred shares because they typically come with certain rights and privileges that common shareholders do not possess such as the right to a fixed dividend, the right to be paid out prior to other shareholders in the event of liquidation, etc. • Certain types of preferred shares could be convertible into common equity after a certain period or triggered by certain events. These are called convertible preferred shares	• Benefits of preferred equity derive from the fact that, unlike lenders of debt, investors take on significant risk alongside the entrepreneur and do not typically take any collateral or guaranteed returns in the event of a downturn. (Hence, the return expectations are also higher than those of debt instruments.) • The risk of preferred equity is that the investor expects some preferred rights. The entrepreneur has to be careful about what these preferred rights could be and should attempt to restrict them to a reasonable minimum

Table 23.1 (continued)

Type	Definition	Characteristics
Convertible debt	• A loan secured from venture capital or angel investors • This is called convertible loan because the lender is able to convert such a loan to a predetermined number of shares of equity in the company typically at the discretion of the lender after a specified period of time	• The entrepreneur should consider a convertible loan if she expects the valuation of the business to increase substantially before the conversion option for the lender kicks in (thus causing minimum dilution) • The key benefits of a convertible loan are that the interest payments are relatively low, and it allows the entrepreneur to raise capital during the early stages of the business without getting heavily diluted • The key risk is that if the company does not perform as projected and the valuation does not increase, the lender could end up owning a large stake in the company
Subordinated debt	• Similar to senior debt except that they are ranked after senior debt in the event of liquidation or bankruptcy. In other words, the company has to repay its senior debt obligations before repaying subordinated debt	• An entrepreneur could use this avenue of capital if they do not have collateral commensurate with the loan they are taking and do not want to raise equity • Subordinated debt is more expensive than a senior debt due to the higher risks; otherwise, benefits and risks are similar
Senior debt	• A loan secured from financial institutions such as banks and micro-finance firms • This is called a senior debt because the company is obliged to repay this debt first in the event of liquidation or bankruptcy, before paying off any other creditors or shareholders • This is typically structured with a predetermined tenor, potentially a grace period before starting repayments, and regular interest payments; and is secured against collateral. The interest payments can be fixed or floating	• The entrepreneur should consider senior debt if the business is generating stable cash flows or is likely to do so in a predictable period of time, *and* if the business has assets that could be pledged as a collateral with the lender The key benefit of a senior debt is that it allows the entrepreneur to preserve her equity (i.e., no dilution) and is usually the cheapest form of financing The key risk is that in the case of default, the lender could liquidate the company in order to regain part or all of their money back

As we move through the table from grants to senior debt, the level of risk to the investor and cost of capital to the company varies significantly. The type of capital a company raises at any stage should be determined by what dilution in her ownership the entrepreneur is willing to accept, what cost of capital the company can afford, what kind of cash flows it has to support repayments, what assets it has to provide collateral, and, finally, whether there is a need for a strategic partner to support or accelerate growth. Furthermore, access to particular types of funds often depends on the status of the project or organization, with only established companies with established revenue history able to access more conservative financing such as senior debt.

Do I Need Capital, and If So, How Much and When?

The answer to this question depends on the stage of development a business is in. We drew upon a framework that was first published in the report "From blueprint to scale: The case for philanthropy in impact investing" [1] to classify the evolution of a business into four stages—blueprint, validate, prepare, and scale. A brief description of these stages and capital needs during each are detailed below.

1. *Blueprint.* This is the earliest stage for a business, when entrepreneurs are drafting their business concept, understanding their customers' needs, and initiating the legal requirements of setting up an enterprise. For most businesses, particularly in the eHealth and mHealth space, the capital needs at this stage are modest. Entrepreneurs typically self-fund or secure small injections of cash from family, friends, or grants to move past this stage.

2. *Validate.* Once the business model has been drafted, key aspects of the model should be tested for viability. The entrepreneur typically conducts market trials, tests business model assumptions, and refines product or business model during this phase. At this stage, capital needs depend on the marketplace, geographical location, and extent and duration of testing. Ideally, the entrepreneur should look to achieve a thorough validation of the critical aspects of the business model with minimal expense. This stage could end up costing a start-up between US$500,000–$2 million. The investors at this stage are usually friends, family, donors, angel investors, and venture capitalists. The investment is typically secured as equity, convertible loans, or grants.

3. *Prepare.* Upon successful validation, the entrepreneur prepares to scale her business. This involves the development of internal systems and processes, hiring an appropriate management team, securing robust supply chains, and stimulating market demand. This is the stage when a business turns to commercial institutional investors such as venture capitalists, private equity funds, and banks for investments ranging from US$1–$5 million. These investments are typically structured as senior loans, convertible loans, preferred equity, or common equity.

4. *Scale.* Finally, if a business makes it this far, this is where companies emerge to scale their activities in order to break into new geographies or rapidly acquire new customers. Many firms may not have the goal to reach this point of scale (i.e., some entrepreneurs would like to run small and medium businesses)—but in the event that entrepreneurs are looking to take this route, scaling companies translates into a more intense environment and requires the building of a well-oiled machine with all aspects of the business tightly under control. At this point, capital needs are usually US$5 million and above, depending on the business. In addition to commercial financial investors, the company could also tap into strategic partners who could bring in benefits such as new technology, access to larger corporate machinery, entry points into a new market, or a business line in addition to capital.

The ideal type of capital for a growing company varies by its size and prospects. Grants and appropriately structured convertible debt are ideal instruments for the company in the blueprint or validate stages, since these are nondilutive or minimally dilutive. At the prepare and scale stages, equity or preferred equity become preferable as the success of earlier stages allows the company to secure reasonable valuation and minimize dilution. Raising equity capital from experienced investors at this stage also helps the company seek their support to grow and further enhance value. As the company reaches stable and predictable cash flows and builds an asset base, it can turn to senior or subordinated debt to fuel its growth alongside equity.

Where Can I Find Capital?

Each type of capital can be obtained from multiple sources.

- *Grants:* available through friends, family, fellowships, business plan competitions, business incubators, and so on.
- *Equity or quasi-equity investments:* available through angel investors, venture capital funds, private equity funds, hedge funds, development finance institutions, and strategic investors.
- *Debt:* commercial banks, development finance institutions, and crowdsourcing.

The need to attract the right investor cannot be overstated, since an investor does not just bring capital but also unique philosophies, compliance requirements, brand equity, and value additions. The entrepreneur needs to assess whether the capital and value additions that a particular investor brings weigh favorably against their compliance requirements and cost of capital, and whether the investor's brand equity and philosophy are in line with the company's own. For instance, it may be better in the long term to refuse a grant from an institution whose philosophy does not align with that of the entrepreneur, and instead opt for more expensive capital from a venture fund that brings significant networks or expertise in the sector of interest to the company.

Table 23.2 contains a list of sources of capital. It is not meant to be exhaustive, but rather illustrative of the resources available that can provide both financial and capacity-building networks. This list is focused on sources of capital that are associated with the social impact landscape.

Commercialization

Having identified and secured funding (and understanding that financing your venture will be an ongoing endeavor), the aspiring entrepreneur can focus on the research, development, and delivery of promising medical technologies. This process has essentially three

Table 23.2

Sources of Capital

Category	Examples
Fellowships and networks	1. Acumen 2. Ashoka 3. Canadian Social Entrepreneurship Foundation 4. Draper Richards Foundation 5. Echoing Green 6. PresenTense Social Entrepreneur Fellowship 7. PopTech 8. Rainer Arnhold Fellows Program 9. REDF Farber Fellowship 10. Skoll Foundation 11. Starting Bloc 12. TED 13. Unreasonable Institute
Student-focused	14. C.V. Starr Social Entrepreneurship Fellowship at Brown University 15. Global Social Entrepreneurship Competition (University of Washington) 16. Global Social Venture Competition 17. Harvard Business School 18. Miken Family Foundation (Tulane University) 19. NYU Reynolds Program 20. Sparkseed 21. Upper Valley Social Entrepreneurship Fellowship (Dartmouth) 22. University of Michigan Social Venture Fund 23. Venture Well 24. Wharton Social Enterprise Fellows program
Grants	25. Chinook Fund 26. DoSomething.org grant database 27. Foundation Center 28. Google grants 29. Grantmakers for Effective Organizations 30. Kauffman Foundation 31. Philanthropy New York 32. Social Innovation Fund 33. The Awesome Foundation 34. The Mulago Foundation 35. USA.gov for nonprofits 36. Clinton Foundation 37. Gates Foundation
Crowdfunding	38. 33needs 39. Buzzbnk 40. CauseVox 41. Indiegogo 42. Change.org 43. Chase Community Giving 44. CrowdRise 45. DonorsChoose.org 46. FirstGiving 47. Kickstarter 48. Kiva 49. Pepsi Refresh Project 50. StartSomeGood

Table 23.2 (continued)

Category	Examples
Angels, venture capital and private equity	51. Blue Ridge Foundation 52. Bamboo Finance 53. Calvert Group 54. CEI Ventures 55. Central Fund 56. Central Fund 57. City Light Capital 58. Clean Technology Fund 59. Community Development Venture Capital Alliance 60. Good Capital 61. Grassroots Business Fund 62. Gray Ghost Ventures 63. Gray Matters Capital 64. Ignia Fund 65. Investors' Circle 66. Joshua Venture Group 67. Mission Markets 68. New Cycle Capital 69. New Profit Inc. 70. Next Street 71. Nonprofit Finance Fund 72. NYC Seed 73. New Schools Ventures Fund 74. Omidyar Network 75. Pacific Community Ventures 76. Pipeline Fund 77. Renewal2 78. Root Capital 79. RSF Social Finance Fund 80. Schwab Foundation 81. Soros Economic Development Fund 82. SME Finance Innovation Fund 83. Sustainable Jobs Fund 84. TBL Capital 85. Savannah Fund 86. Invested Development 87. Fanisi 88. Abraaj Group 89. Jacana Partners 90. Investment Fund for Health in Africa 91. Actis 92. Mara Launch Fund 93. Mango Fund 94. Khosla Impact & Seed Fund 95. LGT Venture Partners 96. GroFin Africa Fund 97. The Hub 98. Village Capital 99. Union Square Ventures 100. New Enterprise Associates 101. Social+Capital Partnership 102. Norwest Venture Partners 103. Kleiner Perkins Caufield & Byers

Table 23.2 (continued)

Category	Examples
	104. Domain Associates
	105. HealthCare Ventures
	106. Foundation Medical Partners
	107. Novartis Venture Fund
	108. MPM Capital
	109. Alta Partners
	110. OrbiMed Advisors
	111. Clarus Ventures
	112. SV Life Sciences Advisors
	113. Sofinnova Ventures
	114. Arch Venture Partners
	115. InterWest Partners
Conferences	116. Cleantech Open
	117. GoBig Network
	118. Green Spaces
	119. Ned.com
	120. Net Impact
	121. Skoll World Forum
	122. Social Capital Markets Conference
	123. Social Enterprise Alliance
	124. Social Enterprise Summit
	125. Social Enterprise World Forum
	127. Social Innovation Camp
	128. Social Investment Forum
	129. Toniic
Loan Providers	130. ACCION
	131. Calvert Foundation
	132. Nonprofits Assistance Fund
	133. Partners for the Common Good
	134. ShoreBank
	135. Small Business Administration
	136. Social Capital Partners
	137. Tridos Bank
	138. The New Resource Bank
	139. Wainwright Bank
	140. Progreso Financiero

Note: This list skews in favor of North American resources and was assembled in March 2014.

parts (some of which will be familiar from the organizational validation study recommended above; see figure 23.1).

1. *Identifying unmet needs and potential solutions:* spending time in the field to truly understand local health issues and the local culture of health.

2. *Localized research and development:* finding a viable solution where the local health system is the center of the design process.

3. *Commercialization:* delivering medical technologies effectively to health systems and patients in developing nations and providing best-in-class customer service.

Fundamental components of emerging market medical device development

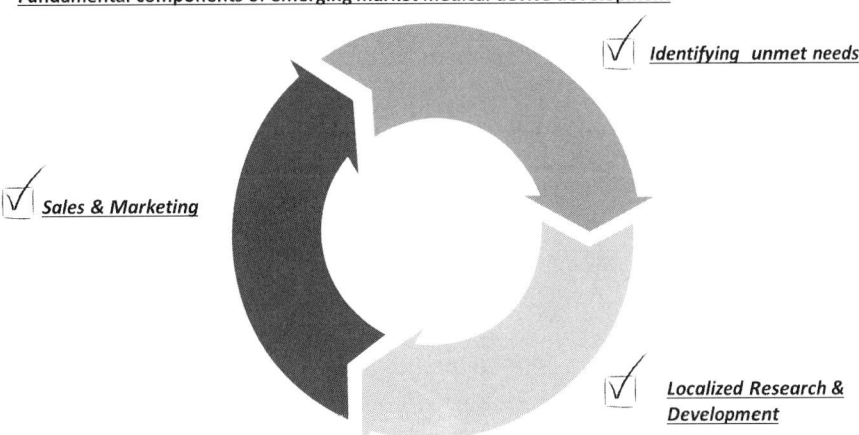

Figure 23.1
Fundamental components of emerging-market medical-device development.

These three key areas are all fundamental to effective medical-technology development and usage in the developing world. We will explore all three in more depth, with a special focus on the third area of commercialization. Developing a product to fit an unmet medical need is important, but can only be successful if you can gain product adoption and distribution, and provide best-in-class service.

Identifying Unmet Needs and Potential Solutions

One of the most fundamental tenets of creating medical devices for the poor in the developing nations is spending a considerable amount of time in the field. This is important for all aspects of the process, but especially for identifying true unmet needs and creating real-world solutions. Many intelligent people can sit in a room together and come up with many great ideas on a whiteboard. However, true understanding of local health systems only occurs when you spend time in the field. It is critical that entrepreneurs spend as much time in the field with patients, physicians, and staff as possible. This is the only way to understand the true health needs of all stakeholders in the health system and appreciate how medicine is actually practiced in the local environment. Entrepreneurs often focus on the limitations of the current gold standard of care in a developing world context, which could include high costs, clinical efficacy, safety, and accessibility; we suggest broadening one's horizons to understand not just limitations, but the full milieu in which a new technology will have to operate.

Spending a large amount of time in the field also provides a better knowledge of the local clinical workflow, which is critical in creating technological solutions that do not disrupt the local practice of medicine to a degree that averts usage of the medical device. In the developing world, the practice of medicine and mindset of patients and providers are often counterintuitive, and thus first-hand interaction with the key stakeholders is the best way to understand these complex health system environments and then creatively generate effective solutions.

Localized Research and Development

Once an unmet health need has been identified, the next step is to develop a product to address the issue. As when identifying the unmet need, the first step for validating the product idea would usually require the entrepreneur again venture into the field and speak with all the relevant stakeholders—physicians, staff, patients—to provide validation that their product idea would address an unmet need or current health system limitation. It is critical to understand current clinical workflow, as new innovations should fit, augment, or improve the workflow without much or any disruption. If the technology veers too much from the current clinical workflow and requires the physician or staff to spend increased time per patient or procedure using the medical device, it will be challenging to have the product adopted.

Once the product concept is formulated, the enterprise can begin using the lean start-up design approach. Once a first minimum viable product is created, the product can be sent to various stakeholders. Interacting closely with these key physicians, other health care staff and patients, the R&D team will receive feedback on how to tweak the prototype to better fit the unmet need. The R&D team continues this lean start-up approach until they feel they the product is ready for a targeted launch.

The venture could then identify a small group of physicians and patients to run a pilot: the product would be launched in a small, controlled setting, with heavy support given to physicians, staff, and patients as they acclimate to the technology. From this pilot, the venture should learn a tremendous amount about how physicians, staff, and patients interact with the device, and what product modifications the R&D team might need to make to further smooth interaction with the new technology.

With the need to interact with local physicians, staff, and patients throughout the entire R&D process, one can see why it is critical for the R&D team to be local and on the ground in the developing country of focus.

Commercialization

The R&D process is extremely important when creating a device to treat an unmet medical need. Equally important is distribution—getting the medical technology in the hands of as many of the right people as possible. Although there are nonprofit ventures that do an effective job creating and distributing medical innovations, in this chapter we assume a for-profit social enterprise. A for-profit social enterprise provides the potential benefits of organic scalability, sustainability, and operational efficiencies, while still maintaining a focus on social impact instead of maximizing profits. We break down commercialization in a for-profit institution into three key components—sales, marketing, and service.

Sales   The art of sales is a unique craft whether one is a sales executive for a Fortune 500 company or a street peddler in a developing country. The fundamentals of sales—trust, credibility, dependability, and asking for business—are true across all verticals. However, there are some key strategic and tactical items that have unique caveats when trying to sell a medical technology in the developing world.

First, and similar to a developed-world business, the early stage venture needs to evaluate different sales channels for its new technology. The key high-level question to ask is: do you use direct channels with your own sales team, or do you leverage indirect channels, such as corporate partnerships or local distributors? Both direct and indirect channels have their own benefits and disadvantages (figure 23.2), and may be utilized variably depending on the developmental stage of your enterprise. Within indirect channels, for the urban distribution of medical devices, partnering with a large multinational to

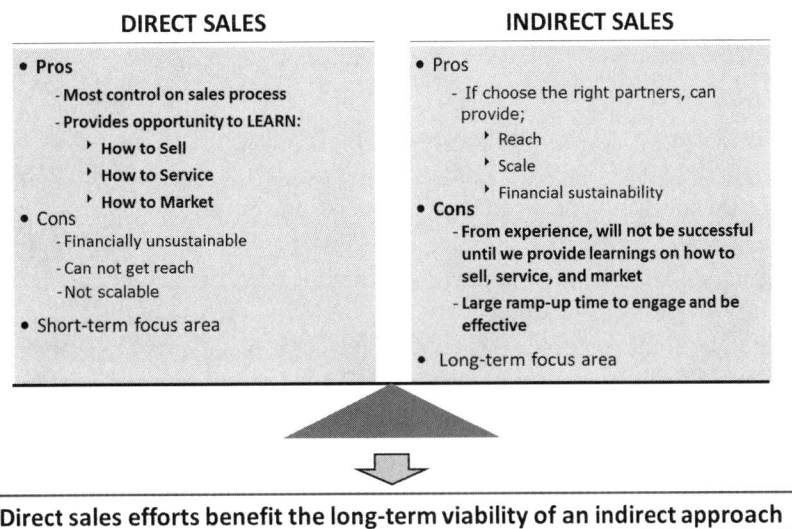

Figure 23.2
Types of sales channels.

leverage their sale and marketing infrastructure may be worth considering. For indirect rural channels, a venture may explore working with local distributors. Managing local distributors and making sure they can maintain their sales volumes can be a challenge, and is an area a venture would need local expertise to manage. Indirect channels can provide the reach, scale, and financial sustainability to cover broad geographical areas, such as India, Africa, or Latin America. Embarking on creating direct-distribution channels needing an internal sales force can be a costly proposition for an early stage venture. The strong benefit of this approach, however, is the ability to control every aspect of the sales process in the critical early days and generate internal knowledge of how to best market and service your product in the context of a developing nation. Many ventures find the right blend of direct distribution channels in the early periods and then transition to indirect channels later.

Assuming one begins with a direct sales channel, the next important step is creating the right sales team—thus targeting the correct sales representative profile for *your* product and *your* environment. This involves matching sales rep capabilities to the clinical and mechanical complexity of your medical device, teaching them the intricacies of the local sales cycles and purchasing process if not already known, and offering them appropriate compensation for the local environment (salary and commission). For example, for a simple-to-use medical device that could be sold directly to patients, working with local village entrepreneurs might be the right sales team profile. For a more complex device that has a more complicated sales cycle via a physician or hospital system, internally recruited and trained sales representatives may be needed.

Finally, one must define the customer interaction. Customer interactions for medical technologies in emerging markets can be very different than in the developed world. The value proposition must be clearly articulated to the potential customer (who likely has significant resource constraints on his or her ability to make new purchases of novel devices or services); crisp messaging for the sales rep to use with the potential customer must be provided and practiced. The organization should create best-in-class sales tools for the sales team, including product and clinical collateral, and provide comprehensive training on how to best use them with customers. Also, the venture should provide training on how to give product demonstrations. Overall, the organization's leadership needs to understand their customer through the lens of a specific emerging market, determine what they would like the interaction to entail, and then provide training to allow the sales team to provide a consistent message to customers.

Marketing   There are many aspects of marketing that also need special focus when trying to commercialize a medical device or service in the developing world. Three key areas that need particular attention are market assessment, developing local physician opinion leaders, and creating lean start-up experiments to find effective marketing programs.

Market assessment can be complicated in the developing world. It is important to understand the local market, segment the market into different types of customers, and then target customer segments that make strategic sense for financial and social mission purposes. Unlike developed countries, where health market information can be found in expensive research reports, these reports either do not exist for emerging markets or are (often) grossly inaccurate. Often the venture needs to create its own market mapping. For example, a venture can have its sales reps profile the different types of local hospitals by revenue, volume, or acuity tiers, as well as the specific names of target physicians within key medical specialties as they enter new towns. The marketing team can use this data to strategically direct the sales team on market leaders or other vital opinion leaders.

Developing relationships with physician key opinion leaders (KOL) in the specialty areas of their medical device is important. For example, if the medical device is for the field of pediatrics, it is important to build relationships with local, regional, and national pediatric thought leaders. Building these relationships may have many benefits, including those following.

- *Drive adoption with mass physician populations.* Physicians are inclined to follow thought leaders whose clinical opinion they respect, which has a strong trickle-down effect in terms of product adoption.

- *Product development.* KOLs can provide expert insights into ongoing R&D, from current product iterations to next-generation product development.

- *Governmental influence.* As health care regulations for every country are constantly evolving, national KOLs can provide a strong voice to provide a better regulatory landscape for your device. For example, if a venture is trying to get their medical device implemented at every community health post, KOLs who support your medical device can provide their clinical opinions to the right medical governmental bodies to support widespread adoption.

Finally, marketing organizations can leverage lean start-up methodologies to determine which marketing programs have the most effective return. Running a series of lean start-up experiments can help find the best programs to encourage technological adoption. For example, assume a venture wanted to run a "text message" marketing campaign, whereby target physicians would be sent informational texts about the product before the sales rep would call on them. The venture could run an experiment to see if the region with the "text message" campaign yielded higher product adoption rates than areas that did not employ the campaign. Through a series of experiments, one can find out which marketing campaigns are most effective for a particular device in a particular distribution or with a specific population.

Service Providing best-in-class service for your medical product is critical in creating product loyalists and champions. Many ventures will cease interaction with the physician or patient once the medical device is sold. In many of these cases, physicians, staff, and patients will not use the device properly or even stop using the device as issues crop up.

Ongoing service and support is required for customers, especially soon after the sale. After the product is delivered, sales reps or other field personal from the company should do regular check-ins to ensure proper device usage by the physician, staff, and patients. Often times, ventures only focus on physician education and overlook the importance of the rest of the health care staff. This is not a wise practice, since it is often the surrounding health care staff who actually use the product and end-up having a strong voice in product adoption.

Furthermore, physicians and allied health care professionals all over the world are usually inundated with different clinical, administrative, and social responsibilities, and ongoing support of a product soon after the sale keeps your product top of mind with the customer. Figure 23.3 illustrates the life cycle of a product from identification of an unmet need to market growth.

By providing best-in-class service, a venture greatly increases the opportunity to create product loyalists, which eventually leads to product champions. This becomes invaluable, as it is the basis for referral business. Product champions are likely to tell their other physician or patient counterparts about the value of the medical device, which is the strongest product-adoption mechanism possible.

Conclusion

While any global health innovation should be linked to clinical outcomes- or clinical quality- improvement, its implementation should also be sustainable to have a widespread

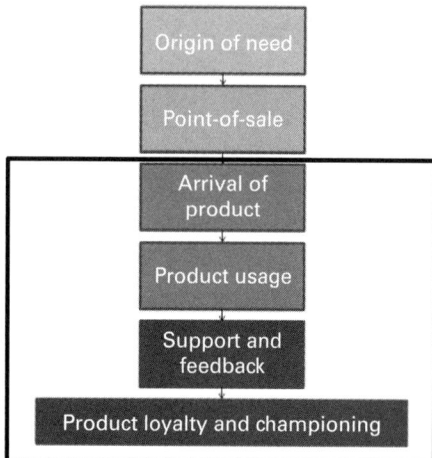

Figure 23.3
Life cycle of a product.

impact. To achieve success in launching a new device or service, innovators need to carefully consider the organizational structure and financing of their venture. Subsequent commercialization should be done prudently, in a stepwise manner, with continuing feedback between the enterprise and its customers and other stakeholders. These tasks can be challenging in the global health setting, but are feasible with clear planning, wise investment, and personal fortitude.

Questions for Discussion

- Evaluate the accomplishments of either your own venture or a venture of your choosing. What stage do you think the venture is in? What are the implications of this in terms of capital needs?
- What are the arguments for or against, and the trade-offs involved, when raising debt over equity—or vice versa?

Reference

1. Koh H, Karamchandani A, Katz R. 2012. From blueprint to scale: The case for philanthropy in impact investing. http://acumen.org/content/uploads/2013/03/From-Blueprint-to-Scale-Case-for-Philanthropy-in-Impact-Investing_Full-report.pdf.

24 Evaluation of Health Information Systems

Hamish S. F. Fraser

Take-Home Messages

- Health information systems (HISs) are increasingly used in low- and middle-income countries, but there is still limited data on their performance and impact.

- Evaluation studies need to examine the whole process of creation of an HIS, from requirements gathering and workflow analysis through development, initial deployment, scale-up and longer-term use, and focus on the needs of a range of stakeholders.

- Individual evaluation studies usually focus on specific aspects of HISs, but may be linked into a multistage evaluation, for example assessing performance, impact, and costs.

- It is important to be aware of the many potential biases in evaluation of HISs, and how these can be minimized with appropriate study designs.

- Rather than focus on a specific technology, studies should be designed to evaluate the underlying principles of HIS interventions, such as access to key data at point of care.

- Data quality is a key issue for all HISs and its regular monitoring and evaluation should be included in all projects.

- While large-scale randomized controlled trials may be required to assess clinical impact, smaller, low-cost studies can provide critical data for design, implementation, and scale-up of systems and help in the design of larger studies.

- Initial results from well-designed clinical trials show that HIS use in low- and middle-income countries can improve key aspects of care, including enrollment and retention in care; access to key laboratory data; time to initiation of lifesaving treatment, adherence to treatment, drug requirement forecasting, and effective disease surveillance.

Summary

Health information systems (HISs) have great potential to improve access to care, quality of care, and management of health systems, as well as impact general health and healthy lifestyles. Despite this potential, there is to date limited evidence that HISs do improve care, especially in low- and middle-income countries (LMIC). Evaluation of HISs builds on the techniques and study designs typically used for other health interventions such as medications, but there are key differences. HISs are usually embedded in the health system and the workflow of patient care, and therefore represent complex interventions that operate through interaction of technology, people, organizations, and infrastructure. Despite these challenges, effective evaluation is possible, and an increasing number of well-designed studies of HISs in LMIC have been published in the last decade. In this chapter, we describe the basic principles of evaluation of HISs and provide examples of effective studies. We review the distinction between formative and summative studies and between quantitative and qualitative studies. We will also briefly discuss qualitative research methods and economic evaluation and discuss examples of effective studies in LMIC. Finally, we will discuss key issues, including data-quality measurement and improvement and the Learning Health System. We also provide a short list of further reading for those interested in learning further about carrying out studies. Readers are encouraged to read chapter 5, "Modern Epidemiology and Global Health in the era of Information Systems and mHealth."

Introduction

Why Evaluate Health Information Systems?

HISs are becoming increasingly widely used worldwide, including in some of the lowest-income countries such as Haiti, Rwanda, and Cambodia. As discussed in earlier chapters, there are many good reasons why these systems are growing in terms of perceived need, improvements in software, and in the availability of smaller, cheaper, more capable hardware that uses a lot less power. However, the deployment and use of HISs should be based on real information needs and on solid evidence that their use improves aspects of health care and patient health more generally. This requires rigorous evaluation studies and publication of evidence to allow development of robust guidance for decision makers. Evaluation studies need to assess a range of parameters—including system performance, usability, stability, and, crucially, data quality—as well as the impact of the systems on patient-care processes and, ideally, clinical outcomes; and finally also examine the costs and cost-effectiveness of such systems. In this chapter, we will discuss the types of evaluations that can performed and the different evaluation methods, with their strengths and weaknesses, as well as give examples of some key evaluation results.

An important point to note is that most HISs do not undergo evaluation at all stages of development, and frequently are not evaluated at all. If the technology used is mature, there may not be a requirement to carry out the evaluation of the earlier stages of software development. However, if there are significant changes, it is important to ensure they have been implemented correctly and assess their impact. Evaluations do not need to be large or complex to yield valuable insights and data that can help the development and implementation process and inform decision makers [1]. A goal of this chapter is to illustrate that evaluation can be carried out by people with a wide range of backgrounds and in a range of environments without necessarily requiring large resources.

Types of Evaluation

HISs are often described as sociotechnical systems—their effect is based on the often-complex interactions of technology, people, organizations, and infrastructure. Therefore, evaluation of such systems must examine the technology, the human elements, and the interactions between them. In practice, this is reflected in study methods, including the division into *quantitative methods* and *qualitative methods*, with the former focusing on numeric measurement of effects, and the latter particularly focusing on the experiences and viewpoints of users.

It is important to address the needs of varied users and to examine systems at each stage, from original requirements gathering to long-term performance. Box 24.1 shows a summary of these stages. In *stage one*, problem definition includes requirements gathering and translation into design and architecture. Mistakes here will clearly impact the ability of the system to address user needs. In *stage two*, bench testing addresses the issue of ensuring the software and hardware combination is stable, usable, and ideally is shown to work well with authentic test data. *Stages three to five* are more conventionally thought of as HIS-evaluation targets, but the distinctions are important here. *Stage three* is based on observing the use of systems in real environments. This is particularly important for environments with poor infrastructure, as often seen in LMIC. Systems need to be *functional* and *used* regularly by staff, and key functions like reports and decision-support tools need to function effectively. *Stage four* is where typical impact studies take place, such as randomized controlled trials. *Stage five* represents monitoring the longer-term use of the system once deployed. With the rapid changes in health systems and technology, a system that works in the initial implementation will not necessarily continue to do so longer term. In addition, the roll-out of a system to new sites often throws up new problems that need to be detected and addressed.

This had led to the development of a variety of evaluation frameworks, one of which is shown in box 24.1.

Box 24.1
Five Levels of Evaluation [2]

1. Problem definition
2. Bench testing
3. Field trials: Observational
4. Field trials: Interventional
5. Long-term follow-up

Formative and Summative Evaluation

A critical first stage in implementing and optimizing an HIS is ensuring that it is developed to address a real need and ensuring that its design and user interface are appropriate. (These issues are discussed in more detail in chapter 4 and chapter 21.) The next stage is ensuring that it functions as expected. This includes stability, speed and responsiveness, usability, usage, and data quality, tested in the real environment with real users, and represents stage three or four in box 24.1. This type of study is often referred to as a *formative evaluation*. It is typically carried out by, or in partnership with, the system developers and results in improvement to the system or implementation. These types of evaluations typically include quantitative and qualitative methods (see below for explanation). An example of a formative evaluation of electronic health record (EHR) system performance is given in the "Data Quality Improvement" section, below.

In contrast, an evaluation study intended to assess the impact of the fully operational HIS is often referred to as a *summative evaluation*. These types of evaluations are usually primarily quantitative and based on study designs intended to assess causality—randomized controlled trials (RCTs) and interrupted time series studies. In summative evaluations, the evaluators are usually more independent of the developers. These studies are usually at stage four and sometimes stage five in box 24.1.

Quantitative Evaluations

The main focus of this chapter in quantitative evaluation. In these studies, the goal is to assess the impact of using an HIS on some measurable endpoints. These could, for example, be the number of errors in drug prescribing or number of missed antenatal clinic appointments. Quantitative evaluations tend to be the best known and most commonly reported in the literature. They can provide rigorous evidence of the impact of the system on care, but may be less effective at explaining the underlying processes and sociotechnical issues that explain results (a key role for qualitative research studies). A range of study types include the following.

- *Demonstration studies.* These assess whether a system behaves as expected based on its design.
- *Comparative studies.* These include intervention and control groups to allow comparison of the intervention and usual care. These are the most common type in the literature.

Control Groups

Scientific studies of the impact of an intervention require a comparison group that stays the same when the intervention is introduced. There are many types of controls:

- historical
- contemporary
- matched
- randomized
- time series.

One of the simplest designs is a "before and after" study of clinical data collection and use, and is carried out when an HIS is implemented. If there are any changes measured in process and outcomes, these may be due to the new system. Unfortunately, these changes may be, and often are, due to unrelated changes in the health system, staffing, other technologies, and so on. Such *historical controls* do not work well for studies of complex interventions, particularly in LMIC where many changes may be happening at once. *Contemporary controls* are other sites, subjects, or groups that are compared to the intervention group. The approach can avoid the biases due to unrelated changes in the health system seen in historical controls, but unfortunately can introduce a different set of potential biases. The other sites may be different from the intervention sites, and therefore not provide a valid comparison. *Matched controls* are selected by statistical comparison with the intervention sites to be similar on key variables such as patient numbers, age, gender, and severity of illness, as well as characteristics like infrastructure, power, networking, and staff IT skills. This approach reduces the risk of bias, but finding good matches is an imprecise process (see chapter 4 for more in-depth discussion of these issues).

Causality: Determining Whether a Health Information System is Responsible for a Change Measured

As noted earlier, when an HIS is implemented, there are likely to be other changes in the health system that may be responsible for any observed differences. The best accepted way to show that changes are due to the HIS is to carry out an RCT. The key features of an RCT are the presence of one or more control groups that don't have the system and the randomization in the selection of these groups. If control subjects or groups are selected by nonrandom methods, it is very difficult to avoid baseline differences between the groups that can lead to bias. In typical RCTs for testing medications, there is an additional feature—double blinding. This means ensuring that neither the patient nor the doctor is aware of whether the patient is receiving the drug or the placebo. This reduces any bias in assessment of the patient. While such an approach could be valuable in studying HIS, it is rarely feasible to hide the use of the HIS.

There are other ways in which it can be possible to attribute causality to an HIS. One example is an *Interrupted Time Series*. In this case a group is studied (e.g., a group of patients) and after a certain period (period 1), the HIS is implemented for a while (period 2), then deactivated (period 3). This may be repeated multiple times. If there are improvements in the study group that are only seen with the HIS, then disappear when it is deactivated, it is likely they are due to the HIS, not other unrelated changes. An example is a decision-support system for chest pain patients incorporated into an ECG machine. In one study, the decision support was switched on and off multiple times [3]. A variant of this approach is studying the roll-out of an HIS such as an EHR to many sites over a period of time in a region or country by examining data submitted to a central site such as a national reporting system (e.g., DHIS2; see chapter 41 in book supplement). If site implementations are carried out on multiple known dates, then any changes in submitted data that occur *consistently* after the HIS is implemented are likely to be due to the system. Other methods for showing causality rely on "natural experiments" when the implementation of the HIS occurs in some site, but not others, due to factors unrelated to the local health system.

Evaluation Matrix: Stakeholders and Possible Evaluation Questions

Table 24.1 breaks down the different evaluation questions and types by the stage of HIS development and implementation and key stakeholders. It is intended to give examples of what type of evaluation study may be useful for a specific project.

Utilization-Focused Evaluation

An important innovation for studies in LMIC is utilization-focused evaluation [4]. This is an approach to ensuring that evaluations are of relevance and use to key stakeholders in the organization implementing the HIS, and are not just focused on questions of interest to, for example, academics and policy makers. The method employs standard stages: (1) identify key stakeholders; (2) determine their evaluation questions; (3) design studies to answer those questions; (4) feedback results to stakeholders. A potential disadvantage of the approach is that involvement of stakeholders may be perceived to bias the study. This may be addressed by involvement of external researchers in the design,

Table 24.1

Matrix of example questions for different stakeholders at each evaluation stage (items may apply to more than one stage)

Stakeholder	Requirements gathering	Design and development	Initial deployment	Scale-up	Long-term use
Clinician	What is the clinical problem? Clinical workflow, quality of care, efficiency of care	User interface, mapping of key activities and workflow, managing risk of errors or failure	Stability, speed, efficiency, security, adaptability, data quality, learnability	Quality of care, reducing errors, effect on speed of care delivery, ease of reporting and administration, evidence of clinical impact	Stability, extensibility, interoperability, maintainability, access to data for clinical care and research
Patient	Access to care, support in care, information, confidentiality	Assessment of information needs, user interface design and testing	Ease of use, quality of explanations, accessibility	Able to cover a range of key issues, delivery of key information like lab results [18], positive feedback from other patients	Good long-term stability and support, growth to new clinical areas
Health service manager	Quality, costs, efficiency	Cost of development, quality of software, suitability of architecture for interoperability and scalability	Stability, speed of implementation, quality of training resources, usage levels and satisfaction, data quality, cost of initial deployment [14], staff job satisfaction	Efficient scale-up and roll-out, compliance with clinical guidelines, evidence of clinical impact, efficient and accurate reporting, data quality, ability to monitor clinics and care processes	Stability, good usage and satisfaction levels, adaptability, total cost of ownership [31]
Developer	Accurate requirements and use cases	Effective software development strategy correctly applied, software testing strategy, user interface testing strategy	Effective implementation plan, training of implementers, formative evaluation of system	Monitoring of roll-out, measurement of stability, usage rates, technical problems	Total cost of ownership, effectiveness of interoperability, ability to support and upgrade system in the field.
MOH	Quality of care, access to care, surveillance, planning	Stability and safety of software, extensibility, interoperability, local support	Implementation plan, usage and acceptability by staff, data quality, reporting quality, and speed	Ability to scale up, scale-up planning, effectiveness of support for national health strategy	Stability, security, extensibility, interoperability, total cost of ownership

implementation, and analysis of the study or following up positive findings in larger and more independent study, or both.

Biases in Evaluation Studies of Health Information Systems

As noted above and in chapter 5, there are a number of potential biases in evaluation of HISs. These discussed in detail in a textbook by Friedman and Wyatt [5] and summarized here. While it is difficult to completely eliminate biases, good design can minimize their effects (+ and – symbols refer to biases that tend to increase or decrease respectively the apparent effect of the HIS).

- *Volunteer effect* (+): recruiting subjects who are keen to use the system and not typical users can lead to better outcomes than those from typical users.
- *Assessment bias* (+/−): in a non-blinded study, participating clinicians may rate intervention patients as healthier or better in some way than the controls when there is no real difference. This can also cause a negative bias.
- *Placebo effect* (+): the presence of the system may change behavior due to user expectations and lead patients to report better outcomes.
- *Checklist effect* (+): structured recording of data on a form can improve data completeness and quality, and therefore improve the processes of care being studied, independent of use of the HIS.
- *Hawthorne effect* (+): monitoring users as part of the study makes them change behavior and potentially try harder to work with the HIS.
- *Carry-over effect* (−): users who have access to decision support for some patients and not others learn from the system and improve care of control patients.
- *Allocation and recruitment bias* (+): evaluators recruit users or patients who are likely to benefit from use of the system.
- *Secular trends (+):* the problem of historical controls; many other changes and improvements are going on at the same time as the study, making improvements hard to attribute to the HIS.

Qualitative Evaluations

These studies focus on the experience of the users of an HIS and assess issues like user satisfaction, ease of use, barriers to effective use of HIS, and social and cultural influences on adoption and use of systems. Clearly, these issues can be of high relevance in LMIC, which have a range of environments and limited experience with information technology. This information is valuable in assessing how users interact with the system and whether those interactions are positive or negative. A key benefit of such studies is understanding how well the HIS fits with the workflow and activities of users and how the system design can be improved. User feedback usually provides important insights into the likelihood that the system will scale and also have a beneficial impact.

Kaplan and Maxwell describe the use of qualitative methods for health informatics in detail [6]. They suggest a qualitative approach can be helpful for the following research questions and situations:

- to determine what might be important to measure or why measured results are as they are; if the subject of study cannot be measured easily.

- to understand not only what happened or what people are responding to, but why; to understand how people think or feel about something and why they think that way, what their perspectives and situations are and how those influence what is happening; to understand and explore what a technology (e.g., a newborn nursery telemonitoring system) or practice (e.g., using a computer to access health information) means to people.

- to investigate the influence of social, organizational, and cultural context on the area of study, and vice versa.

- to examine causal processes, and not simply what causal relationships exist.

- to study processes as they develop and emerge, rather than in outcomes or impacts; for example, to investigate the development process for the application under study in parallel with that process so that you can improve the application development as it progresses.

Methods used in qualitative studies of HIS include semi-structured questionnaires to elicit user views and experiences, focus groups, and observation of users interacting with systems under real-world or experimental conditions. Rose et al. describe the use of "qualitative studies to improve the usability" of an EHR, emphasizing the importance of assessing user needs and experiences with a "results manager" component of an EHR. They used task analysis and focus groups and combined the results to make recommendations for improving the design of the results manager [7]. In another example, Zakane et al. used semi-structured interviews to study the "needs of and attitudes towards a computerized clinical decision-support system in rural Burkina Faso." They found interest in and support for an HIS and decision-support systems to improve maternal and child health, but concerns that the systems would be difficult to learn and might increase work load [8].

These methods also help researchers to understand the meaning and context of items being studied and the underlying dynamics of the processes and the way they impact users. Chapter 6 discusses some of the consequences of implementing health interventions in LMIC and the importance of studying the broader consequences and potential risks. Related to these ideas, Farach and colleagues used semi-structured interviews conducted mainly by Skype to assess the impact of HIS initiatives in addressing the health needs of underserved populations in Latin America and the Caribbean. They reported that HISs can benefit the health needs of such populations [9].

Some researchers go as far as arguing that quantitative, sometimes called "objectivist" studies cannot capture the important sociotechnical interactions that are the real determinants of success and failure of HISs, and therefore are not valid without qualitative studies [10]. There are many examples of technically sound HIS projects that failed due to sociocultural issues. Conversely, there are many projects that failed due to poor design, development, and implementation of software or infrastructure weaknesses. As this chapter should make clear, there are a range of factors that need to be considered in effective evaluation studies, and qualitative research methods are a key element in the mix. While there is not space here to provide an in-depth discussion of the principles and techniques of qualitative research, readers are encouraged to consult the reading list and also consider collaborating with qualitative researchers in their studies.

Economic Evaluation

One area of HIS deployment in LMIC that currently has very little evaluation evidence is the cost of these systems. There are several key principles that are important in assessing the real costs of an HIS and comparing those with evidence of benefits. Readers are encouraged to explore this important topic in more detail (e.g., in references [11] and [12]).

Accurately measuring the true cost of an HIS requires assessing the following items required for *initial implementation*:

• hardware and IT costs

• improvements needed in infrastructure, such as building work, power, networking, and air conditioning

• software development or purchase, including all adaptation and improvement costs

• implementation costs, including staff time for training and reduced productivity during changeover

• training of users and support staff

• IT support staff.

In addition, the costs of *running the system over several years* must be measured. These include:

• ongoing staff costs for IT support, training, data management, analysis, and so on

• replacement hardware such as servers, clients, and networking

• supplies and monthly costs such as printing, network subscriptions, and power

- ongoing software costs, which could include licenses, essential improvements, upgrades, and security fixes.

Combining these items creates the *total cost of ownership*. This figure is critical in assessing which HIS projects make most sense, since initial costs may give a misleading impression of the longer-term costs. This is especially true with proprietary software with high license fees and projects dependent on reliable network connections, which may be expensive (and possibly unreliable despite the cost).

More advanced economic evaluations take into account the impact of the HIS as well as the cost. These include *cost-effectiveness* analysis, where the total cost of ownership is combined with measured benefits of the HIS to show the cost of a specific, measured improvement per specific health outcome, patient, or health facility. *Cost-benefit* analysis is similar, except that it considers an array of benefits and assigns a financial value to each—a more difficult and controversial approach, especially in LMIC. Both techniques rely on an accurate evaluation of the actual benefits of the HIS, so must be combined with rigorous outcome studies.

Two examples of costing studies illustrate some of these key principles. Saronga and colleagues examined the cost of implementing a decision-support system for maternal care in Tanzania. They detail the many items that need to be costed, including vehicles and transport, computers and IT hardware, furniture, buildings, software, personnel, training, and supplies and communication. These were grouped into "installation and operation costs; capital and recurrent costs; and fixed and variable costs." The total cost reported was $185,927, with 77% incurred in the installation phase. Training and software were the largest cost items, at 33% and 32% of total cost, respectively [13].

A study by Driessen and colleagues looked at the potential cost savings from implementing an EHR system in a hospital in Lilongwe, Malawi [14]. They costed both the implementation of the EHR and the running cost over 3–5 years. They also modeled the costs that could be saved by improving efficiency of processes, such as the labeling and tracking of laboratory samples. The hospital typically had substantial losses due to discarded samples and repeating tests due to poor labeling. This problem was addressed by the creation of bar-coded ID labels and cards from the EHR system. An actual prospective evaluation is required to assess the true costs and savings.

Examples of Key Studies in LMIC

There are an increasing number of studies of HISs in LMIC being published over the last decade. An early systematic review of the literature in 2010 showed initial evidence of benefits of these systems in a number of areas [15]. These benefits have been largely confirmed by more recent and rigorous studies, some of which are enumerated below:

- tracking patients through treatment initiation and monitoring adherence, then detecting those at risk for loss to follow-up (e.g., text messages to increase antenatal clinic adherence [16] and to encourage HIV-positive patients to return for treatment [17])

- decreasing time to create administrative reports (many unpublished studies)

- tools to label or register samples and patients (such as labeling and tracking of samples in a hospital in Malawi [14])

- collection of clinical or research data using personal digital assistants (now confirmed in a number of mHealth projects)

- reduction in errors in laboratory and medication data [18,19]

- reminding patients of health care actions (such as text-messaging reminders for HIV treatment [20,21], although there are also some negative studies of these approaches)

More recent systematic reviews have examined the impact of mHealth systems on health service delivery processes [22], and on care of patients with HIV [23]. They have shown progress in certain areas such as text-messaging reminders to patients to take medications for HIV, but emphasized the need for more and better studies. Based on the experience of this study, Free et al. also note the importance of clearer descriptions of the underlying interventions to better understand what was done and how to reproduce it.

In 2011, there was a meeting in Bellagio, Italy, to encourage more and better evaluation studies in LMIC. This led to the development of a call to action for eHealth evaluation and a set of nine principles to do so (see the recommendations for further reading at the end of this chapter).

Data Quality Improvement

Good data quality is absolutely fundamental to achieving positive benefits from HISs. Worldwide, all HISs have challenges with data quality, though these are often greater in LMIC.

Data quality is primarily defined by the following three metrics.

- Data completeness (is there missing data?)

- Data timeliness (is data entered in time for required uses?)

- Data accuracy (is data a true reflection of the real-world items being measured?)

A useful principle is to determine if the data is "fit for purpose." This metric will differ depending on the type of use. So, for example, data for clinical care or research needs to be highly accurate, but timeliness requirements may vary. It may be acceptable for research data to be entered sometime after the patient is seen, but clinical data needs to be available as soon as possible, especially in a hospital setting. While it is unlikely that HIS projects can completely eliminate poor data, there are several strategies that should be applied to improve it:

1. ensure that staff collecting and entering data can see how it is used and, in general, get benefit from their own data. When clinical staff and other health care workers enter data directly, they should be able to see what they entered and summaries or reports created from it. Many public health projects in LMIC have a "one-way ticket" with staff who are required to collect data, for example for a monthly report on HIV patient care, sending it off on forms to be used at district or national levels and never seeing the results [24].

2. provide training to staff collecting and entering data to help them maintain high accuracy. This should be supplemented with tools to measure data quality and opportunities for staff to recommend ways to improve data quality.

3. ensure that the HIS is well designed and tested, possesses a good user interface and clear methods for coding and export of data, and runs on stable hardware and networks. For direct data entry by clinical staff, the system must be available during all clinic hours. Significant down time is highly disruptive and will result in loss of confidence in the system and likely reduced use.

4. ensure that a unique ID is issued for each patient and used for all entries in the EHR. This will reduce errors, for example, mis-entry of data into the wrong record, duplicate entries that are not easily found by clinicians, and poor naming of lab samples leading to lost results.

5. automate uploading data from other systems where possible. This is particularly valuable for laboratory data. Many EHR systems can upload lab data using open interoperability standards like HL7.

6. resist the temptation to collect more than the essential data needed for clinical care, or if additional data is required for example for research, add extra staff and resources.

Most importantly, data quality must be measured regularly—ideally, daily, and action taken promptly to fix problems. Several studies have shown significant improvements in data quality for care of HIV, multidrug-resistant TB, and maternal health patients with the implementation of HISs in LMIC, via the use of better tools and training [18, 25–27].

Example: Real-Time Assessment of System Performance and Data Quality

An example of monitoring and evaluation of system performance and data quality is being implemented in Rwanda as part of an evaluation of the impact of an EHR system (OpenMRS) that has been rolled out to over 300 clinic sites by the Rwandan Ministry of Health. Many sites have limited or unstable power, and Internet access is variable and sometimes completely unavailable. To ensure intervention sites are performing well, each will have the following metrics measured:

1. EHR system uptime and downtime, both frequency and total duration
2. EHR data completeness for key variables
3. EHR system usage, including viewing of key pages and data entry into forms by staff.

These metrics are being measured with a custom software module, and results will be transmitted to a central server on a daily basis (via the mobile network in many sites). In addition, periodic site visits will be made to assess data quality in the EHR versus paper records or other data sources. The study will also survey users on their experience using the EHR and what improvements may be required. This will be supplemented by a qualitative research study interviewing a subset of users and observing them working with the HIS. This study can be classed as a formative evaluation of system performance (or sometimes a Process Evaluation) and will be followed by actions to improve sites where performance falls below certain thresholds on one or more metrics.

The Learning Health System

A range of new initiatives are bringing together many of the key initiatives described in this chapter and more broadly in the book to create a system for continuous measurement and quality improvement in health systems. Entitled the Learning Health System, part A (figure 24.1) combines the processes of data collection and analysis with the development of new knowledge. This part of the process may lead to publication of clinical insights. Part B describes the process by which the insights into clinical care and workflow are turned into guidelines and clinical decision-support tools (or other health care improvements) to support improved quality of care.

Critical to these processes are the feedback loops that support clinical care. Loop 1 is use of clinical data for direct care, an essential part of ensuring clinician buy-in and oversight of data quality. Loop 2 is the development of knowledge based on analysis of multiple records (Part B above). Loop 3 is the publication of new knowledge that informs broader health care initiatives. By combining all three processes based on routine clinical data collection, resources can be shared for data-quality control processes.

Conclusion and Future Directions

Evaluation studies are intimately linked to methods and processes to improve the quality of HIS projects. Working through the different stages of evaluation and addressing the needs of key stakeholders should ensure that appropriately targeted, well-designed and programmed HISs are created that are also easy to use and viewed as helpful by users.

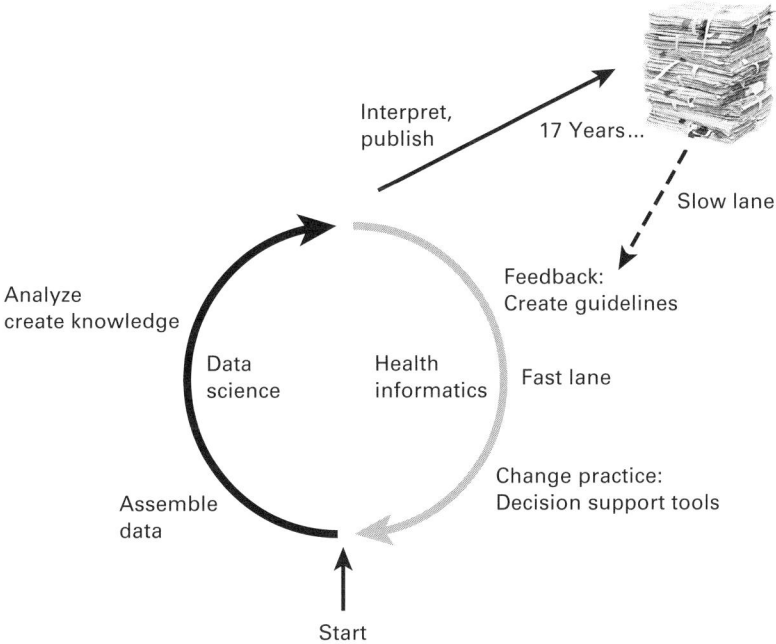

Figure 24.1
The learning health system (adapted from Friedman [28]).

A high-quality HIS of this sort will not guarantee success in all projects, since the complexities of different organizations and cultures may lead to unanticipated problems. However, most big failures of HISs are attributable to major errors in requirements gathering, design, programming, or implementation—known and preventable problems [29]. Frequently, systems are not complete or not designed for the purpose and workflow for which they are being used, or they are difficult to use and lack user testing. A particular challenge in LMIC are HISs that require much better infrastructure than is available, including power, networking, Internet, and effective IT support. The process of monitoring daily usage of an HIS, including uptime, page views, and data completeness, goes a long way to ensure that failures are detected early—offering opportunities to correct the problem or in some cases cancel the project and go back to the drawing board.

Another strategy for successful system implementation is to combine "bottom-up" and "top-down" approaches. The bottom-up approach ensures that HIS projects address clinical needs and problems, focus on local ownership and priorities, and prioritize data quality. These approaches help to ensure the project works well in the original site. The top-down approach includes planning for wide use, a horizontal approach to health care delivery where systems can cover a whole range of diseases and clinical problems, along with a focus on creating a core dataset and supporting open standards and interoperability. Both approaches should be married, along with a focus on evaluation and evidence-based decision making.

Finding the resources, expertise, and time to carry out effective evaluation of an HIS remains a concern for many organizations, but, as described here, there are many different approaches that can be applied. In addition, even small, formative evaluations can be very useful, both for the implementing organization and as lessons for the wider community [30]. The alternative cost of avoiding evaluation can be very high—large-scale projects that fail in expensive and embarrassing ways due to elementary and preventable errors.

Questions for Discussion

• Choose a project you are familiar with and critically examine what tools are in place to monitor and improve data quality. What else should be done to maximize data quality

• Choose a specific evaluation question and list all the stakeholders likely to be interested in it. At what stage or stages in the life cycle of a health information system is it most relevant to carry out an evaluation?

• Taking the example from the previous question, what biases are likely to be important in the evaluation study you have in mind?

• A randomized controlled trial performed a decade ago showed that a web-based health information system can improve the timeliness of, access to, and quality of laboratory data. Is that result likely to be relevant today for a project planning to use an mHealth application to support laboratory reporting? What is different, and what is likely to be similar?

Further Reading

The following articles and books provide additional depth for readers interested in carrying out evaluation studies.

• Friedman CP, Wyatt J. *Evaluation Methods in Biomedical Informatics*. Springer Science and Business Media; 2006. Textbook providing a comprehensive overview of the subject and how to perform evaluations studies, third edition due to be published 2015.

• Bellagio eHealth Evaluation Group. 2011. Call to Action on Global eHealth Evaluation. Consensus Statement of the WHO Global eHealth Evaluation Meeting, Bellagio, Italy, September.
https://www.ghdonline.org/uploads/The_Bellagio_eHealth_Evaluation_Call_to_Action
-Release.docx.

- Were MC, Nyandiko WM, Huang KT, Slaven JE, Shen C, Tierney WM, Vreeman RC. 2013. Computer-generated reminders and quality of pediatric HIV care in a resource-limited setting. *Pediatrics* 131(3): e789–e796.
  A key study showing use of RCT methodology to demonstrate impact of eHealth system on quality of HIV care in Kenya.

- Blaya JA, Shin SS, Yagui M, Contreras C, Cegielski P, Yale G, Suarez C, et al. 2014. Reducing communication delays and improving quality of care with a tuberculosis laboratory information system in resource poor environments: A cluster randomized controlled trial. *PLoS ONE* 9(4): e90110.
  A key study showing use of RCT methodology to demonstrate impact of eHealth system on access to critical laboratory data to improve management of drug resistant TB in Peru.

- Nykanen P, Brender J, Talmon J, de Keizer N, Rigby M, Beuscart-Zephir MC, et al. 2011. Guideline for good evaluation practice in health informatics (GEP-HI). *Int J Med Inform* 80(12): 815–827.
  A valuable framework for carrying out and documenting evaluation studies in Health Informatics.

- Aqil A, Lippeveld T, Hozumi D. 2009. PRISM framework: A paradigm shift for designing, strengthening and evaluating routine health information systems. *Health Policy Plan* 24(3): 217–228.
  This article describes a classic evaluation framework for health information systems with a focus on LMIC and patient-level data.

References

1. Fraser HSF, Blaya J, Choi SS, Bonilla C, and Jazayeri D. 2006. Evaluating the impact and costs of deploying an electronic medical record system to support TB treatment in Peru. *AMIA Annu Symp Proc* 2006: 264–268.

2. Stead WW, Haynes RB, Fuller S, Friedman CP, Travis LE, Beck JR, et al. 1994. Designing medical informatics research and library—resource projects to increase what is learned. *J Am Med Inform Assoc* 1(1): 28.

3. Selker, HP, Beshansky JR, Griffith JL, Aufderheide TP, Ballin DS, Bernard SA, et al. Use of the acute cardiac ischemia time-insensitive predictive instrument (ACI-TIPI) to assist with triage of patients with chest pain or other symptoms suggestive of acute cardiac ischemia: A multicenter, controlled clinical trial. *Ann Intern Med* 129(11): 845–855.

4. Patton MQ. *Utilization-Focused Evaluation.* Sage Publications; 2008.

5. Friedman CP, Wyatt J. *Evaluation Methods in Biomedical Informatics.* Springer Science and Business Media; 2006.

6. Kaplan B, Maxwell JA. Qualitative research methods for evaluating computer information systems. In Anderson JG, Aydin CE, eds. *Evaluating the Organizational Impact of Heathcare Information Systems*. 2nd ed. New York: Springer; 2005: 30–55.

7. Rose AF, Schnipper JL, Park ER, Poon EG, Li Q, Middleton B. 2005. Using qualitative studies to improve the usability of an EMR. *J Biomed Inform* 38(1): 51–60.

8. Zakane SA, Gustafsson LL, Tomson G, Loukanova S, Sié A, Nasiell J, et al. 2014. Guidelines for maternal and neonatal point of care: Needs of and attitudes toward a computerized clinical decision support system in rural Burkina Faso. *Int J Med Inform* 83(6): 459–469.

9. Farach N, Faba G, Julian S, Mejía F, Cabieses B, D'Agostino M, Cortinois AA. 2015. Stories from the field: The use of information and communication technologies to address the health needs of underserved populations in Latin America and the Caribbean. *JMIR Public Health and Surveillance* 1(1): E1.

10. Greenhalgh T, Russell J. 2010. Why do evaluations of eHealth programs fail? An alternative set of guiding principles. *PLoS Med* 7(11): E1000360. doi:10.1371/journal.pmed.1000360.

11. Levin H, McEwan P. 2001. *Cost-effectiveness analysis: Methods and applications* . Thousand Oaks, CA: Sage Publications.

12. Tan-Torres Edejer T, Baltussen R, Adam T, Hutubessy R, Acharya A, Evans DB, et al., eds. 2012. Making choices in health: WHO guide to cost-effectiveness analysis. Geneva, Switzerland: World Health Organization. http://www.who.int/choice/publications/p_2003_generalized_cea.pdf?ua=1.

13. Saronga HP, Dalaba MA, Dong H, Leshabari M, Sauerborn R, Sukums F, et al. 2015. Cost of installing and operating an electronic clinical decision support system for maternal health care: Case of Tanzania rural primary health centers. *BMC Health Serv Res* 15(1): 132.

14. Driessen J, Cioffi M, Alide N, Landis-Lewis Z, Gamadzi G, Gadabu OJ, et al. 2013. Modeling return on investment for an electronic medical record system in Lilongwe, Malawi. *J Am Med Inform Assoc* 20(4): 743–748.

15. Fraser HSF, Blaya J. 2010. Implementing medical information systems in developing countries, what works and what doesn't. *Proc AMIA Symp* 2010: 232–236.

16. Lund S, Nielsen BB, Hemed M, Boas IM, Said A, Said K, et al. 2014. Mobile phones improve antenatal care attendance in Zanzibar: A cluster randomized controlled trial. *BMC Pregnancy Childbirth* 14(1): 29.

17. Siedner MJ, Lankowski AJ, Kanyesigye M, Bwana MB, Haberer JE, Bangsberg DR. 2015. A combination SMS and transportation reimbursement intervention to improve

HIV care following abnormal CD4 test results in rural Uganda: A prospective observational cohort study. *BMC Med* 13(1): 160.

18. Blaya JA, Shin SS, Yagui M, Contreras C, Cegielski P, Yale G, et al. 2014. Reducing communication delays and improving quality of care with a tuberculosis laboratory information system in resource poor environments: A cluster randomized controlled trial. *PLoS One* 9(4): E90110.

19. Choi S, Jazayeri D, Mitnick C, Chalco K, Pachao F, Bayona J, et al. 2004. A web-based nurse order entry system for multidrug-resistant tuberculosis patients in Peru. *Proc. Medinfo* 11: 202–206.

20. Lester RT, Ritvo P, Mills EJ, Kariri A, Karanja S, Chung MH, et al. 2010. Effects of a mobile phone short message service on antiretroviral treatment adherence in Kenya (WelTel Kenya1): A randomised trial. *Lancet* 376(9755): 1838–1845.

21. Pop-Eleches C, Thirumurthy H, Habyarimana JP, Zivin JG, Goldstein MP, De Walque D, et al. 2011. Mobile phone technologies improve adherence to antiretroviral treatment in a resource-limited setting: A randomized controlled trial of text message reminders. *AIDS* 25(6): 825.

22. Free C, Phillips G, Watson L, Galli L, Felix L, Edwards P, et al. 2013. The effectiveness of mobile-health technologies to improve health care service delivery processes: A systematic review and meta-analysis. *PLoS Med* 10(1): E1001363.

23. Catalani C., Philbrick W, Fraser H, Mechael P, Israelski DM. 2013. mHealth for HIV treatment and prevention: A systematic review of the literature. *Open AIDS J* 7: 17–41.

24. Mate KS, Bennett B, Mphatswe W, Barker P, Rollins N. 2009. Challenges for routine health system data management in a large public programme to prevent mother-to-child HIV transmission in South Africa. *PLoS One* 4(5): E5483.

25. Amoroso C, Akimana B, Wise B, Fraser HSF. 2010. Using electronic medical records for HIV Care in rural Rwanda. *Stud Health Technol Inform* 160: 337–341.

26. Blaya JA, Cohen T, Rodríguez P, Kim J, Fraser HSF. 2009. Personal digital assistants to collect tuberculosis bacteriology data in Peru reduce delays, errors, and workload, and are acceptable to users: Cluster randomized controlled trial. *Int J Infect Dis* 13(3): 410–418.

27. Haskew J, Rø G, Saito K, Turner K, Odhiambo G, Wamae A, et al. 2015. Implementation of a cloud-based electronic medical record for maternal and child health in rural Kenya. *Int J Med Inform* 84(5): 349–354.

28. Learning Healthcare Project. http://www.learninghealthcareproject.org/section/background/learning-healthcare-system. Accessed 28/11/2016

29. Coiera E. 2013. Why e-health is so hard. *Med J Aust* 198(4): 178–179.

30. Fraser HSF, Blaya J, Choi SS, Bonilla C, and Jazayeri D. 2006. Evaluating the impact and costs of deploying an electronic medical record system to support TB treatment in Peru. *AMIA Annu Symp Proc* 2006: 264–268.

31. Dalaba MA, Akweongo P, Aborigo RA, Saronga HP, Williams J, Blank A, et al. 2015. Cost-effectiveness of clinical decision support system in improving maternal health care in Ghana. *PLoS One* 10(5): E0125920. doi:10.1371/journal.pone.0125920.

IV DIGITAL HEALTH APPLICATIONS

In the first three sections of this book, we focused on core concepts related to global health, health information technology, and management. In this section, we will bring these key ideas together by exploring potential opportunities for digital health applications. The section is not comprehensive—the potential areas within health care that may benefit from technology are unlimited and each year we are discovering more opportunities. For example, scheduling and appointment reminders, behavior change applications, artificial intelligence, and medical financial software were omitted simply because the size of this book could not permit us to illustrate all examples. We will, however, cover many of the fundamental digital health applications used today, such as tele-medicine and decision-support systems as well as areas that are ripe to be transformed by technology, such as supply-chain management and medication compliance.

There is some overlap between this section and part II, "Introduction to Health Information Technology." Some concepts in section two could have been placed in this section, such as electronic health records, registries, security, and secondary use of health data. However, they were placed in part II because these concepts are core to most health information technology systems. In addition, having a basic understanding of these concepts is critical for anyone who wishes to work in the field.

25 Mobile-Enhanced Telemedicine: Transcending Barriers to Access and Care with Wireless Communications Technologies

Lavanya Vasudevan and Alain Labrique

Take-Home Messages

- Telemedicine, the provision of remote medical assistance using information and communication technologies, seeks to improve access to medical care, extend continuity of care beyond the boundaries of health facilities, and improve patient outcomes while lowering costs.
- Mobile telemedicine leverages the growing global mobile-cellular subscriptions to increase the reach and scale of telemedicine programs and permit task shifting to nonclinical staff.
- Several challenges exist in mainstreaming mobile telemedicine, including adapting telemedicine applications to rapidly evolving information and communication technologies, the need for new standards and guidelines governing the use of these new technologies for medical care, and the need for evidence on impact of telemedicine applications on cost-effectiveness and patient health.

Introduction

In today's digital age, rapid advances in information and communications technologies (ICTs) are creating profound paradigm shifts in the way health information and medical care can be delivered to patients. With the advent of smartphones and increasing global mobile phone penetration, the field of telemedicine—the provision of remote medical care and health information to patients—is undergoing radical transformations. The ability of wearable sensors and handheld wireless communication devices to capture patient biometrics and behaviors continuously is enabling real-time monitoring and analysis of patient health status, allowing the provision of timely intervention but also improved self-efficacy and patient empowerment. Mobile technologies have extended the practicality and reach of telemedicine by reducing (in many instances), the need for specialized equipment or dependence on tethered landlines. This new era of mobile-enhanced telemedicine brings renewed promise of improved access to quality medical care and health information despite barriers that may prevent patients from physically interacting with clinical care providers, or increasing the frequency and reducing the costs of follow-up. In this chapter, we explore the expanding domain of mobile telemedicine, briefly review the history and evolution of the field, describe recent applications, and discuss future opportunities and challenges.

What Is Telemedicine?

Although there may not be a universally accepted definition of telemedicine (box 25.1), it classically has referred to the provision of remote medical care and exchange of health information over communication networks [1–6]. The requisite properties of telemedicine applications include (1) physical separation between the patient and the health provider, or between two or more health providers; and (2) use of information and communication technologies for collecting, storing, and disseminating health or medical information [4,7]. The goals of telemedicine systems are to improve access to care, extend continuity of care beyond the boundaries of health facilities, and, overall, seek improvements in patient outcomes while lowering costs [8]. Although classically, telemedicine use cases have been largely constrained to being extensions of fixed-site facility care, the ubiquity of mobile networks has led to the development of independent telemedicine services as a first point of care for areas where facility care coverage is extremely low (e.g., the mDoctor system in Bangladesh; or the Mera Doctor system in India, which allows patients to videoconference with doctors on demand through a smartphone application and receive prescriptions on their phones instantaneously, bypassing the need to travel to a health facility) [3,9,10].

The term telemedicine is sometimes used interchangeably with other domains of ICTs for health, namely telehealth and mHealth (box 25.1) [1–6]. Bashshur et al. proposed, in 2011, a possible taxonomic classification for these branches of ICT for health [1]. A recent framework to describe mHealth strategies for health-systems strengthening incorporates applications that some may be considered integral to mobile telemedicine—sensors and point-of-care diagnostics, (remote) data collection and reporting, electronic health records, electronic decision support, provider-provider communication, and provider training and education (figure 25.1) [11]. It is likely that the definitions of ICT for health subdomains will continue to evolve in the coming years in parallel with innovations and discovery of novel uses of mobile and wireless technologies in health care. (See chapter 7 for a detailed discussion of ICT for health taxonomy.)

Box 25.1
Definitions

Telemedicine (aka Telematics)

"The practice of medicine by means of an interactive audio-video communications system without the usual physician-patient confrontation." —Bird KT, 1971

"The use of medical information exchanged from one site to another via electronic communications to improve a patient's clinical health status. Telemedicine includes a growing variety of applications and services using two-way video, e-mail, smart phones, wireless tools and other forms of telecommunications technology." —American Telemedicine Association

"The delivery of health care services, where distance is a critical factor, by all health care professionals using information and communication technologies for the exchange of valid information for diagnosis, treatment and prevention of disease and injuries, research and evaluation, and for the continuing education of health care provides, all in the interests of advancing the health of individuals and their communities." —World Health Organization

Telehealth

"A broader range of health-related activities, including patient and provider education and administration, as well as patient care." —Bennett AM, 1978

mHealth

"Medical and public health practice supported by mobile devices, such as mobile phones, patient monitoring devices, personal digital assistants (PDAs), and other wireless devices." —World Health Organization

---

History of Telemedicine

Telemedicine emerged as a field, in part, from attempts to provide medical care where such services were sparse—in battlefields, on remote seas, and even in outer space (box 25.2) [2,7,12–14]. While early attempts at telemedicine involved experimentation with the transmission of medical information using technology and one-on-one demonstrations of remote medical care, classical telemedicine as we know it began in the 1960s, when remote medical care was provided to wider populations and in a variety of settings [2,7]. Early examples of classical telemedicine projects are [7,14]

- the Logan Airport Telemedicine Project, linking travelers to remote medical care at the Massachusetts General Hospital in Boston.
- the INTERACT system connecting seven northern England institutions providing a range of services such as speech therapy and dermatology consultations.

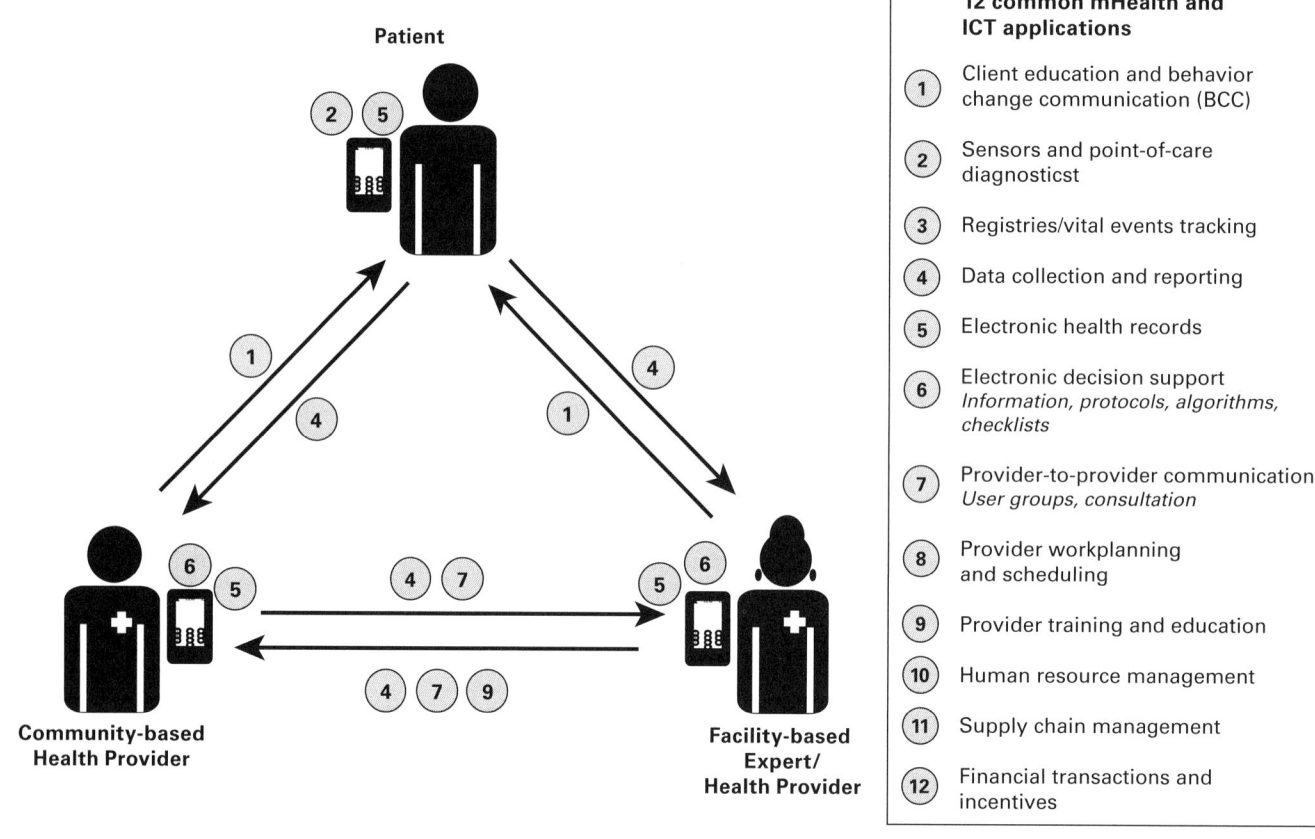

Figure 25.1
Illustration of the 12 common mHealth and information and communication technology applications in the context of a mobile telemedicine patient, community-based health provider, and facility-based expert/health provider communication triad.

- the Space Technology Applied to Rural Papago Advanced Health Care, or STARPAHC, telemedicine collaboration between NASA and the Indian Health Service to provide remote health care to the Papago reservation in Arizona.

Advances in web-based global communications networks ushered in the current digital era of telemedicine (1990–present) as communications technologies became cheaper, more ubiquitous, computationally more powerful and smaller in size, all the while enabling the integration of higher-quality images, audio, and text [7]. Mobile telemedicine (2003–present) represents the newest wave in a continued evolution of telemedicine, leveraging handheld, wireless devices such as mobile phones, tablets, or PDAs to facilitate delivery of health information and bolster medical care. In many cases, these devices are used in

Box 25.2
Evolution of Telemedicine with Advances in Information and Communications Technologies

1860–1905	Telegraph used to relay information to facilitate medical care management of wounded soldiers during the US civil war (1861–1865) and the Russian-Japanese war (1904–1905)
1905	William Einthoven transmits the first remote ECG signal from a distance of 1,500 meters between his laboratory and the academic hospital in Leiden
1920s	Radio transmissions used to communicate remote medical assistance to seafaring crews
1949	Invention of the color television enables first medical full-color videoconference
1957	The United States and Soviet Union develop wireless monitoring technologies to support telemetry in space; a dog named Laika aboard Sputnik 2 becomes first mammal monitored using telemetry in space
1965	Dr. Michael DeBakey, inventor of the artificial heart, performs first live transatlantic demonstration of aortal valve implantation
1967	Patients at the Logan Airport receive remote medical diagnosis by physicians at the Massachusetts General Hospital as part of the Logan Airport Telemedicine Project in Boston; Bird publishes first definition of telemedicine
2014	The number of mobile-cellular subscriptions in the world equals the world's population of 7 billion; wearable sensors and smartphone technology allow individuals to capture and share their physiological and behavioral data in real time

conjunction with sensors and other point-of-care diagnostic devices capable of capturing patients' vitals as well as other sociobehavioral and contextual metrics, irrespective of their physical location, to assist with monitoring, medical diagnoses, and subsequent pathways of care.

Current Applications in Mobile Telemedicine

Clinical implementations of mobile telemedicine cover a range of applications, including primary care and specialist referral services, remote patient monitoring (e.g., during home-based care), and medical education [3]. Typically, these implementations involve either asynchronous/store-and-forward approaches or synchronous/real-time interactions between patients and providers [4,13].

Store-and-Forward (Asynchronous) Approaches

Store-and-forward approaches represent the capture and storage of patient medical information (e.g., blood glucose readings, pictures of suspicious skin lesions) for consultation with a health provider at a later time. Most common applications of store-and-forward approaches are seen in radiology, pathology, oncology, ophthalmology and dermatology, and other situations where real-time interactions may not be necessary or practical [13]. The ubiquitous availability of camera phones and other portable diagnostic technologies are enabling applications involving store-and-forward approaches to become more commonplace. An example of a store-and-forward approach is AliveCor's FDA-approved EKG monitor, which clips on to the back of smartphones to provide EKG readings on demand with an accuracy similar to standard EKG machines, but at a lower cost [15]. The readings may be shared with the doctor for further clinical action. For store-and-forward approaches, transmission of stored information may occur through e-mails, over the Internet, or thorough multimedia messaging on mobile phones from remote sites.

Real-Time (Synchronous) Approaches

Real-time interactions in telemedicine are more common in psychiatry, rehabilitation, cardiology, neurology, and gerontology, where live patient consultations occur routinely and diagnoses may be dependent on verbal interactions with patients. An example of real-time telemedicine interactions is the use of robotic intensive care unit telemedicine technologies to reduce delays in consultation with experts during neurological deterioration or strokes [16]. Real-time systems can also be used to provide instantaneous feedback to medical trainees in the prevention of medical errors and support continuing medical education [16].

Using Mobile Telemedicine to Facilitate Task Shifting in Resource-Limited Settings   The arena of global health has, perhaps, seen the most explosive growth in mobile telemedicine applications in the last decade, due to the ever-expanding mobile phone ownership and connectivity across the world [17]. In many countries, front-line community health workers serve as the only link to the health system for clients residing in rural or remote locations in the face of the global shortage of trained medical professionals [18]. While clients in these settings are constrained by the costs, time, and large distances to attend medical facilities, community health workers often work in isolation from the health system they are meant to serve, under the constraints of poor communications infrastructure, and with little to no formal medical training [19–21]. Mobile telemedicine has helped ameliorate these constraints in task shifting by enhancing nonclinical staff's capacity to identify, stabilize, and refer patients through the use mobile technology for provision of job aids, clinical decision-support algorithms, remote consultations, and data sharing [19–21]. Mobile devices have also been used as a medium for continuing medical education among health providers and community health workers in resource-limited settings. Mobile telemedicine applications have been demonstrated in supporting paramedical professionals in ambulances, mobile telemedicine units, and for providing remote medical assistance during disaster management. Examples of these task-shifting applications include:

- OScan, a scanning tool integrated with a camera phone, that can be used to document oral lesions. Images can be taken by health workers with basic knowledge of camera phones, and shared wirelessly with remote experts for diagnosis of oral cancer [22].

- eC3, a mobile phone camera—based cervical cancer screening tool that allows local health workers to capture images of suspicious cervical lesions and share them with remote experts for cervical cancer diagnosis [23].

- small portable ultrasounds (e.g., General Electric's VScan, Mobisante's MobiUS SP1, and Signostics' Sinos portable ultrasound device) with handheld touchscreen monitors or the ability to link to smartphones to permit on-the-go imaging by health workers at a fraction of the cost of traditional facility-based ultrasound machines [24–26].

- the *Chipatala Cha Pa Foni* 24-hour hotline service in Malawi, which allows health workers to use a decision-support software and electronic medical records to provide maternal and child health information, advice, and referrals to clients with access to mobile phones, potentially reducing time and costs of unnecessary travel to distant medical facilities for clients seeking health care [27].

- mobile technology platforms such as Sana, which link to electronic medical records and offer a programmable workflow interface for sharing medical information (e.g., audio, images, location-based data, text) and decision support. Sana has been used in rural South India to provide decision support to front-line health workers screening for pre-cancerous and cancerous oral lesions, and linking them to specialists at dental hospitals [28,29].

- closed user groups, such as Switchboard's MDNet in Ghana and Liberia, which empower different cadres of health providers to communicate, and hence improve their ability to provide quality medical care to patients in under-resourced settings [30].

- the eMocha TB Detect application, which streams multimedia education content and provides tuberculosis screening tools that can be accessed via mobile phones in resource-limited settings [31].

- the use of mobile phones to transmit images of patient X-rays and wounds during the 2010 earthquake in Haiti for consultation with medical experts in the United States [32].

These examples of task shifting illustrate how mobile telemedicine can be leveraged to allow lesser-trained workers to perform early phases of screening, thereby reducing the burden on advanced clinical staff, who may be in short supply in low-resource settings.

Challenges in Mobile Telemedicine

The ICTs underlying the implementation of mobile telemedicine are rapidly evolving [8,33]. Wearable tech and smartphones have taken the place of personal digital assistants and Blackberries just in the matter of the last decade. While evolution in technology has been accompanied by an increase in efficiency and quality, it also implies new costs and efforts in upgrading existing infrastructures, the need for standards and guidelines governing the use of new technologies for medical care, and the need for new methodologies for their evaluation. Many challenges remain in the implementation and testing of telemedicine programs, as described below.

- Despite the long history of telemedicine, there are few systematic evaluations of its efficacy and cost-effectiveness. Currently, the data to support clinical and cost-effectiveness of classical and mobile telemedicine interventions are mixed, although the benefits of these interventions as a substitute for in-person care are well accepted [8,34–37].

- While many patients welcome the opportunity to be connected to medical care or information irrespective of their location, others find this substitution to be impersonal and less trustworthy compared to a face-to-face encounter with the medical provider, especially in instances when medical prognosis is poor [38], However, there is data to suggest that the acceptability for using personal mobile devices for receiving health information and medical care is high, particularly among younger generations [34,39].

- Acceptability of mobile telemedicine among health providers also remains a challenge. Mainstream medicine has been slow to adopt telemedicine services due to lack of standards and guidelines for remote medical care, issues with reimbursements, and licensure and legal challenges surrounding the practice of telemedicine across state and national boundaries, to name a few. The future of mobile telemedicine relies on the development and implementation of standards and legislation that overcome barriers to the sustainable integration of such services within mainstream medicine [7,8,33,34,36,37,40].

- There is no doubt that the evidence base for mobile telemedicine is being strengthened through research efforts. However, there is still a lingering skepticism regarding its scalability and sustainability as few mobile telemedicine projects have been demonstrated at scale to date beyond initial periods of funding [34,35,41–44].

- Other challenges in the mainstream adoption of mobile telemedicine include patient privacy and security of medical data being transmitted wirelessly [36]. Access to data is also an issue, with the current system of electronic medical records being inaccessible to patients involved in disease self-management [40]. Data portability and software interoperability between different applications is another important challenge if telemedicine applications are to be used universally, highlighting the critical need for uniform data dictionaries and standards.

Several experts argue that mobile telemedicine programs will continue to play a critical role in health systems, despite the many challenges in implementing and testing such programs [8,36,45]. While the road to ubiquitous health care may be long, with increasing mobile phone coverage and reducing costs of communication technologies, especially in the developing world, the promise of putting health information and medical care at the fingertips of every human being on earth is slowly coming to fruition [7,17].

Questions for Discussion

- How has the rapid evolution of information and communication technologies impacted the maturity of telemedicine as a practical solution to health care needs?
- What are important regulatory challenges and concerns around mainstreaming telemedicine?

References

1. Bashshur R, Shannon G, Krupinski E, Grigsby J. 2011. The taxonomy of telemedicine. *Telemed J E Health* 17: 484 494.

2. Dumanskyy YV, Vladzymyrskyy AV, Lobas VM, Lievens F. 2013. *Atlas of the Telemedicine History*. Donetsk, Ukraine: International Society for Telemedicine and eHealth.

3. American Telemedicine Association. 2014. What is telemedicine?

4. World Health Organization. 2010. Telemedicine: Opportunities and developments in member states. Global observatory for eHealth series, Vol. 2. Geneva, Switzerland: World Health Organization.

5. World Health Organization. 2011. mHealth: New horizons for health through mobile technologies: Second survey on eHealth, Vol. 3.

6. Bennett AM, Rappaport WH, Skinner EL. 1978. *Telehealth Handbook*. PHS publication No. 79–3210. Washington, DC: US Department of Health, Education, and Welfare.

7. Bashshur RL, Reardon TG, Shannon GW. 2000. Telemedicine: A new health care delivery system. *Annu Rev Public Health* 21: 613–637.

8. Bashshur RL, Shannon G, Krupinski EA, Grigsby J. 2013. Sustaining and realizing the promise of telemedicine. *Telemed J E Health* 19: 339–345.

9. mHealth Ventures India Pvt. Ltd. 2015. Mera Doctor. http://www.meradoctor.com/.

10. ITmedicus. 2015. mDoctor. http://www.mdoctorbd.com/.

11. Labrique AB, Vasudevan L, Kochi E, Fabricant R, Mehl G. 2013. 12 common applications and a visual framework. *Glob Health Sci Pract* 1: 160–171.

12. Doarn CR, Merrell RC. 2014. Telemedicine in space medicine and extreme terrestrial analogs. *Telemed J E Health* 20: 405–407.

13. Moore M. 1999. The evolution of telemedicine. *Future Gener Comput Syst* 15: 245–254.

14. Higgins C, Dunn E, Conrath D. 1984. Telemedicine : An historical perspective. *Telecomm Policy* 8(4): 307-313.

15. AliveCor. Take control of your heart health.

16. Lilly CM, Zubrow MT, Kempner KM, Reynolds HN, Subramanian S, Eriksson E, et al. 2014. Critical care telemedicine: Evolution and state of the art. *Crit Care Med* 42: 2429–2436.

17. International Telecommunications Union. 2014. The world in 2014: ICT facts and figures. Geneva, Switzerland: International Telecommunications Union.

18. World Health Organization. 2007. Taking stock: Task shifting to tackle health worker shortages.

19. Global Health Workforce Alliance. 2010. Global experience of community health workers for delivery of health related millennium development goals : A systematic review, country case studies and recommendations for integration into national health systems. Geneva, Switzerland: World Health Organization.

20. Willis-Shattuck M, Bidwell P, Thomas S, Wyness L, Blaauw D, Ditlopo P. 2008. Motivation and retention of health workers in developing countries: A systematic review. *BMC Health Serv Res* 8: 247.

21. Källander K, Tibenderana JK, Akpogheneta OJ, Strachan DL, Hill Z, ten Asbroek AHA, et al. 2013. Mobile health (mHealth) approaches and lessons for increased performance and retention of community health workers in low- and middle-income countries: A review. *J Med Internet Res* 15: E17.

22. Prakash Lab. Date unknown. OScan: Screening tool for oral lesions. Stanford University. http://web.stanford.edu/~manup/Oscan/.

23. Parham GP, Mwanahamuntu MH, Pfaendler KS, Sahasrabuddhe VV, Myung D, Mkumba G, et al. 2010. eC3—a modern telecommunications matrix for cervical cancer prevention in Zambia. *J Low Genit Tract Dis* 14: 167–173.

24. GE Healthcare... VScan.

25. MobiSante: Imaging at the point of care. Date unknown. Smartphone ultrasound: The MobiUS SP1 system.

26. Signostics. Date unknown. Signos real-time personal ultrasound.

27. Crawford J, Larsen-Cooper E, Jezman Z, Cunningham SC, Bancroft E. 2014. SMS versus voice messaging to deliver MNCH communication in rural Malawi: Assessment of delivery success and user experience. *Glob Health Sci Pract* 2: 35–46.

28. Sana. Date unknown. Sana technology platform.

29. Celi LA. Date unknown. Sana mobile health platform. GSMA Mob Heal.

30. Switchboard. 2014. Switchboard: Mobilizing global health.

31. Johns Hopkins Center for Clinical Global Health Education. Date unknown. eMocha TB Detect. The Johns Hopkins Center for TB Research.

32. Louden K. 2010. Telemedicine connects earthquake-ravaged Haiti to the world. *Medscape Med News*, February 18.

33. Doarn CR, Merrell RC. 2014. Standards and guidelines for telemedicine — an evolution. *Telemed J E Health* 20: 187–189.

34. Ekeland AG, Bowes A, Flottorp S. 2010. Effectiveness of telemedicine: A systematic review of reviews. *Int J Med Inform* 79: 736–771.

35. Kim H-S, Hwang Y, Lee J-H, Oh HY, Kim Y-J, Kwon HY, et al. 2014. Future prospects of health management systems using cellular phones. *Telemed J E Health* 20: 544–551.

36. Newton MJ. 2014. The promise of telemedicine. *Surv Ophthalmol* 59(5): 559-567.

37. Nepal S, Li J, Jang-Jaccard J, Alem L. 2014. A framework for telehealth program evaluation. *Telemed J E Health* 20: 393–404.

38. Wyatt SN, Rhoads SJ, Green AL, Ott RE, Sandlin AT, Magann EF. 2013. Maternal response to high-risk obstetric telemedicine consults when perinatal prognosis is poor. *Aust New Zeal J Obstet Gynaecol* 53(5): 494-497.

39. Sankaranarayanan J. 2013. Rural patients' access to mobile phones and willingness to receive mobile phone-based pharmacy and other health technology services: A pilot study. *Telemed J E Health* 20(2): 182–185.

40. Bashshur RL. 2013. Compelling issues in telemedicine [guest editorial]. *Telemed J E Health* 19: 330–332.

41. Labrique A, Vasudevan L, Chang LW, Mehl GH. 2013. H_pe for mHealth: More "y" or "o" on the horizon? *Int J Med Inform* 82: 467–469.

42. Whittaker R, Mcrobbie H, Bullen C, Borland R, Rodgers A, Gu Y. 2012. Mobile phone-based interventions for smoking cessation. *Cochrane Database Syst Rev* 11: CD006611.

43. Free C, Phillips G, Watson L, Galli L, Felix L, Edwards P, et al. 2013. The effectiveness of mobile-health technologies to improve health care service delivery processes: A systematic review and meta-analysis. *PLoS Med* 10: E1001363.

44. Tomlinson M, Rotheram-Borus MJ, Swartz L, Tsai AC. 2013. Scaling up mHealth: Where is the evidence? *PLoS Med* 10: E1001382.

45. Merrell RC, Doarn CR. 2014. m-Health. *Telemed J E Health* 20: 99–101.

26 Clinical Decision Support

Jonathan M. Teich

Take-Home Messages

- Clinical decision support (CDS), whether embedded into electronic health record systems or in other contexts, is a key function of health information systems, facilitating improved quality, safety, and efficiency of health care.
- CDS can be very powerful in conjunction with electronic health records; the extensive clinical data present in those systems supports more comprehensive analysis, more detailed clinical knowledge models, and more sophisticated logic to provide highly precise, specific recommendations.
- CDS can be classified into ten basic types, each of which groups and presents information in different ways. Different clinical settings and tasks call for the use of different types of CDS. Care should be taken to avoid overuse of alerts, which can disrupt the workflow and cause user frustration when used excessively.
- CDS systems need to be built on sound scientific knowledge and models, and must be well designed, tested, and evaluated clinically.
- CDS has many applications in low- and middle-income countries. It is well suited to common clinical problems such as infectious disease and chronic care management, and provides extra knowledge support where there are shortages of skilled health care workers.

Introduction

Humans are excellent at certain tasks. Humans are notably superior to computers in making strategic decisions, recognizing patterns, planning, noticing unusual events, doing procedures, providing empathy. At the same time, humans make mistakes, and we make them in repeatable patterns. We miss details, we forget individual facts, we cannot always recall the most significant pieces of information at the time they are needed. In health care, this human failing leads to errors of commission, such as incorrect dosing, and of omission, such as forgetting to provide timely drug therapy or vaccination. It also leads to inefficiencies, such as redoing tests more frequently than necessary. These errors can lead to adverse events and suboptimal outcomes. We know, for example, that fewer than 55% of all patients in the best medical centers get all of the available recommended preventive care management tests and vaccinations [1]. We also know that hundreds of thousands of hospitalized patients die each year from adverse events, many of which are preventable [2,3].

Clinical decision support (CDS) can help prevent these human errors and facilitate the consistent use of best clinical practices. CDS is a process for ensuring that health-related decisions and actions are informed by pertinent patient information and clinical knowledge to enhance health and health care delivery [4]. CDS entails providing clinicians and patients with a combination of clinical knowledge and patient data, intelligently filtered or presented at appropriate times, to help make the best decision at a given point in time for a given patient.

To get a sense of this concept, think of the GPS routing apps found on many smartphones or installed in motor vehicles. Behind the scenes, these apps combine an impressive collection of technology: a satellite-derived fix on your current location (data), a map of every street in the area, and a routing algorithm to find the best route between any two points (domain knowledge). But to the user, the result of all this is filtered and presented in the clearest way: a picture of a street, an arrow, a voice saying "turn right." The GPS provides you with the precise information you need, in the most actionable format. Well-designed and implemented CDS provides much the same service, helping clinicians and patients decide which way to turn at any step in their management of a medical issue.

Types of Clinical Decision Support

One of the most recognizable CDS interventions is an allergy warning, a member of the *alert* CDS type (figure 26.1). In this instance, the clinician has started to enter an order for the antibiotic cefuroxime. The patient is allergic to penicillins, which can also indicate an allergy to the related cephalosporin drug class that includes cefuroxime. The clinician forgot or didn't know this about the patient, but the computer has kept track because that allergy was previously entered into the record. As soon as the drug name is entered, an alert screen appears, declaring that this order may be hazardous because of the patient's possible allergy. Supplemental decision-making information is provided to the clinician, specifically that the patient develops hives when exposed to penicillins, suggesting a more serious allergy. Importantly, at the bottom of the window the clinician can immediately make the decision and act on it: to cancel the order because of concerns about the allergy, or to override the recommendation, perhaps because the clinician knows that this patient has tolerated this medication in the past. Providing clear and precise information and

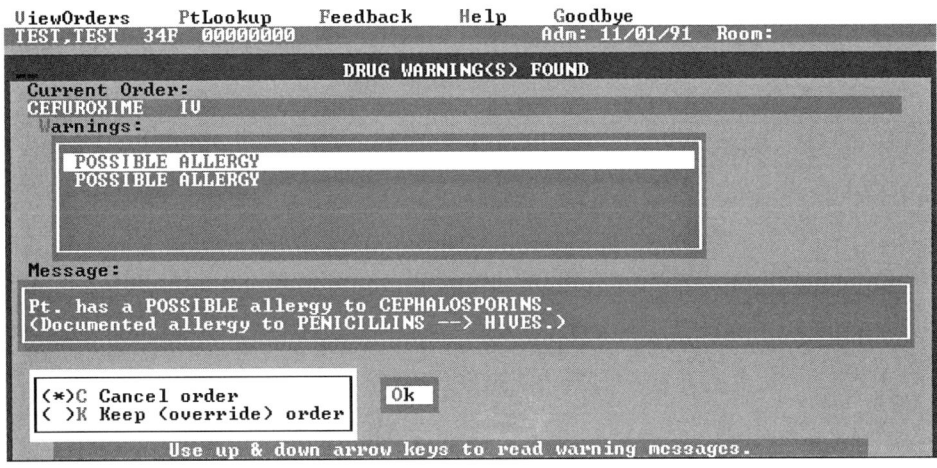

Figure 26.1
A standard allergy alert.

allowing the resulting decision to be executed right away are two features associated with successful, well-accepted CDS.

Alerts are an important and well-recognized form of CDS intervention, but must be handled with care. In fact, an increasing body of evidence suggests that alerts are often overused and that they disrupt the clinician's workflow too frequently (alert fatigue). As a result, clinicians may try to subvert the alerting process, learning quickly what buttons they have to press to make an alert go away rather than paying close attention to its clinical meaning [5].

In fact, there are 10 types of CDS interventions, each one suited for a particular point in the workflow and a particular clinical objective [6]. Some particularly important ones are described in detail in box 26.1.

An *order set* is a collection of prewritten orders suitable for a given clinical situation. For example, when admitting a patient with pneumonia, normally the clinician should order a chest X-ray, one or more antibiotics, perhaps blood cultures and certain other lab tests. Rather than making the clinician go through the time-consuming process of determining, selecting, and entering each of these orders individually (whether on paper or in a computerized order entry system), an order set can speed up the ordering process greatly, while also ensuring that the clinician sees the most recommended orders (as determined by the person or group that wrote the order set, often a hospital's quality committee) and has every opportunity to utilize those for the patient. Because ordering is a task that a clinician must do anyway, and because order sets are usually faster than individual order selection, they are generally well appreciated and well used by clinicians.

Box 26.1
Ten Key Types (Presentations) of Clinical Decision Support

1. Immediate alerts: Warnings and critiques
2. Event-driven alerts and reminders
3. Order sets, care plans, and protocols
4. Parameter guidance
5. Smart documentation forms
6. Relevant data summaries (single-patient)
7. Multi-patient monitors and dashboards
8. Predictive and retrospective analytics
9. Filtered reference information and knowledge resources
10. Expert workup advisors

Relevant data summaries provide the clinician with a subset of the patient's data, a subset chosen to facilitate one particular decision or to illustrate one particular clinical issue. For example, in a tuberculosis treatment program, a relevant data display may show all of the anti-TB antibiotics that have been used alongside the patient's culture results and clinical status indicators for the same time period. Figure 26.2 shows such a display in OpenMRS for multidrug-resistant TB (MDR-TB) patients, used in Haiti and other low- and middle-income countries (LMICs). The clinician can easily see and process this cluster of information without having to extract it from the clutter of all the other medications, tests, and findings in the record. Relevant data displays have been shown to significantly reduce medical errors in such areas as patient care handoffs from one clinician to another [7].

Filtered reference information can be especially useful when doing initial patient assessment or trying to understand a particular clinical issue or medical problem. If a clinician is seeing a patient with an unfamiliar illness, the clinician may need to pause, find a library reference, find the right section, and scan through that to get the information needed to further evaluate the patient. In the CDS version, the reference information is directly within the electronic health record, often in the form of a carefully placed hyperlink or "infobutton," and is pre-selected to be suited to the current situation and likely questions. The whole process is much faster, making it much more likely that the clinician will actually take the time to read and benefit from the information.

Analytics is coming into greater prominence as larger and more sophisticated databases come available. Analytic engines can combine dozens of parameters to make a decision, whereas traditional decision-support, and traditional human brains, normally can only handle a few factors at a time. As a result, analytics can allow us to make much more

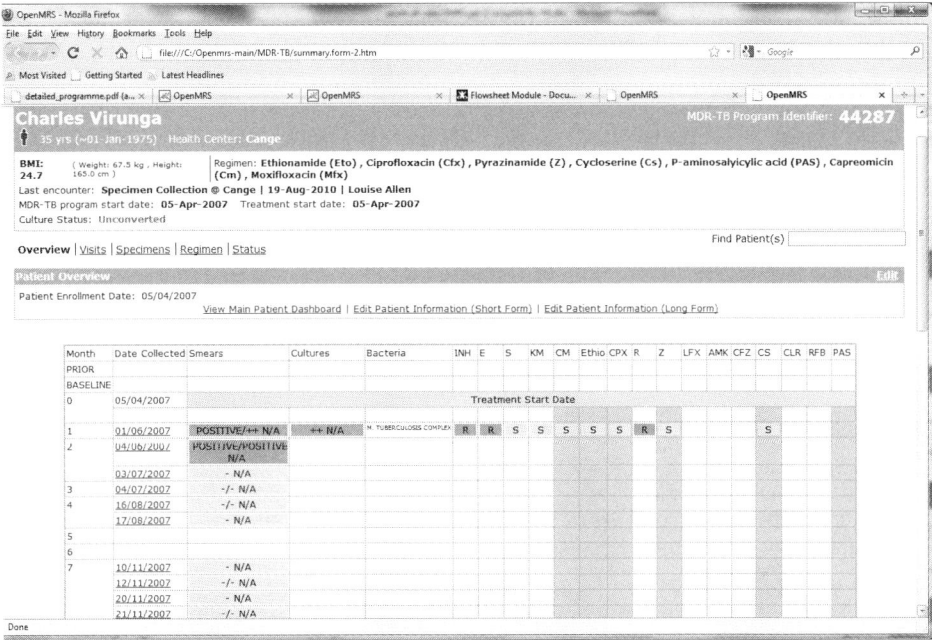

Figure 26.2
Display of key laboratory data for multidrug-resistant TB patient in Haiti using the OpenMRS-TB system (not real patient details). From Fraser HS, et al. 2013. E-health systems for management of MDR-TB in resource-poor environments: A decade of experience and recommendations for future work. *Stud Health Technol Inform* 192: 627–631.

specific recommendations and to separate similar but nonidentical patients much more precisely. New applications of analytics include selecting precise cancer treatments for individual patients and customizing management of chronic medical conditions such as congestive heart failure and diabetes (see chapter 15 for more information on clinical data analysis).

These different CDS presentation types are best suited to different processes and needs. Figure 26.3 is a general diagram describing the different stages of workflow and information used in any clinical patient encounter, from initial intake and assessment through diagnosis and treatment all the way to discharge and patient self-care at home. Each step has its own particular information needs and each lends itself to particular kinds of CDS. For example, in step C, when forming the overall plan of care, interactive reference can present evidence-based guidelines, outlining the specific diagnostic and therapeutic actions the clinician should take and the rationale behind those choices. When test results come back on step H, alerts and prompts can notify the clinician of abnormal or concerning results. Toward discharge, patient education and patient self-care guidance tools can be the most valuable.

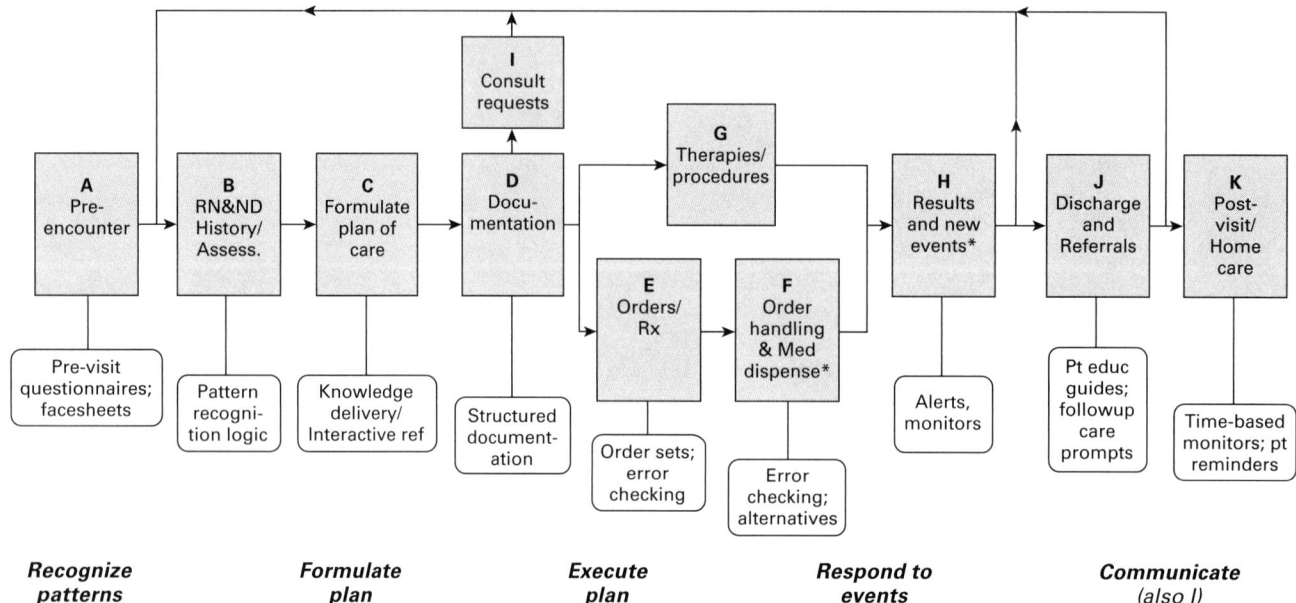

Figure 26.3
Stages of workflow and information use in a clinical encounter. From Osheroff JA, et al. Improving Outcomes with Clinical Decision Support: An Implementers' Guide, 2nd ed. Chicago: HIMSS Press, 2012. Reproduced with permission.

Key Elements of a Clinical Decision Support Intervention

Regardless of the type of CDS used, there are common design elements that need to be designed properly to ensure ease of implementation, acceptance by clinicians, and effectiveness in improving quality and safety (figure 26.4). Any type of intervention starts with a *trigger*—the initial event, action or passage of time that suggests that the logic of a particular CDS intervention should be checked. Examples of triggers include a lab test result prompting the computer to check for an abnormal-lab alert; a new diagnosis triggering a potential order set; an admission event prompting review of the patient's vaccination status; a discharge event triggering automatic suggestions for patient self-care materials, or the passage of time suggesting that a check should be run for missed drug doses.

Once triggered, the intervention *logic* goes into action to interpret the available data. The logic could simply determine that no new information needs to be presented at this time (e.g., if the lab test is abnormal but actually improving, the required dose has been given, or no new orders are needed). If the logic determines that there are alerts, suggested orders, or other information important enough to present to the clinician or patient, then the CDS system presents that information in one of the 10 forms described above. At

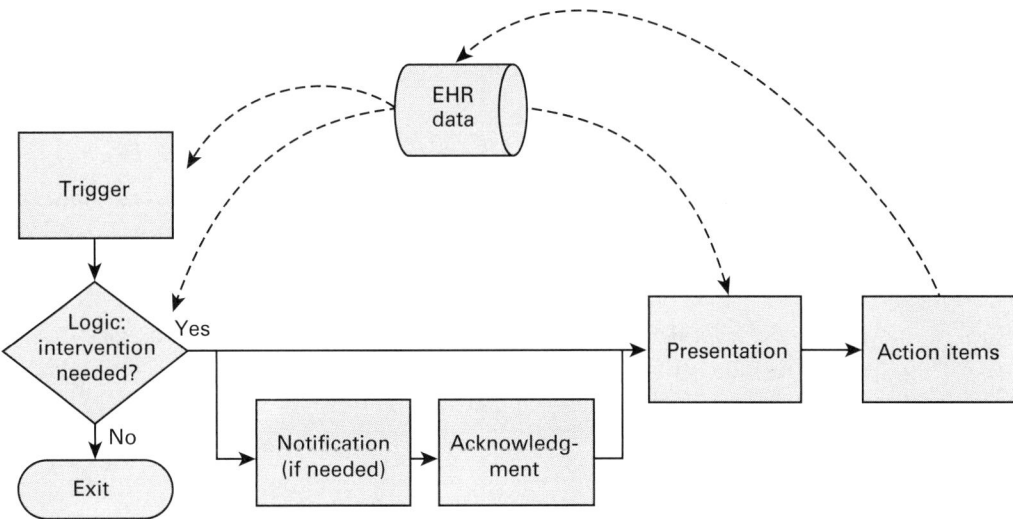

Figure 26.4
Core components of a CDS intervention. From Osheroff JA, et al. Improving Outcomes with Clinical Decision Support: An Implementers' Guide, 2nd ed. Chicago: HIMSS Press, 2012. Reproduced with permission.

that point, the clinician may select one or more *actions*. Actions typically include new orders, changing or stopping orders, viewing new information, posting a fact to the medical record, or, importantly, posting an exception—that is, a reason why the clinician chooses not to accept this particular CDS suggestion.

As a routine matter, a record should be made of all CDS interventions considered and presented and the clinical actions taken in response. This generates a database that is invaluable for short-term and long-term CDS evaluation studies, which will lead to much more precise and effective CDS in the future. Such a database is also an important tool for understanding patterns of illness progression and comparing effectiveness of different treatment approaches.

Impact of Clinical Decision Support

Properly designed and implemented, CDS can have a profound beneficial impact on process measures and on patient outcomes. Studies showed early on [8,9] that CDS could prevent 80% of errors and 55% of adverse events in a hospital service. Other studies have demonstrated significant reductions in incorrect dosing, increased use of guidelines, and reduction in readmissions.

On the other hand, some studies have shown that electronic medical record use (not CDS in particular) can be a contributing cause of new errors [10,11]. These errors were frequently due to awkward workflows or difficult-to-read information on the screen that led to, for example, writing orders for the wrong patient or selecting incorrect doses. Other CDS interventions could potentially be put in place to eliminate some of these problems. However, a key takeaway lesson is that CDS does not produce beneficial impact automatically; careful attention to design, communication, implementation, and usability for all health information technology is important if CDS is to make health care better and not worse. Another lesson from these studies is that CDS success depends on people factors—gaining support of key clinicians, strong communication with medical leadership, responsiveness to concerns and complaints—as much or more than it does on system design.

Overall, several reviews [12–14] have shown a net positive impact from CDS implementation and use, and improved usability and design will continue to increase its benefit for health care quality, safety, and cost.

Clinical Decision Support and Global Health

Much of the published literature on CDS systems comes from industrialized countries, which have had more time to evolve health information technology and more money and time to devote to CDS. However, the benefit that CDS can provide may be even greater in LMICs, where basic health needs are so great and where basic quality infrastructure may not yet be fully implemented. CDS tools that may be highly beneficial in LMIC include:

• vaccination reminder systems
• tracking and missed-event detection systems for field workers administering complicated drug treatments for infectious diseases such as MDR-TB [15]
• interactive reference guides for complex, unfamiliar, or unusual problems
• automatic printing of patient self-care materials for nutrition, hydration, chronic condition self-care, and more.

The recent Ebola outbreak in West Africa illustrates where effective CDS could make a real difference [16]. The recommended treatment regimen changed as the crisis progressed; this could be addressed with order sets and interactive reference clarifying the changes. As the endemic areas shifted, surveillance tools could be directed to the most critical areas. Contact-tracing systems could be matched against census information to ensure the best possible results. In developed countries where fear of importing cases of Ebola was very high, CDS was used to provide continually updated screening tools [17]. As new medications and vaccines for Ebola come into play, alerting systems could prompt clinicians in both developed and developing countries to be aware of these new treatment possibilities when they are seeing a patient with possible Ebola infection.

LMICs often have serious shortages of trained medical and nursing staff, leading to task shifting of clinical diagnosis and management to less skilled staff. The potential benefits of CDS are increased even more in these settings. Well-designed CDS systems can provide knowledge of optimal care patterns embedded into order sets, care plans, and smart documentation tools, while also providing expert situational awareness through alerts and reminders. Such tools have been beneficial, for examples, for nurses managing HIV patients in Kenya [18]; MDR-TB patients in Peru [15]; or community health care workers managing malaria in East Africa [19].

New Directions in Clinical Decision Support

New technologies and new health priorities make CDS available more widely, more rapidly, and in more forms than ever before. A few examples follow.

Genomics. Practical clinical applications of genomics are rapidly increasing. A key example in LMICs is the use of genomic information to detect mutations associated with drug resistance in a patient's particular HIV virus strain; the system could use this and other clinical data to provide recommendations for alternative regimens. The rapid advances in genomics over the past decade have led to enormous databases of gene variations, matched to corresponding phenotypic differences; this information is so dense that finding usable clinical meaning demands very skillful filtering and presentation—exactly the hallmarks of good CDS. The key challenge for CDS is to take a genome analysis, involving thousands of genes and billions of base pairs, and to bring back just enough information to the clinician and the patient that is actionable and not overwhelming. Sometimes this will mean that a medium-priority recommendation is worth showing for one patient but will add too much information clutter when applied to another—a social and psychological challenge as well as a technical one.

Big data and crowdsourced data. Even outside of genomics, big data and crowdsourcing are very interesting sources of CDS. Google Flu Trends [20] was an attempt to provide early analytic detection of spread of influenza into a new geographic region, based on the number of people in the region who were searching for topics such as "fever" and "headache." The first time this was tried during a large flu outbreak, it did not perform very accurately; it turned out there were many confounders, making it impossible to use the simple searching analysis hypothesized by the experimenters. However, with each experiment comes improved results; Google and other researchers are continuing to develop this form of analytic CDS to see if its predictive value can be improved.

Mobile clinical and self-care apps. These rapidly proliferating tools include portable drug-dosing applications, skin rash guides, smart documentation tools, and interactive reference for clinicians from large companies and research institutions that have traditionally provided similar information in other forms. They also include thousands of apps built by small companies or individuals that provide access to health records, fitness and nutrition guidance, pill-taking reminders, self-assessment for patients with chronic conditions, and many more. With billions of cell phones—many of them smartphones—active in nearly every country on the planet, the technology to support mobile CDS apps in every community and every practice is available to a far greater degree than existed even five years ago. However, there are concerns about the quality of the design, content, and logic for many health-related apps and the lack of effective evaluation [21]. An example of particular concern was an app designed to detect malignant melanoma that missed many cases, and therefore potentially discouraged patients from seeking lifesaving care. This highlights the importance of basing clinically important apps on sound evidence and clinical knowledge, and of carrying out rigorous evaluation studies.

Question answering. Medical errors and suboptimal care are often due to lack of immediately available best knowledge. Perhaps the needed knowledge was something that the clinician simply didn't recall and didn't have time to look up; perhaps it was new information recently published and adopted, so the clinician did not even know there was important information available. With millions of pages of new medical research published each year, there is no way for any individual to absorb all the relevant information that might be needed. Active research is being devoted to addressing this information overload in several ways:

- to understand the questions that are typically asked in clinical care and self-care (studies suggest that a doctor typically only asks 80 or 90 types of questions [22]) and to provide focused, accurate, and evidence-based answers, quickly enough that the clinician or patient can comfortably ask the question and make use of the answer.

- to make it easy for a clinician to become aware, when seeing a patient, that there is new information—that the treatment that he or she has always confidently used has been supplanted by a new recommended best practice.

- to make it easy to translate new primary research studies into usable guidelines much more quickly and effectively than we can do today.

Sharing of CDS. Once a new medication is invented and approved, it is easy to implement in a health care practice: systems are in place to register, procure, and store the new medication, add it to the drug database, and make it available in the ordering system. Even in low-income countries, procurement systems and supply chains are improving rapidly. When a new CDS intervention is developed and shown to be effective in one setting, though, it is currently very difficult to transfer it to another. Because of lack of interoperability standards, the same data element can have different vocabulary entries and different meanings from one place to another (for example, the status of being a "cigarette smoker" may be interpreted in different locations as being a heavy, moderate, occasional, or former smoker of cigarettes, cigars, pipes, or electronic cigarettes). Because there is currently no generally used standard for representing the 10 types of CDS from one electronic health record vendor to another, even the framework of the same desired intervention may vary widely, let alone the actual computer code.

There are ongoing projects to establish CDS intervention standards, and repositories or services that will make it easier to take effective, well-designed, quality-improving CDS from one hospital or practice to another one quickly and painlessly, even across different electronic health record (EHR) manufacturers and different clinical settings [23]; a number of these are making their way through standards bodies such as HL7. Another approach is to have a common EHR framework that is widely implemented so that CDS can be shared across a common code and standards base. The OpenMRS system (see chapter 40 in the online supplement to this book) includes a standardized concept dictionary of all clinical data items and standardized data structures. One goal of standardizing the dictionary is to allow decision-support tools, reports, and patient summaries to work on OpenMRS EHR systems implemented by different organizations. Work is currently under way to share clinical guidelines for HIV care in Rwanda, as part of a CDC funded evaluation study of the impact of EHR use on HIV care.

Conclusion

Fundamentally, merging the computer's talent for memory and logic with the human's natural skill in perceiving and planning should make the combination much better at improving health care decisions. Indeed, CDS has improved the quality, safety, and cost-effectiveness of health care in many settings. A number of challenges still need to be solved to make CDS completely reliable, consistently effective, and widely available; but even at this stage of evolution it is vital for all health care workers to consider how CDS can be planned, implemented, and used daily in their own setting, for the benefit of their patients and their practices.

Question for Discussion

- Explain three ways clinical decision support has the ability to change health care.

References

1. McGlynn EA, Asch SM, Adams J, Keesey J, Hicks J, DeCristofaro A, et al. 2003. The quality of health care delivered to adults in the United States. *N Engl J Med* 348(26): 2635–2645.

2. James JT. 2013. A new, evidence-based estimate of patient harms associated with hospital care. *J Patient Saf* 9(3): 122–128.

3. Kohn LT, Corrigan JM, Donaldson MS. 2000 *To err is human: Building a safer health system.* Washington, DC: National Academies Press.

4. Osheroff JA, Teich JM, Middleton B, Steen EB, Wright A, Detmer DE. 2007. A roadmap for national action on clinical decision support. *J Am Med Inform Assoc* 14: 141–145.

5. Sittig DF, Teich JM, Osheroff JA, Singh H. 2009. Improving clinical quality indicators through electronic health records: It takes more than just a reminder. *Pediatrics* 124(1): 375–377.

6. Osheroff JA, Teich JM, Levick D, Saldana L, Velasco F, Sittig DF, et al. 2012 *Improving Outcomes with Clinical Decision Support: An Implementers' Guide*, 2nd ed. Chicago: HIMSS Press.

7. Petersen LA, Orav EJ, Teich JM, O'Neil AC, Brennan TA. 1998. Using a computerized sign-out to improve continuity of inpatient care and prevent adverse events. *Jt Comm J Qual Improv* 24(2): 77–87.

8. Bates DW, Leape LL, Cullen DJ, Laird N, Petersen LA, Teich JM, et al. 1998. Effect of computerized physician order entry and a team intervention on prevention of serious medication errors. *JAMA* 280(15): 1311–1316.

9. Bates DW, Teich JM, Lee J, Seger D, Kuperman GJ, Ma'Luf N, et al. 1999. The impact of computerized physician order entry on medication error prevention. *J Am Med Inform Assoc* 6(4): 313–321.

10. Schiff GD, Amato MG, Eguale T, Boehne JJ, Wright A, Koppel R, et al. 2015. Computerized physician order entry-related medication errors: Analysis of reported errors and vulnerability testing of current systems. *BMJ Qual Saf* 24(4): 264–271.

11. Koppel R, Metlay JP, Cohen A, Abaluck B, Localio AR, Kimmel SE, et al. 2005. Role of computerized physician order entry systems in facilitating medication errors. *JAMA* 293(10): 1197–1203.

12. Amarasingham R, Plantinga L, Diener-West M, Gaskin DJ, Powe NR. 2009. Clinical information technologies and inpatient outcomes: A multiple hospital study. *Arch Intern Med* 169(2): 108–114. doi:10.1001/archinternmed.2008.520.

13. Kawamoto K, Houlihan CA, Balas EA, Lobach DF. 2005. Improving clinical practice using clinical decision support systems: A systematic review of trials to identify features critical to success. *BMJ* 330: 765.

14. Garg AX, Adhikari NKJ, McDonald H, Rosas-Arellano MP, Devereaux PJ, Beyene J, et al. 2005. Effects of computerized clinical decision support systems on practitioner performance and patient outcomes: A systematic review. *JAMA* 293(10): 1223–1238.

15. Choi S, Jazayeri D, Mitnick C, Chalco K, Pachao F, Bayona J, et al. 2004. A web-based nurse order entry system for multidrug-resistant tuberculosis patients in Peru. *Proc Medinfo* 11: 202–206.

16. Jazayeri D, Oza S, Ramos G, Fraser H, Teich JM, Kanter AS, et al. 2015. Design and development of an EMR for Ebola Treatment Centers in Sierra Leone using OpenMRS. *Stud Health Technol Inform* 216: 916.

17. Landman AB, Goralnick E, Teich JM. 2015. Clinical decision support in the management of patients with suspected Ebola infection. *Disaster Med Public Health Prep* 9(5): 591–594.

18. Were MC, Nyandiko WM, Huang KT, Slaven JE, Shen C, Tierney WM, et al. 2013. Computer-generated reminders and quality of pediatric HIV care in a resource-limited setting. *Pediatrics* 131(3): E789–e796.

19. Zurovac D, Sudoi RK, Akhwale WS, Ndiritu M, Hamer DH, Rowe AK, et al. 2011. The effect of mobile phone text-message reminders on Kenyan health workers' adherence to malaria treatment guidelines: A cluster randomized trial. *Lancet* 378 9793.: 795–803.

20. Ginsberg J, Mohebbi MH, Patel RS, Brammer L, Smolinski MS, Brilliant L. 2009. Detecting influenza epidemics using search engine query data. *Nature* 457: 1012–1014.

21. Lewis TL, Wyatt JC. 2014. mHealth and mobile medical Apps: A framework to assess risk and promote safer use. *J Med Internet Res* 16(9): e210.

22. Ely JW, Osheroff JA, Gorman PN, Ebell MH, Chambliss ML, Pifer EA, et al. 2000. A taxonomy of generic clinical questions: Classification study. *BMJ* 321 7258.: 429–432.

23. Kawamoto K, Hongsermeier T, Wright A, Lewis J, Bell DS, Middleton B. 2013. Key principles for a national clinical decision support knowledge sharing framework: Synthesis of insights from leading subject matter experts. *J Am Med Inform Assoc* 20(1): 199–207.

27 Pharmacy Systems and Global Health

Raymond Francis Sarmiento and Alvin B. Marcelo

Take-Home Messages

- Pharmacy systems play an important role in quality of care and patient safety improvement.
- An integrated pharmacy system is crucial for the successful implementation of adverse event monitoring in patients, syndromic surveillance using real-time data, and outbreak response plans.
- This chapter describes the burden of medical errors, particularly medication errors, in health care systems; the role of pharmacy systems in improving patient safety and reducing medication errors; the effect of implementing an integrated pharmacy system on public health surveillance; emerging solutions that may be useful in addressing the complexities of medication management; and the global health challenges surrounding the production, consumption, use, and regulation of medicines.

Introduction

In 1999, the Institute of Medicine (IOM) published the seminal paper entitled "To err is human: Building a safer health care system", which reported that as many as 98,000 people die every year because of medical errors [1]. Though generally believed to be a conservative estimate, this report increased the level of awareness on the severity of medical errors as a problem. As a consequence, numerous efforts toward improving patient safety were initiated. However, there have been reports that this trend has worsened over time. A recent study published in the *Journal of Patient Safety* estimates that each year, between 210,000 and 440,000 patients cared for at US hospitals experience some form of preventable adverse event that contributes to their death [2]. Medical errors that result in actual harm have also proven to be costly. In 2008, medical errors cost the United States approximately $17 billion on ancillary services, prescription drug services, and additional patient care, aside from $1.1 billion and $1.4 billion due to lost productivity and increased mortality, respectively [3]. Furthermore, when quality-adjusted life years are taken into consideration, economic losses of up to $98 billion have been estimated [3].

The majority of medication errors happen in hospital settings. Studies have shown that 33% of all hospital errors may be attributed to medication errors [4], with 33% to 66% of hospital admissions having unintended medication-related discrepancies [5–7]. An IOM report released in 2007 [8] found that drug-related errors were the most common medical errors and happen at every stage of the medication-use process, from prescribing to dispensing to administering to monitoring [8–9]. Although the majority of these errors do not harm the patient, on average each hospital patient is still exposed to at least one drug error every day [8–9].

In addition, costs due to medication errors have become prohibitive. In 2014, Samp et al. [10] developed a decision model to estimate the cost of medication errors as reported by clinical pharmacists in the Medication Error Detection, Amelioration and Prevention (MEDAP) study. The authors found that the mean expected cost of a medication error in a base case was $88.57, the additional cost per hospitalization due to a medication error was $32.59 to $136.40, and the additional cost per patient death due to medication errors was $81.83 to $95.31 [10]. If we use these numbers to compute for the estimated cost per patient death due to medication errors, the annual amount would be between $17 million and nearly $42 million. This burden of medication errors has prompted hospitals to employ several interventions to reduce these errors, but with mixed results. In addition to improving drug-labeling efforts and performing medication reconciliation [11–13], pharmacy systems have been implemented to help reduce risks and inefficiencies as well as enhance patient safety.

Pharmacy systems, also called pharmacy information systems, are computerized systems designed to meet the business needs of pharmacy departments for the efficient provision and utilization of pharmacy services, including inpatient and outpatient order entry, management, and dispensing; inventory and purchasing management; reporting; clinical monitoring; manufacturing and compounding; intervention management; medication administration; and pricing, charging, and billing [14]. As part of an integrated hospital information system, pharmacy systems play a significant role in improving the quality and safety of services being administered to patients by providing updated medication information at the point of care [15].

Safer Health Care Delivery Using Pharmacy Systems

Over the years, pharmacists have seen their roles increase when delivering patient care services in a wide range of practice settings. The US federal government has recognized this change and has subsequently adopted and implemented a health care delivery model where pharmacists, through collaborative practice agreements with physicians or as part of a health care team, assess patients, prescribe medications to manage disease, order and interpret laboratory tests, and formulate treatment plans [16]. This expansion in roles has prompted pharmacists to rely on health information technology (IT) as a solution to help fulfill their jobs more effectively.

Since 2011, the Meaningful Use program, through the Health Information Technology for Economic and Clinical Health (or HITECH) Act of 2009, has incentivized and thus increased the adoption of electronic health records (EHRs) in health care settings. One of the intended outcomes of this implementation was the reduction, or possibly the elimination, of injuries and other adverse events caused by medical errors. Widespread EHR use has helped pharmacists practice pharmacy informatics [17], a specialized field that utilizes health IT to enhance the efficiency and accuracy of medication administration, streamline patient care, and improve patient safety outcomes. The Cleveland Clinic and the Veterans Administration are examples of institutions that benefit from the effective use of pharmacy systems [18]. At the Cleveland Clinic, the implementation of smart infusion pumps enhanced medication safety at the bedside by reducing the risk for infusion pump errors related to high-risk medications while reducing the burden of nurses and pharmacists with unnecessary alerts [19]. The use of drug libraries or close reduction error software in these smart pumps allow clinicians to select medications from customizable pre-loaded lists. When integrated with pharmacy systems, computerized provider order entry (CPOE) systems, and EHRs, smart pumps facilitate safe medication administration by assisting health care providers in calculating doses and programming delivery rates [20,21]. Meanwhile, CPOE systems at the Veterans Administration allow users to have better control over prescriptions for controlled substances by requiring two-factor authentication [18].

Pharmacy systems can have a positive impact on medication reconciliation. In medication reconciliation, the most accurate list of medications for the patient is identified by comparing the patient's medication history in the medical record to an external list obtained from the hospital, a provider, or the patient himself [22]. Medication reconciliation is vital, particularly in transitions of care, when any discrepancy between medication lists must be resolved quickly. Studies have shown that medication reconciliation improves patient outcomes by reducing the occurrence of adverse drug events (ADEs) [23] and decreasing the unintended discrepancies in medication reconciliation at transfers of care [11–13]. With the use of pharmacy systems, providers may be able to implement medication reconciliation faster and more efficiently.

Establishing an enterprise architecture that contains a pharmacy system integrated with core clinical systems such as CPOE, barcode or QR code technology, and EHRs will be critical in addressing patient safety concerns because it will guide the development of clinical decision support (CDS) tools that will help keep patients safe and save lives.

Pharmacy Systems and Public Health

Traditionally, disease-related data from the field is sent to public health officials when a pattern begins to be perceived among individuals with similar symptoms in a given locality. Health care facilities share clinical data with public health agencies, who then conduct investigations in order to verify if there is an emerging cluster or an imminent outbreak in the area. Once confirmed, public health actions are taken and disease trends are monitored to evaluate the status of the outbreak and effectiveness of any interventions. Syndromic surveillance is used for the early detection of outbreaks, to determine their size and spread, to monitor trends in disease incidence, and to implement and evaluate response plans [24–25]. Syndromic surveillance systems use real-time health data on disease trends and health-seeking behaviors to identify and analyze existing and potential outbreaks in a timely fashion [24]. Currently, inpatient and ambulatory care data have been used in developing surveillance systems [26]. But with the increase in EHR adoption in recent years, investigators now have more tools at their disposal to perform more efficient syndromic surveillance. Patient-specific EHR data transmitted using electronic-messaging standards such as HL7 can be useful when shared for syndromic surveillance and can help guide response plans in public health emergencies.

Pharmacy systems, especially those integrated with EHRs, can also play a critical role in improving public health through syndromic surveillance. For example, geographic and temporal trends in infectious outbreaks may be identified through commercial pharmacy systems, such as when a sudden increase in over-the-counter sales of anti-diarrheal medication may indicate an emerging outbreak in a specific community [27]. When hospital pharmacy systems are integrated with EHRs, these data can be correlated clinically based on data from patient encounters. In addition, real-time data analysis on the medications prescribed for a single disease may be used as an indicator of the number of symptomatic patients [28].

Data from pharmacy systems that use standard drug code sets such as RxNorm may be used to develop prescription behavior surveillance systems [29] and controlled-substance surveillance systems [30]. Analyzing de-identified, longitudinal prescription drug–monitoring data may help in developing early warning systems and intervention programs to reduce prescription drug abuse by describing the rates and patterns of prescribing and dispensing, the risk of overdose, and the presence of a drug abuse epidemic in a community [29]. Prescription drug overdose surveillance systems can be developed by linking data from pharmacy systems with other clinical and nonclinical sources of data to track cases of drug overdose deaths and injuries and design effective public health interventions [31].

Other Emerging Solutions to Address Medication Management Complexities

Many institutions have now implemented CPOE and e-prescribing systems through EHRs with CDS capabilities in an attempt to reduce medication errors, improve care delivery, and lower costs. With the advent of these systems, poor handwriting or errors in the transcription of medication orders have decreased [32–35]. Often used in tandem, CPOE and e-prescribing systems allow providers to flag the priority of an order if needed for stat administration. These also alert clinicians to particular drug-drug interactions, medication allergies, or other ADEs in a patient [36]. Moreover, as recommended by the IOM, CDS triggers for excessively high dosages, drug-laboratory issues, and pregnancy-related issues should be included in these systems [37].

A meta-analysis conducted in 2008 by Ammenwerth et al. found that 23 out of 25 studies on the effects of CPOEs showed significant relative risk reductions of 13% to 99% on medication error rates; 30% to 84% relative risk reductions in ADEs in four of seven studies but with one study showing a non-significant increase of 9%; and 35% to 98% relative risk reductions in potential ADEs in six of nine studies but with another study showing a statistically significant risk increase of 29% [38]. However, it is important to note that CPOEs alone may not be enough to reduce medication errors, so implementing a CDS that works *in sync* with CPOEs and e-prescribing systems is recommended [36,39]. CPOE and e-prescribing are two of 13 objectives required in the core measures for achieving meaningful use [40]. Another important point worth noting is that not all CPOE systems are created the same. As with any software, the success of the end CPOE solution depends on several factors such as user interface, speed, connectivity, among others.

Facility registries provide a database of prescribing facilities and dispensing pharmacies. Implementing local, regional, and national health facilities registries helps improve health outcomes, especially in resource-limited settings, by providing the ability to collect, curate, store, distribute, and track standardized and current facility and resource data to health system networks in a country [41]. Reliable and efficient patient referrals are facilitated using accurate and up-to-date information on the geographic distribution of health care infrastructure and services.

Provider registries can be used to identify who can prescribe and who can dispense such as pharmacists and pharmacy technicians. In the United States, covered health care providers, health plans, and health care clearinghouses are assigned by the Centers for Medicare & Medicaid Services with unique 10-digit identification numbers called the National Provider Identifier using the National Plan and Provider Enumeration System [42,43]. The identifier is a Health Insurance Portability and Accountability Act Administrative Simplification Standard for use in administrative and financial transactions [42].

Global Health Needs and Challenges

Most of the challenges related to pharmacy systems, particularly in developing countries, stem from the complexity of the pharmacy management process. However, several factors outside of the health system pharmacy are also critical to the successful adoption and implementation of pharmacy systems. These include (1) the advancement of the pharmacy workforce; (2) the implementation of national data registries; and (3) the development of a strong governance framework. When properly established, these factors significantly contribute to improved quality of care and patient safety.

Due to the rapid growth of the health care and pharmaceutical industries, the demand for skilled pharmacy professionals has been on the rise. However, in the United States alone, it has been estimated that there will be a shortage of 157,000 pharmacists by the year 2020 [44]. Addressing the lack of human resources in the pharmacy field will considerably improve health services delivery. Findings from the 2012 Global Pharmacy Workforce Report emphasized the importance of collaboration between a country's ministries of health and education, academic institutions, and professional associations in advancing a pharmacy workforce responsive to the needs of the people [45]. Establishing a sufficient number of skilled pharmacy human resources and building their capacity in using pharmacy systems will be crucial in delivering quality of care and improving patient safety outcomes. A coordinated action of the global pharmacy workforce that results in increased feminization, continuous monitoring and evaluation of clinical governance measures, increased job satisfaction, and decreased medication therapy complexities and burden of increased prescriptions is therefore essential [46].

Implementing national data registries such as chronic disease patient registries, facility registries, and provider registries will aid monitoring and surveillance efforts to help ensure that patients receive the appropriate care and follow-up they need, especially when these registries are linked to pharmacy systems and EHRs. In addition, a good civil registry system linked to these data registries will help countries to successfully provide universal health care coverage. Establishing an effective and functional civil registration and vital statistics system [47–48], one that provides timely and accurate reporting to a national statistics system, will enhance the capacity of governments, especially those from low- to middle-income countries, to deliver health services by identifying who needs what kind of services.

Extensive system changes that take into account cognitive and social factors are needed to address pharmacy management issues. From registration, procurement, prescription, dispensing, and administration to adverse reporting, areas for improvement exist, because each step of the pharmacy management process commonly operates in silos. Often, appropriate handoff mechanisms are not in place. Therefore, establishing a clear governance framework is necessary to manage conflicting goals and to control complexities within the whole pharmacy management process. IT governance frameworks such as COBIT5 [49], ISO 38500 [50], and ISO TR 14639 [51] offer systematic organization of resources to ensure that investments in pharmacy systems are able to address the key objectives of the organization. These resources include having a shared enterprise architecture among stakeholders and a monitoring system to supervise compliance.

Developing a strong governance framework, building workforce capacity, and implementing an enterprise architecture that includes a robust pharmacy information system are key ingredients to success.

Conclusion

Pharmacy systems play an important role in delivering quality care and improving patient safety as related to the provision, dispensing, maintenance, and monitoring of medications. Managing a pharmacy system efficiently and effectively is critical for reducing and preventing medical errors and safety hazards. Integrating a pharmacy system with core clinical systems is recommended to carry out successful monitoring of adverse events in patients, syndromic surveillance using real-time data, and outbreak response implementation.

Questions for Discussion

- How can pharmacy systems be used to improve the quality and safety of health care services?
- How can the effective and meaningful use of pharmacy systems help address current global health needs and challenges?
- In your opinion, what is the value and impact of pharmacy systems outside of the hospital setting?

References

1. Kohn LT, Corrigan JM, Donaldson MS, eds. *To Err Is Human: Building a Safer Health Care System*. Washington, DC: National Academies Press; 2000.

2. James JTA. 2013. New, evidence-based estimate of patient harms associated with hospital care. *J Patient Saf* 9(3): 122–128. doi:10.1097/PTS.0b013e3182948a69.

3. Andel C, Davidow SL, Hollander M, Moreno DA. 2012. The economics of health care quality and medical errors. *J Health Care Finance* 39(1): 39–50.

4. Milch CE, Salem DN, Pauker SG, Lundquist TG, Kumar S, Chen J. 2006. Voluntary electronic reporting of medical errors and adverse events. An analysis of 92,547 reports from 26 acute care hospitals. *J Gen Intern Med* 21: 165–170.

5. Gleason KM, McDaniel MR, Feinglass J, Baker DW, Lindquist L, Liss D, et al. 2010. Results of the Medications at Transitions and Clinical Handoffs (MATCH) study: An analysis of medication reconciliation errors and risk factors at hospital admission. *J Gen Intern Med* 25: 441–447.

6. Caglar S, Henneman PL, Blank FS, Smithline HA, Henneman EA. 2011. Emergency department medication lists are not accurate. *J Emerg Med* 40: 613–616. doi:10.1016/j.jemermed.2008.02.060.

7. Tam VC, Knowles SR, Cornish PL, Fine N, Marchesano R, Etchells EE. 2005. Frequency, type and clinical importance of medication history errors at admission to hospital: A systematic review. *CMAJ* 173: 510–515.

8. Aspden P, Wolcott J, Bootman JL, Cronenwett LR, eds. *Preventing Medication Errors.* Quality Chasm Series. Washington, DC: National Academies Press; 1999.

9. Roehr B. 2006. Institute of Medicine report strives to reduce medication errors. *BMJ* 333(7561): 220. doi:10.1136/bmj.333.7561.220-f.

10. Samp JC, Touchette DR, Marinac JS, Kuo GM. 2014. Economic evaluation of the impact of medication errors reported by U.S. clinical pharmacists. *Pharmacotherapy* 34(4): 350–357. doi:10.1002/phar.1370.

11. Mueller SK, Sponsler KC, Kripalani S, Schnipper JL. 2012. Hospital-based medication reconciliation practices: A systematic review. *Arch Intern Med* 172: 1057–1069.

12. Gardella JE, Cardwell TB, Nnadi M. 2012. Improving medication safety with accurate preadmission medication lists and postdischarge education. *Jt Comm J Qual Patient Saf* 38: 452–458.

13. Hron JD, Manzi S, Dionne R, Chiang VW, Brostoff M, Altavilla SA, et al. 2015. Electronic medication reconciliation and medication errors. *Int J Qual Health Care* 27(4): 314–319.

14. Troiano D. 1999. A primer on pharmacy information systems. *J Healthc Inf Manag* 13(3): 41–52. Accessed August 3, 2015.

15. Saghaeiannejad-Isfahani S, Mirzaeian R, Jannesari H, Ehteshami A, Feizi A, Raeisi A. 2014. Evaluation of pharmacy information system in teaching, private and social services hospitals in 2011. *J Educ Health Promot* 3: 39. doi:10.4103/2277-9531.131919.

16. Giberson S, Yoder S, Lee MP. 2011. Improving patient and health system outcomes through advanced pharmacy practice: A report to the US Surgeon General. Office of the Chief Pharmacist, US Public Health Service. December. http://www.accp.com/docs/positions/misc/improving_patient_and_health_system_outcomes.pdf. Accessed July 20, 2015.

17. American Society of Health-System Pharmacists. 2007. ASHP statement on the pharmacist's role in informatics. *Am J Health Syst Pharm* 64: 200–203.

18. Morsani College of Medicine, University of Florida. Date unknown. Pharmacy informatics creating a safer healthcare system: Automating the medication-use process can reduce errors and improve patient care. http://www.usfhealthonline.com/resources/key-concepts/pharmacy-informatics-creating-a-safer-healthcare-system/#.VaQW3XYpDIX. Accessed July 20, 2015.

19. Guarino B. 2013. For safer smart pumps, setting harder drug dose limits urged. *Pharmacy Practice News*, 40. http://www.pharmacypracticenews.com/ViewArticle.aspx?d=Technology&d_id=52&i=December+2013&i_id=1022&a_id=24560. Accessed July 20, 2015.

20. Wilson K, Sullivan M. 2004. Preventing medication errors with smart infusion technology. *Am J Health Syst Pharm* 61(2): 177–183.

21. Institute for Safe Medication Practices. 2009. Proceedings from the ISMP Summit on the use of smart infusion pumps: Guidelines for safe implementation and use. Philadelphia, PA: Institute for Safe Medication Practices. http://www.ismp.org/tools/guidelines/smartpumps/printerVersion.pdf. Accessed August 3, 2015.

22. Centers for Medicare and Medicaid Services. 2014. Eligible professional meaningful use menu set measures. Measure 6 of 9. EHR Incentive Program. http://www.cms.gov/Regulations-and-Guidance/Legislation/EHRIncentivePrograms/downloads/7_Medication_Reconciliation.pdf. Accessed July 20, 2015.

23. Schnipper JL, Hamann C, Ndumele CD, Liang CL, Carty MG, Karson AS, et al. 2009. Effect of an electronic medication reconciliation application and process redesign on potential adverse drug events: A cluster-randomized trial. *Arch Intern Med* 169: 771–780.

24. Henning KJ. 2004. What is syndromic surveillance? *MMWR Morb Mortal Wkly Rep* 53(Suppl): 5–11.

25. Van den Wijngaard CC, van Pelt W, Nagelkerke NJ, et al. 2011. Evaluation of syndromic surveillance in the Netherlands: Its added value and recommendations for implementation. *Euro Surveill* 16: 9.

26. Mandl KD, Overhage JM, Wagner MM, Lober WB, Sebastiani P, Mostashari F, et al. 2004. Implementing syndromic surveillance: A practical guide informed by the early experience. *J Am Med Inform Assoc* 11(2): 141–150.

27. American Pharmacists Association. 2015. Improving public health through syndromic surveillance. *Pharmacy Today*, January 1. http://www.pharmacist.com/improving-public-health-through-syndromic-surveillance. Accessed July 20, 2015.

28. Sugawara T, Ohkusa Y, Ibuka Y, Kawanohara H, Taniguchi K, Okabe N. 2012. Real-time prescription surveillance and its application to monitoring seasonal influenza activity in Japan. *J Med Internet Res* 14(1): E14. doi:10.2196/jmir.1881.

29. PDMP Center of Excellence. COE prescription behavior surveillance system: Using PDMP data for early warning and evaluation. Brandeis University. http://www.pdmpexcellence.org/content/coe-prescription-behavior-surveillance-system-using-pdmp-data-early-warning-and-evaluation. Accessed July 20, 2015.

30. Wellman GS, Hammond RL, Talmage R. 2001. Computerized controlled-substance surveillance: Application involving automated storage and distribution cabinets. *Am J Health Syst Pharm* 58(19): 1830–1835.

31. Centers for Disease Control and Prevention. Drug overdose prevention. http://www.cdc.gov/injury/pdfs/budget/fy2016_pres_budget_final_drug-overdose-prevention.pdf. Accessed August 7, 2015.

32. Devine EB, Hansen RN, Wilson-Norton JL, Lawless NM, Fisk AW, Blough DK, et al. 2010. The impact of computerized provider order entry on medication errors in a multispecialty group practice. *J Am Med Inform Assoc* 17(1): 78–84.

33. Kaushal R, Kern LM, Barro'n Y, Quaresimo J, Abramson EL. 2010. Electronic prescribing improves medication safety in community-based office practices. *J Gen Intern Med* 25(6): 530–536.

34. Abramson EL, Barro'n Y, Quaresimo J, Kaushal R. 2011. Electronic prescribing within an electronic health record reduces ambulatory prescribing errors. *Jt Comm J Qual Patient Saf* 37(10): 470–478.

35. Kannry J. 2011. Effect of e-prescribing systems on patient safety. *Mt Sinai J Med* 78(6): 827–833.

36. Wolfstadt JI, Gurwitz JH, Field TS, Lee M, Kalkar S, Wu W, et al. 2008. The effect of computerized physician order entry with clinical decision support on the rates of adverse drug events: A systematic review. *J Gen Intern Med* 23(4): 451–458.

37. Young D. 2006. IOM advises CPOE, other technology for preventing medication errors. *Am J Health Syst Pharm* 63(17): 1578, 1580.

38. Ammenwerth E, Schnell-Inderst P, Machan C, Siebert U. 2008. The effect of electronic prescribing on medication errors and adverse drug events: A systematic review. *J Am Med Inform Assoc* 15: 585–600.

39. Sethuraman U, Kannikeswaran N, Murray KP, Zidan MA, Chamberlain JM. 2015. Prescription errors before and after introduction of electronic medication alert system in a pediatric emergency department. *Acad Emerg Med* 22(6): 714–719. doi:10.1111/acem.12678.

40. Centers for Medicare and Medicaid Services. 2014. Eligible professional meaningful use table of contents core and menu set objectives. http://cms.gov/Regulations-and-Guidance/Legislation/EHRIncentivePrograms/Downloads/EP_MU_TableOf Contents.pdf. Accessed July 20, 2015.

41. Open Health Information Exchange. Date unknown. Facility registry community. https://ohie.org/facility-registry/. Accessed July 20, 2015.

42. Centers for Medicare and Medicaid Services. 2015. National provider identifier standard. https://www.cms.gov/Regulations-and-Guidance/HIPAA-Administrative -Simplification/NationalProvIdentStand/index.html?redirect=/NationalProvIdent Stand/. Accessed July 20, 2015.

43. Centers for Medicare and Medicaid Services. National provider identifier. National plan and provider enumeration system. https://nppes.cms.hhs.gov/NPPES/Welcome.do . Accessed July 20, 2015.

44. American Association of Colleges of Pharmacy. 2013. Job outlook for pharmacists. http://www.aacp.org/resources/student/pharmacyforyou/Pages/joboutlook.aspx . Accessed August 11, 2015.

45. Gal, D, Bates I, eds. 2012. Global pharmacy workforce report. Pharmacy Workforce Report Working Group, International Pharmaceutical Federation. www.fip.org/files/ members/library/FIP_workforce_Report_2012.pdf. Accessed July 20, 2015.

46. Hawthorne N, Anderson C. 2009. The global pharmacy workforce: A systematic review of the literature. *Hum Resour Health* 7: 48. doi:10.1186/1478-4491-7-48.

47. World Health Organization. 2013. Global Summit on Civil Registration and Vital Statistics, April 18–19, Bangkok, Thailand. http://www.globalsummitoncrvs.org/crvs .html. Accessed July 20, 2015.

48. The World Bank. Global civil registration and vital statistics scaling up investment plan 2015–2024. http://www.worldbank.org/en/topic/health/publication/global-civil -registration-vital-statistics-scaling-up-investment. Accessed July 20, 2015.

49. TechRepublic. 2013. COBIT 5 for information security: The underlying principles. http://www.techrepublic.com/blog/it-security/cobit-5-for-information-security-the -underlying-principles. September 4. Accessed July 31, 2015.

50. International Organization for Standardization. Information technology—governance of IT for the organization. ISO/IEC 38500:2015. http://www.iso.org/iso/catalogue _detail.htm?csnumber=62816. Accessed July 31, 2015.

51. International Organization for Standardization. Health informatics—capacity-based eHealth architecture roadmap. Part 1: Overview of national eHealth initiatives. ISO/TR 14639–1:2012. http://www.iso.org/iso/catalogue_detail?csnumber=54902. Accessed July 31, 2015.

28 Medication Adherence

Peter K. Olds and Jessica E. Haberer

Drugs don't work in patients who don't take them.

—C. Everett Koop, former US Surgeon General

Take-Home Messages

- Medication adherence measurement and improvement should not be taken for granted or considered as optional or a bonus. Adherence is critical for evaluating and improving individual health, for interpreting clinical trial data, and for estimating health care costs at the population level. In the case of infectious diseases, it may also impact public health. Failure to pay attention to adherence can undermine efforts to improve outcomes of any disease, especially in resource-limited settings.
- Individuals usually face multiple barriers to adherence. Effective interventions are therefore often multifaceted and should be individualized where possible, taking into account the resources available and the relevant cultural context.
- Innovative technology solutions that provide an opportunity to strengthen adherence and help overcome barriers should be explored.

Introduction

While the importance of medications in achieving better health outcomes is generally well known, the challenges in attaining adequate levels of adherence to medications are often underappreciated. Most individuals prescribed medication face competing priorities and a multitude of barriers, and may not have sufficient access to facilitators to overcome those barriers, especially in developing countries. Additionally, many health care providers, researchers, and policy makers do not realize the extent of the problem. Per the World Health

Organization, "Adherence to long-term therapy for chronic illnesses in developed countries averages 50%. In developing countries, the rates are even lower" [1]. Adherence data is important not only for the health of the individual prescribed the medication, but also for interpreting findings in clinical trials [2] and estimating health care costs at a population level [3]. In the case of infectious diseases, it may also impact public health [4].

Key aspects of adherence can be divided into three main areas, which are closely intertwined: measurement, barriers, and interventions. Technology can play a role in the advancement of each of these three areas. Accurate measurement is critical for identifying those individuals who are doing well with adherence and learning from their successes. It is also vital for identifying those who are struggling and learning how to support them. Unfortunately, all measures of adherence are imperfect, and no gold standard exists. This chapter provides an overview of the strengths and weaknesses of each approach currently in use, as well as highlights novel developments in adherence measurement. It also presents common barriers to adherence and approaches to intervention. While not a systematic review, the chapter raises key issues for consideration in multiple conditions and settings and frames an evidence-based understanding of medication adherence. With such an understanding, opportunities for technology to play a role in improving adherence can be discovered.

Adherence Measurement

Multiple subjective and objective adherence measurement tools are listed in table 28.1.

Subjective Adherence Measurement

Self-Report Self-reported adherence is the oldest and most commonly used adherence measurement tool. It is easy to administer and inexpensive, and is therefore particularly prevalent in developing settings. Self-report exists in numerous permutations regarding question type, administration, and time frame. Questions can be global and ask about the ability to adhere (e.g., poor or well) or the frequency of high adherence (e.g., rarely or often). Alternatively, they may be more specific (e.g., number of doses taken or missed). This type of adherence measurement can be obtained from patients directly, or indirectly through a family member or caregiver (e.g., in the setting of pediatric adherence). Self-reported adherence questions may be administered in person or across a wide array of platforms (e.g., questionnaires, SMS, or interactive voice response [IVR]). A visual analog scale (e.g., a line with an empty medication bottle on one end and a full medication bottle on the other) may be used for assessing adherence in individuals with lower education levels [5]. Finally, the time period may range from that day to several months in the past. Shorter recall periods tend to be more accurate [6], although longer recall periods better capture day-to-day variation.

Table 28.1

Adherence Measurement Tools

Measure	Strengths	Weaknesses
Subjective		
Self-report	Easy to collect; inexpensive; specific	Often overestimates adherence (social desirability and recall bias)
Objective		
Announced, clinic-based pill counts	Quantifiable; easy to perform; inexpensive	Susceptible to manipulation (i.e., pill dumping before visits)
Unannounced home-based pill counts	Less susceptible to pill dumping	Resource-intensive; may be challenging to conduct (e.g., stigma, logistics)
Pharmacy refill	Relatively easy to obtain	Requires a closed pharmacy system and good record keeping; refill is not equivalent to medication ingestion
Electronic monitoring devices (EMDs)	Potential for high accuracy; track patterns of adherence	Requires adherence to the EMD; subject to misclassification of openings (e.g., curiosity openings, pocket doses); expensive
Drug concentrations	Highly sensitive in detecting ingestion of drug	Resource-intensive; plasma levels subject to "white coat" effect; subject to behavioral (dose timing) and biological variation (pharmacokinetics)

Because of the subjective nature of self-report, it assumes that the patient can reliably understand the question, remember the doses that were taken (or missed), and respond appropriately. The potential biases that may arise include recall bias (especially among individuals with cognitive deficits that impair memory); differential response bias (i.e., interpreting the meaning of the question differently); and social desirability bias (i.e., describing falsely elevated adherence to please the interviewer). Social desirability bias may be a particular problem when negative consequences result from reporting poor adherence or the patient feels judged.

Objective Adherence Measurement

Pill Counts   As the name implies, pill counts refer to counting the balance of pills at a particular point in a patient's prescription. Pill counts typically occur at clinic, pharmacy, or study visits, but may also be performed unannounced (e.g., at the individual's home [7] or by phone [8]). They are calculated as follows:

$$\% \text{ adherence} = \frac{(\text{pills dispensed} - \text{pills counted}) * 100}{(\text{pills prescribed per day}) * (\text{days between dispensing and count})}$$

This calculation makes several assumptions: (1) no pills are lost, given away, or sold in the interim; (2) the patient has only one source of medication; (3) the pharmacy prescription and refill records are complete and accurate.

Pill counts are an objective means of measuring adherence and inexpensive to perform; however, much like self-reported adherence, social desirability can affect the accuracy of pill counts. Patients may dispose of excess medication to appear more adherent (called "pill dumping"; [9]). Moreover, any deviations from the above-noted assumptions could introduce inaccuracy in the measure. Unannounced pill counts lessen the opportunity for pill dumping; however, they are much more resource-intensive to conduct and are generally not practical for most clinical settings.

Pharmacy Refill   This approach to adherence measurement is derived from pharmacy records and the medication prescription. It indicates the amount of drug picked up and therefore available to a patient, and is calculated as follows:

$$\% \text{ adherence} = \frac{\text{observed \# of days of medication supply in a given interval (i.e., between two refills)} * 100}{\text{actual \# of days in the interval}}$$

Pharmacy refill adherence relies on objective data and is relatively easy to obtain, making it attractive for developing settings; however, it requires knowledge of all utilized pharmacies and accurate, complete records. Moreover, it indicates the maximal predicted adherence, since an individual may or may not ingest the medication.

Electronic Monitoring Devices   Electronic monitoring devices (EMDs) are typically medication containers that record each opening as a proxy for medication ingestion, usually accomplished by a microprocessor in the container cap that records the date and time of opening. This data can then be either downloaded at periodic intervals or transmitted through cellular networks depending on the device [10,11].

EMDs offer objective adherence data with a granularity that other methods of adherence monitoring do not offer. They provide a dose-by-dose assessment that can be used to understand patterns of adherence rather than a summary of adherence over a given time period. Patterns may be important for certain conditions, like HIV/AIDS, in which drug resistance can develop during a short gap in adherence, despite otherwise high adherence overall [12]. EMDs may be particularly helpful in populations where cognitive impairments or inadequate development (e.g., young children) might decrease the feasibility or accuracy of other measurement tools.

EMDs, however, are expensive and often rely on the premise that each opening represents medication dosing. Patients may open their device without pill removal (called "curiosity openings"), or take multiple pills at once for later dosing (called "pocket doses"). While adjustments can be made for these limitations, they rely on self-reported data, which have the limitations of recall and social desirability bias as noted above.

Technological advancements have allowed for various designs of EMDs. For example, some EMDs measure the amount of medication in the bottle using sensors, while some use facial recognition with smartphones to help measure adherence.

Drug Concentrations Drug concentrations can be determined from multiple biological sources (e.g., plasma, dried blood spots, urine, hair, saliva) and present an objective measure of medication ingestion [13–17]. The drug concentration is influenced by the pharmacokinetics of the drug, timing of the dose, and the individual's metabolism. Plasma concentrations typically reflect a few days, whereas hair and dried blood spots tend to reflect weeks to months of medication use. Drug concentrations are used most commonly in clinical practice for medication dose titration (e.g., lithium for bipolar disorder [18]) and to assess for controlled-substance use [15], rather than measure adherence per se. In clinical trials, they are useful as confirmation of ingestion [19,20]. Drug concentrations, however, can only be obtained periodically and do not indicate patterns of adherence. Hair and dried blood spots are being assessed for more frequent drug concentration assessment, given relative ease and safety of collection and the ability to ship them for centralized laboratory analysis [21,22].

Novel Approaches to Adherence Measurement through Technology The real-time approaches to adherence monitoring noted above (i.e., interactive voice response–based and SMS-based self-report surveys, and EMDs that transmit data via cellular networks) are becoming more common, although techniques for achieving optimal feasibility, acceptability, and validity are active areas of research [11,23,24]. Additional technology advances in adherence monitoring have expanded into the development of ingestion event monitors. Some, for example, rely on edible tracers (e.g., microchips attached to pills detected by an external sensor [25]) and taggants (e.g., drug metabolite detected through a breathalyzer or urine test [26]). Ongoing research is needed to determine the feasibility, acceptability, and validity of these approaches as well.

Although technology costs tend to decrease over time, cost is a major consideration for most novel approaches to adherence measurement and may limit their use, particularly in developing settings. One notable exception, however, are the cellular-based technologies, such as SMS, which leverage the wide availability of mobile phones globally and can overcome widely dispersed populations in rural areas. Moreover, nontraditional approaches to diagnostics, such as dried blood spots, could make drug-level monitoring more feasible; however, the cost of the drug-level determination itself is still cost-prohibitive. Further efforts, potentially through groups such as Diagnostics For All (which create low-cost, easy-to-use, point-of-care laboratory testing tools), are needed to develop accurate, objective adherence measurement tools for resource-limited settings.

Principles for Measuring Adherence

The Hawthorne Effect   The Hawthorne effect describes an increase in adherence that arises because an individual knows he or she is being monitored. It is primarily the result of social desirability, may bias an adherence measurement, and may persist for several weeks before returning to baseline [27]. This scenario has also been called the "white coat" effect in reference to increased adherence prior to a clinic appointment [28–30].

Determination of Validity   As noted above, each adherence measure has limitations, which raise questions about validity. Two strategies are commonly used to assess validity. The first is measuring the concordance of a measurement tool with an objective outcome. While improved health status or a cure would be ideal, they are often not achieved for long periods of time and are not solely dependent on adherence. Intermediate markers (e.g., HIV RNA level—also called viral load—in the case of HIV antiretroviral therapy [ART] or hemoglobin A1C for diabetes) are therefore typically employed. The second strategy is measuring the concordance among multiple measures of adherence [31–33] under the assumption that true adherence likely lies among the different estimates.

Numerous studies comparing adherence measurements have been conducted for HIV ART given the well-known relationship between adherence, HIV RNA levels, and clinical outcomes [7]. For example, while correlated with HIV RNA levels, self-report generally overestimates adherence when compared to EDMs [34]. Global assessments (e.g., ability rating), however, may be more accurate compared to specific missed doses [35]. Pharmacy refill was found to predict suppression of HIV RNA with patients tracked within a closed pharmacy system [36], and a single untimed plasma drug level has been shown to be sensitive in identifying very low adherence [37]. EDMs typically provide the highest correlations with HIV RNA levels [38,39].

Choice of Adherence Measure   The strengths and limitations of the various adherence measures should be carefully considered when designing a research study or clinical program. Key factors include validity; feasibility with available resources (including human capacity, technology, and funding); and cultural acceptability, especially when contemplating the use of novel measurement approaches. When possible, use of at least one objective measure will likely improve the accuracy of adherence estimates.

Adherence Barriers

Barriers to adherence can arise from numerous sources and vary widely (table 28.2). Generally, they can be categorized as relating to the individual, medication regimen, medical condition, and health care system [40–42]. Barriers may be more complex in certain populations, such as children and individuals with disabilities [43]. They also often

Table 28.2

Common Barriers to Adherence

Barriers to Adherence	References
The individual	
Belief in the medication, illness, or health care system	[97–99]
Limitations in cognition, poor health literacy	[100–102]
Concurrent mental illness (especially depression)	[103–105]
Substance use	[105–107]
Poverty (e.g., no means to pick up medications), food insecurity	[83,108,109]
The medication	
Side effects	[110–112]
Treatment regimen complexity	[113–115]
The medical condition	
Stigma, fear of disclosure	[116]
Severity of illness	[117]
Response to treatment (i.e., asymptomatic disease)	[114,118]
Health care system	
Distance to clinic and cost of transportation	[119,120]
Therapeutic relationship with provider	[121,122]
Overburdened health care system	[123]
Availability and cost of medication	[124,125]

reflect local resources and standards, such as pharmacy stock-outs in resource-limited settings and stigma with certain diseases, like HIV/AIDS. Structural barriers, such as transportation to clinic, also tend to be common in resource-limited settings. While forgetfulness is commonly listed as a barrier to adherence by patients, it may reflect a more complex constellation of factors that make remembering difficult, including stigma, depression, drug and alcohol use, and lack of social support [44].

Adherence Interventions

As listed in table 28.3, adherence interventions can generally be divided into the following categories: cognitive, behavioral, affective, structural, and medical. Theory-based interventions tend to have more significant effects [45], such as those based on the health beliefs model [46] and social cognitive theory [47,48]. Not all interventions prove successful across different diseases and most have modest effect sizes [49], and the use of multiple interventions and individualization of interventions may lead to more significant improvements [44,50–52]. Examples of each category of intervention are provided below.

Table 28.3
Examples of Adherence Interventions

Intervention	Examples	Evidence
Cognitive		
Reminders	Alarms; SMS or cell phone reminders; beepers; wrist alarms	HIV/AIDS [55,56]
Educational materials	Monthly letters	Depression [126]
Behavioral		
Directly observed therapy	Daily or weekly home visits; video conferencing	Tuberculosis [127]
Cash incentives	Lotteries, voucher reinforcement	HIV/AIDS [128]
Affective		
Counseling	Cognitive behavioral therapy; telephone interventions; positive psychology	HIV/AIDS [129]; heart failure [130]; diabetes [131]
Treatment supporters	Help with directly observed therapy; Provide social support (emotional, instrumental)	HIV/AIDS [132]
Structural		
Transit time and expense	Mobile clinics or health workers; virtual clinics	Osteoporosis [133]
Case management	In combination with intensive interdisciplinary assessment; collaborative care	HIV/AIDS [134]
Reduced medication costs	Making medications free of charge (especially in HIV care); improved insurance coverage.	Cardiovascular disease [135]; diabetes [136]
Medical		
Education	In the clinic, over the phone, or interactive web-based education modules	Hypertension [137]
Medication regimen simplification	Decreasing number of medications	HIV/AIDS [89]
Pill boxes	Blister packaging; EMDs with dosing reminders	Hypertension [138], HIV/AIDS [11]

Cognitive Intervention

The most common cognitive intervention is a reminder to take medication. Strategies such as pillboxes and medication planners have been successful [53,54], as have SMS reminders [55–57]. Mobile technology currently shows promise for cognitive interventions, including dosing and appointment reminders. This approach is particularly promising for the management of chronic illnesses and in resource-limited settings [58]. Importantly, however, SMS reminders have not improved adherence in all settings [59,60], suggesting that the mechanism by which reminders function may go beyond cognition and include other factors like social support and enhanced provider communication [61,62].

Additionally, understanding the requirements of a given medication can be difficult, especially in the setting of complex diseases like cancer. Interventions to provide patient education have been effective in diverse settings [63]. Mobile technology can also be harnessed for delivery of self-care education, such as providing "just in time" instructions and health status monitoring and feedback [64–66].

Behavioral Intervention

A well-known form of behavioral intervention is directly observed therapy, in which a health care worker or someone chosen by the patient is present and observes medication dosing [67,68]. While resource intensive, feasibility is improved through the use of lay health care workers (e.g. community health workers) and potentially through cell phones [55,69], which may be attractive for developing settings. Effectiveness has been shown for tuberculosis, but has been mixed for HIV/AIDS [70,71].

Another example of behavioral intervention derives from behavioral economics and includes cash incentives in exchange for adherence and other forms of contingency management [72–74]. Sustainability is a concern, however, and techniques such as lotteries may help reduce overall costs.

Affective Intervention

Depression is very common, especially in individuals with other chronic illnesses, and is often overlooked in settings with limited health care infrastructure. Depression has been shown to impact adherence to medication regimens for numerous health conditions, including HIV/AIDS and diabetes [75,76]. Counseling interventions using cognitive behavioral therapy can be effective in overcoming both depression and adherence challenges, with enduring and clinically meaningful benefits [77]. Other interventions aim to provide affective support through treatment supporters, which have been successful for HIV ART in sub-Saharan Africa [78–80].

Structural Intervention

Poverty and other social determinants of health can have a major impact on adherence both in developing and developed settings [81,82], and are exacerbated by poor patient-clinician relationships, untreated depression, and substance abuse [40]. Interventions to bring care to patients (e.g., mobile clinics) or overcome transportation barriers have been effective [83,84]. In developed countries, case management and reduced out-of-pocket expenses (e.g., improved insurance coverage) are also beneficial [85–87].

Medical Intervention

Medication formulations can be simplified to improve adherence. For example, higher adherence has been associated with a lower pill burden (e.g., as achieved through sustained-release formulations and fixed-dose combinations of HIV ART [88,89]). Long-acting formulations, such as injectables, have been proposed as another means for improved adherence; however, results have been mixed in treatment of schizophrenia [90].

Technology and Future Directions for Adherence Interventions

Intervention effectiveness varies across individuals, populations, settings, and medical conditions, and barriers to care are often multi-factorial [44,49,91]. Interventions that are personalized and targeted to those with known adherence challenges are therefore most likely to be effective [92]. Additionally, allowing patients to personalize a portion of the intervention can lead to improved engagement in care and further improved rates of adherence [51,93]. Importantly, since adherence is often not well measured, targeted interventions may prove difficult to implement.

Technology may play an increasing role in adherence both as novel interventions and as means to adapt and improve existing interventions. In addition to the SMS reminders noted above, interactive web-based platforms and SMS are being used for education and counseling [51]. Peer and social support, both identified with improved adherence in sub-Saharan Africa [94], can be provided through web- and cell phone-based social networking tools [95]. When combined with real-time adherence measurement, interventions can now be administered when and where they are needed most.

Adherence also needs to be viewed in the context of the management of medications within the health system. Medication stock-outs due to poor local record keeping and communication, poor management of forecasting and procurement at national levels, or suboptimal transport and storage affects many clinics in low- and middle-income countries. In addition, substandard or counterfeit medication is also common [96] and may weaken or negate the benefits of the medication or even harm the patient. Better measurement and management at all levels in the medication supply chain and usage workflow can pay dividends for patients and health systems alike. A comprehensive set of eHealth solutions could improve many aspects of the key health system function and allow better monitoring of adherence based on dispensing, pill counts, and other methods. These issues are covered in chapter 34 in this section.

Conclusion

Adherence to medication is frequently suboptimal, which has implications for individual and potentially public health, interpretation of clinical trial data, and estimating health care costs at the population level. Technology holds promise to improve adherence, but in order to effectively develop a technology solution, it is important to understand the current adherence landscape as it relates to measurement, barriers, and interventions. Measuring and improvement of adherence should be considered in population health management; failure to do so will undermine efforts to improve outcomes of any disease. Adherence can only be understood well if it is measured well, and each measurement tool has limitations and advantages. Choice of adherence measure(s) for any given setting or study will depend on numerous factors, including validity, feasibility, and acceptability. Adherence barriers arise from numerous sources and can be categorized as relating to the individual, medication, medical condition, and health care system. Adherence interventions generally take one or more of the following approaches: cognitive, affective, behavioral, structural, and medical. Adherence barriers and interventions should be tailored to the available resources and cultural context. To date, most interventions have had modest success, partly due to untargeted use. Better measurements, including eHealth tools with real-time capacity, may facilitate effective and tailored intervention delivery when support is most needed. SMS may be a particularly effective platform for developing settings. Finally, integration of tools for monitoring and improving adherence into the broader processes of medication procurement, supply chain, and dispensing are critical for supporting adherence at a systems level.

Questions for Discussion

- You are implementing a clinical asthma program for children in rural Peru. How would you measure adherence? How would you determine the barriers?
- What types of interventions would you consider and why? How would your answers differ if you were establishing a tuberculosis program for adults in urban India?

References

1. Sabaté E. *Adherence to Long-Term Therapies: Evidence for Action.* Geneva: World Health Organization; 2003: xv.

2. Weiss HA, Wasserheit JN, Barnabas RV, Hayes RJ, Abu-Raddad LJ. 2008. Persisting with prevention: The importance of adherence for HIV prevention. *Emerg Themes Epidem0069ol* 5: 8.

3. Iuga AO, McGuire MJ. 2014. Adherence and health care costs. *Risk Manag Healthc Policy* 7: 35–44.

4. Safren SA, Mayer KH, Ou SS, McCauley M, Grinsztejn B, Hosseinipour MC, et al.; HPTN 052 Study Team. 2015. Adherence to early antiretroviral therapy: Results from HPTN 052, a phase III, multinational randomized trial of ART to prevent HIV-1 sexual transmission in serodiscordant couples. *J Acquir Immune Defic Syndr* 69(2): 234–240.

5. Amico KR, Fisher WA, Cornman DH, Shuper PA, Redding CG, Konkle-Parker DJ, et al. 2006. Visual analog scale of ART adherence: Association with 3-day self-report and adherence barriers. *J Acquir Immune Defic Syndr* 42(4): 455–459.

6. Wilson IB, Carter AE, Berg KM. 2009. Improving the self-report of HIV antiretroviral medication adherence: Is the glass half full or half empty? *Curr HIV/AIDS Rep* 6(4): 177–186.

7. Bangsberg DR, Hecht FM, Charlebois ED, Zolopa AR, Holodniy M, Sheiner L, et al. 2000. Adherence to protease inhibitors, HIV-1 viral load, and development of drug resistance in an indigent population. *AIDS* 14(4): 357–366.

8. Kalichman SC, Amaral CM, Stearns H, White D, Flanagan J, et al. 2007. Adherence to antiretroviral therapy assessed by unannounced pill counts conducted by telephone. *J Gen Intern Med* 22(7): 1003–1006.

9. Turner BJ. 2002. Adherence to antiretroviral therapy by human immunodeficiency virus-infected patients. *J Infect Dis* 185(Suppl 2): S143–S151.

10. Matsui D, Hermmann C, Braudo M, Ito S, Olivieri N, Koren G. 1992. Clinical use of the Medication Event Monitoring System: A new window into pediatric compliance. *Clin Pharmacol Ther* 52(1): 102–103.

11. Haberer JE, Kahane J, Kigozi I, Emenyonu N, Hunt P, Martin J, et al. 2010. Real-time adherence monitoring for HIV antiretroviral therapy. *AIDS Behav* 14(6): 1340–1346.

12. Oyugi JH, Byakika-Tusiime J, Ragland K, Laeyendecker O, Mugerwa R, Kityo C, et al. 2007. Treatment interruptions predict resistance in HIV-positive individuals purchasing fixed-dose combination antiretroviral therapy in Kampala, Uganda. *AIDS* 21(8): 965–971.

13. Gifford AL, Bormann JE, Shively MJ, Wright BC, Richman DD, Bozzette SA. 2000. Predictors of self-reported adherence and plasma HIV concentrations in patients on multidrug antiretroviral regimens. *J Acquir Immune Defic Syndr* 23(5): 386–395.

14. Edelbroek PM, van der Heijden J, Stolk LM. 2009. Dried blood spot methods in therapeutic drug monitoring: Methods, assays, and pitfalls. *Ther Drug Monit* 31(3): 327–336.

15. Linares OA, Daly D, Stefanovski D, Boston RC. 2013. A new model for using quantitative urine testing as a diagnostic tool for oxycodone treatment and compliance. *J Pain Palliat Care Pharmacother* 27(3): 244–254.

16. Gandhi M, Ameli N, Bacchetti P, Anastos K, Gange SJ, Minkoff H, et al. 2011. Atazanavir concentration in hair is the strongest predictor of outcomes on antiretroviral therapy. *Clin Infect Dis* 52(10): 1267–1275.

17. Pichini S, Papaseit E, Joya X, Vall O, Farré M, Garcia-Algar O, et al. 2009. Pharmacokinetics and therapeutic drug monitoring of psychotropic drugs in pediatrics. *Ther Drug Monit* 31(3): 283–318.

18. Sienaert P, Geeraerts I, Wyckaert S. 2013. How to initiate lithium therapy: A systematic review of dose estimation and level prediction methods. *J Affect Disord* 146(1): 15–33.

19. Farmer KC. 1999. Methods for measuring and monitoring medication regimen adherence in clinical trials and clinical practice. *Clin Ther* 21(6): 1074–1090, discussion 1073.

20. Kastrissios H, Suárez JR, Hammer S, Katzenstein D, Blaschke TF. 1998. The extent of non-adherence in a large AIDS clinical trial using plasma dideoxynucleoside concentrations as a marker. *AIDS* 12(17): 2305–2311.

21. Huang Y, Yang Q, Yoon K, Lei Y, Shi R, Gee W, et al. 2011. Microanalysis of the antiretroviral nevirapine in human hair from HIV-infected patients by liquid chromatography-tandem mass spectrometry. *Anal Bioanal Chem* 401(6): 1923–1933.

22. Roberts T, Bygrave H, Fajardo E, Ford N. 2012. Challenges and opportunities for the implementation of virological testing in resource-limited settings. *J Int AIDS Soc* 15(2): 17324.

23. Patel K, Foster NR, Farrell A, Le-Lindqwister NA, Mathew J, Costello B, et al. 2013. Oral cancer chemotherapy adherence and adherence assessment tools: A report from North Central Cancer Group Trial N0747 and a systematic review of the literature. *J Cancer Educ* 28(4): 770–776.

24. Choo PW, Rand CS, Inui TS, Lee ML, Cain E, Cordeiro-Breault M, et al. 1999. Validation of patient reports, automated pharmacy records, and pill counts with electronic monitoring of adherence to antihypertensive therapy. *Med Care* 37(9): 846–857.

25. Kane JM, Perlis RH, DiCarlo LA, Au-Yeung K, Duong J, Petrides G. 2013. First experience with a wireless system incorporating physiologic assessments and direct confirmation of digital tablet ingestions in ambulatory patients with schizophrenia or bipolar disorder. *J Clin Psychiatry* 74(6): e533–540.

26. Morey TE, Wasdo S, Wishin J, Quinn B, Van Der Straten A, Booth M, et al. 2013. Feasibility of a breath test for monitoring adherence to vaginal administration of antiretroviral microbicide gels. *J Clin Pharmacol* 53(1): 103–111.

27. Deschamps AE, Van Wijngaerden E, Denhaerynck K, De Geest S, Vandamme AM. 2006. Use of electronic monitoring induces a 40-day intervention effect in HIV patients. *J Acquir Immune Defic Syndr* 43(2): 247–248.

28. Feinstein AR. 1990. On white-coat effects and the electronic monitoring of compliance. *Arch Intern Med* 150(7): 1377–1378.

29. Cramer JA, Scheyer RD, Mattson RH. 1990. Compliance declines between clinic visits. *Arch Intern Med* 150(7): 1509–1510.

30. Podsadecki TJ, Vrijens BC, Tousset EP, Rode RA, Hanna GJ. 2008. "White coat compliance" limits the reliability of therapeutic drug monitoring in HIV-1-infected patients. *HIV Clin Trials* 9(4): 238–246.

31. Skeppholm M, Friberg L. 2014. Adherence to warfarin treatment among patients with atrial fibrillation. *Clin Res Cardiol* 103(12): 998–1005.

32. Campagna EJ, Muser E, Parks J, Morrato EH. 2014. Methodological considerations in estimating adherence and persistence for a long-acting injectable medication. *J Manag Care Pharm* 20(7): 756–766.

33. Bangsberg DR, Hecht FM, Clague H, Charlebois ED, Ciccarone D, Chesney M. 2001. Provider assessment of adherence to HIV antiretroviral therapy. *J Acquir Immune Defic Syndr* 26(5): 435–442.

34. Simoni JM, Kurth AE, Pearson CR, Pantalone DW, Merrill JO, Frick PA. 2006. Self-report measures of antiretroviral therapy adherence: A review with recommendations for HIV research and clinical management. *AIDS Behav* 10(3): 227–245.

35. Lu M, Safren SA, Skolnik PR, Rogers WH, Coady W, Hardy H, et al. 2008. Optimal recall period and response task for self-reported HIV medication adherence. *AIDS Behav* 12(1): 86–94.

36. Bisson GP, Gross R, Bellamy S, Chittams J, Hislop M, Regensberg L, et al. 2008. Pharmacy refill adherence compared with CD4 count changes for monitoring HIV-infected adults on antiretroviral therapy. *PLoS Med* 5(5): E109.

37. Liechty CA, Alexander CS, Harrigan PR, Guzman JD, Charlebois ED, Moss AR, et al. 2004. Are untimed antiretroviral drug levels useful predictors of adherence behavior? *AIDS* 18(1): 127–129.

38. Bangsberg DR. 2008. Preventing HIV antiretroviral resistance through better monitoring of treatment adherence. *J Infect Dis* 197(Suppl 3): S272–S278.

39. Berg KM, Arnsten JH. 2006. Practical and conceptual challenges in measuring antiretroviral adherence. *J Acquir Immune Defic Syndr* 43(Suppl 1): S79–S87.

40. Mills EJ, Nachega JB, Buchan I, Orbinski J, Attaran A, Singh S, et al. 2006. Adherence to antiretroviral therapy in sub-Saharan Africa and North America: A meta-analysis. *JAMA* 296(6): 679–690.

41. Posse M, Meheus F, van Asten H, van der Ven A, Baltussen R. 2008. Barriers to access to antiretroviral treatment in developing countries: A review. *Trop Med Int Health* 13(7): 904–913.

42. Munro SA, Lewin SA, Smith HJ, Engel ME, Fretheim A, Volmink J. 2007. Patient adherence to tuberculosis treatment: A systematic review of qualitative research. *PLoS Med* 4(7): E238.

43. Haberer J, Mellins C. 2009. Pediatric adherence to HIV antiretroviral therapy. *Curr HIV/AIDS Rep* 6(4): 194–200.

44. Saberi P, Johnson MO. 2011. Technology-based self-care methods of improving antiretroviral adherence: A systematic review. *PLoS One* 6(11): E27533.

45. Lopez LM, Tolley EE, Grimes DA, Chen-Mok M. 2013. Theory-based interventions for contraception. *Cochrane Database Syst Rev* 8: CD007249.

46. Jones CJ, Smith H, Llewellyn C. 2014. Evaluating the effectiveness of health belief model interventions in improving adherence: A systematic review. *Health Psychol Rev* 8(3): 253–269.

47. Marinik EL, Kelleher S, Savla J, Winett RA, Davy BM. 2014. The Resist Diabetes trial: Rationale, design, and methods of a hybrid efficacy/effectiveness intervention trial for resistance training maintenance to improve glucose homeostasis in older prediabetic adults. *Contemp Clin Trials* 37(1): 19–32.

48. Smith SR, Rublein JC, Marcus C, Brock TP, Chesney MA. 2003. A medication self-management program to improve adherence to HIV therapy regimens. *Patient Educ Couns* 50(2): 187–199.

49. Viswanathan M, Golin CE, Jones CD, Ashok M, Blalock SJ, Wines RC, et al. 2012. Interventions to improve adherence to self-administered medications for chronic diseases in the United States: A systematic review. *Ann Intern Med* 157(11): 785–795.

50. Haynes RB, McKibbon KA, Kanani R. 1996. Systematic review of randomized trials of interventions to assist patients to follow prescriptions for medications. *Lancet* 348 (9024): 383–386.

51. Simoni JM, Huh D, Frick PA, Pearson CR, Andrasik MP, Dunbar PJ, et al. 2009. Peer support and pager messaging to promote antiretroviral modifying therapy in Seattle: A randomized controlled trial. *J Acquir Immune Defic Syndr* 52(4): 465–473.

52. Chaiyachati KH, Ogbuoji O, Price M, Suthar AB, Negussie EK, Bärnighausen T. 2014. Interventions to improve adherence to antiretroviral therapy: A rapid systematic review. *AIDS* 28(Suppl 2): S187–S204.

53. Petersen ML, Wang Y, van der Laan MJ, Guzman D, Riley E, Bangsberg DR. 2007. Pillbox organizers are associated with improved adherence to HIV antiretroviral therapy and viral suppression: A marginal structural model analysis. *Clin Infect Dis* 45(7): 908–915.

54. Mahtani KR, Heneghan CJ, Glasziou PP, Perera R. 2011. Reminder packaging for improving adherence to self-administered long-term medications. *Cochrane Database Syst Rev* (9): CD005025.

55. Lester RT, Ritvo P, Mills EJ, Kariri A, Karanja S, Chung MH, et al. 2010. Effects of a mobile phone short message service on antiretroviral treatment adherence in Kenya (WelTel Kenya1): A randomized trial. *Lancet* 376 (9755): 1838–1845.

56. Pop-Eleches C, Thirumurthy H, Habyarimana JP, Zivin JG, Goldstein MP, de Walque D, et al. 2011. Mobile phone technologies improve adherence to antiretroviral treatment in a resource-limited setting: A randomized controlled trial of text message reminders. *AIDS* 25(6): 825–834.

57. Castano PM, Bynum JY, Andrés R, Lara M, Westhoff C. 2012. Effect of daily text messages on oral contraceptive continuation: A randomized controlled trial. *Obstet Gynecol* 119(1): 14–20.

58. Piette JD, Mendoza-Avelares MO, Milton EC, Lange I, Fajardo R. 2010. Access to mobile communication technology and willingness to participate in automated telemedicine calls among chronically ill patients in Honduras. *Telemed J E Health* 16(10): 1030–1041.

59. Mbuagbaw L, Thabane L, Ongolo-Zogo P, Lester RT, Mills EJ, Smieja M, et al. 2012. The Cameroon Mobile Phone SMS (CAMPS) trial: A randomized trial of text messaging versus usual care for adherence to antiretroviral therapy. *PLoS One* 7(12): E46909.

60. Hou MY, Hurwitz S, Kavanagh E, Fortin J, Goldberg AB. 2010. Using daily text-message reminders to improve adherence with oral contraceptives: A randomized controlled trial. *Obstet Gynecol* 116(3): 633–640.

61. Van der Kop ML, Karanja S, Thabane L, Marra C, Chung MH, Gelmon L, et al. 2012. In-depth analysis of patient-clinician cell phone communication during the WelTel Kenya1 antiretroviral adherence trial. *PLoS One* 7(9): E46033.

62. Smillie K, Van Borek N, Abaki J, Pick N, Maan EJ, Friesen K, et al. 2014. A qualitative study investigating the use of a mobile phone short message service designed to improve HIV adherence and retention in care in Canada (WelTel BC1). *J Assoc Nurses AIDS Care* 25(6): 614–625.

63. Ciciriello S, Johnston RV, Osborne RH, Wicks I, deKroo T, Clerehan R, et al. 2013. Multimedia educational interventions for consumers about prescribed and over-the-counter medications. *Cochrane Database Syst Rev* 4: CD008416.

64. Chueh H, Barnett GO. 1997. "Just-in-time" clinical information. *Acad Med* 72(6): 512–517.

65. Murtaugh CM, Pezzin LE, McDonald MV, Feldman PH, Peng TR. 2005. Just-in-time evidence-based e-mail "reminders" in home health care: Impact on nurse practices. *Health Serv Res* 40(3): 849–864.

66. Intille SS, Kukla C, Farzanfar R, Bakr W. 2003. Just-in-time technology to encourage incremental, dietary behavior change. *AMIA Annu Symp Proc* 2003: 874.

67. Farmer P, Kim JY. 1998. Community based approaches to the control of multidrug resistant tuberculosis: Introducing "DOTS-plus". *BMJ* 317(7159): 671–674.

68. Farmer P, Léandre F, Mukherjee JS, Claude M, Nevil P, Smith-Fawzi MC, et al. 2001. Community-based approaches to HIV treatment in resource-poor settings. *Lancet* 358(9279): 404–409.

69. Mitnick C, Bayona J, Palacios E, Shin S, Furin J, Alcántara F, et al. 2003. Community-based therapy for multidrug-resistant tuberculosis in Lima, Peru. *N Engl J Med* 348(2): 119–128.

70. Ford N, Nachega JB, Engel ME, Mills EH. 2009. Directly observed antiretroviral therapy: A systematic review and meta-analysis of randomized clinical trials. *Lancet* 374 (9707): 2064–2071.

71. Nachega JB, Chaisson RE, Goliath R, Efron A, Chaudhary MA, Ram M, et al. 2010. Randomized controlled trial of trained patient-nominated treatment supporters providing partial directly observed antiretroviral therapy. *AIDS* 24(9): 1273–1280.

72. Rosen MI, Dieckhaus K, McMahon TJ, Valdes B, Petry NM, Cramer J, et al. 2007. Improved adherence with contingency management. *AIDS Patient Care STDS* 21(1): 30–40.

73. Meredith SE, Jarvis BP, Raiff BR, Rojewski AM, Kurti A, Cassidy RN, et al. 2014. The ABCs of incentive-based treatment in health care: A behavior analytic framework to inform research and practice. *Psychol Res Behav Manag* 7: 103–114.

74. Loewenstein G, Asch DA, Volpp KG. 2013. Behavioral economics holds potential to deliver better results for patients, insurers, and employers. *Health Aff (Millwood)* 32(7): 1244–1250.

75. Mayston R, Kinyanda E, Chishinga N, Prince M, Patel V. 2012. Mental disorder and the outcome of HIV/AIDS in low-income and middle-income countries: A systematic review. *AIDS* 26(Suppl 2): S117–S135.

76. Gonzalez JS, Esbitt SA. 2010. Depression and treatment nonadherence in type 2 diabetes: Assessment issues and an integrative treatment approach. *Epidemiol Psychiatr Soc* 19(2): 110–115.

77. Safren SA, Gonzalez JS, Wexler DJ, Psaros C, Delahanty LM, Blashill AJ, et al. 2014. A randomized controlled trial of cognitive behavioral therapy for adherence and depression (CBT-AD) in patients with uncontrolled type 2 diabetes. *Diabetes Care* 37(3): 625–633.

78. Stubbs BA, Micek MA, Pfeiffer JT, Montoya P, Gloyd S. 2009. Treatment partners and adherence to HAART in Central Mozambique. *AIDS Care* 21(11): 1412–1419.

79. Chang LW, Kagaayi J, Nakigozi G, Ssempijja V, Packer AH, Serwadda D, et al. 2010. Effect of peer health workers on AIDS care in Rakai, Uganda: A cluster-randomized trial. *PLoS One* 5(6): E10923.

80. Kabore I, Bloem J, Etheredge G, Obiero W, Wanless S, Doykos P, et al. 2010. The effect of community-based support services on clinical efficacy and health-related quality of life in HIV/AIDS patients in resource-limited settings in sub-Saharan Africa. *AIDS Patient Care STDS* 24(9): 581–594.

81. Farmer PE, Nizeye B, Stulac S, Keshavjee S. 2006. Structural violence and clinical medicine. *PLoS Med* 3(10): E449.

82. Mukherjee JS, Ivers L, Leandre F, Farmer P, Behforouz H. 2006. Antiretroviral therapy in resource-poor settings. Decreasing barriers to access and promoting adherence. *J Acquir Immune Defic Syndr* 43(Suppl 1): S123–S126.

83. Weidle PJ, Wamai N, Solberg P, Liechty C, Sendagala S, Were W, et al. 2006. Adherence to antiretroviral therapy in a home-based AIDS care programme in rural Uganda. *Lancet* 368(9547): 1587–1594.

84. Pienaar DML, Cleary S, Coetzee D, Michaels D, Cloete K, Schneider H, et al. *Models of Care for Antiretroviral Service Delivery.* Cape Town : University of Cape Town; 2006.

85. Mann BS, Barnieh L, Tang K, Campbell DJT, Clement F, Hemmelgarn B, et al. 2014. Association between drug insurance cost sharing strategies and outcomes in patients with chronic diseases: A systematic review. *PLoS One* 9(3): E89168.

86. Maciejewski ML, Farley JF, Parker J, Wansink D. 2010. Copayment reductions generate greater medication adherence in targeted patients. *Health Aff (Millwood)* 29(11): 2002–2008.

87. Zhang Y, Lave JR, Donohue JM, Fischer MA, Chernew ME, Newhouse JP. 2010. The impact of Medicare Part D on medication adherence among older adults enrolled in Medicare-Advantage products. *Med Care* 48(5): 409–417.

88. Bangsberg DR, Ragland K, Monk A, Deeks SG. 2010. A single tablet regimen is associated with higher adherence and viral suppression than multiple tablet regimens in HIV+ homeless and marginally housed people. *AIDS* 24(18): 2835–2840.

89. Nachega JB, Parienti J-J, Uthman OA, Gross R, Dowdy DW, Sax PE, et al. 2014. Lower pill burden and once-daily antiretroviral treatment regimens for HIV infection: A meta-analysis of randomized controlled trials. *Clin Infect Dis* 58(9): 1297–1307.

90. Kishimoto T, Nitta M, Borenstein M, Kane JM, Correll CU. 2013. Long-acting injectable versus oral antipsychotics in schizophrenia: A systematic review and meta-analysis of mirror-image studies. *J Clin Psychiatry* 74(10): 957–965.

91. Barnighausen T, Chaiyachati K, Chimbindi N, Peoples A, Haberer J, Newell M-L. 2011. Interventions to increase antiretroviral adherence in sub-Saharan Africa: A systematic review of evaluation studies. *Lancet Infect Dis* 11(12): 942–951.

92. Amico KR, Harman JJ, Johnson BT. 2006. Efficacy of antiretroviral therapy adherence interventions: A research synthesis of trials, 1996 to 2004. *J Acquir Immune Defic Syndr* 41(3): 285–297.

93. Simoni JM, Chen W-T, Huh D, Fredriksen-Goldsen KI, Pearson C, Zhao H, et al. 2011. A preliminary randomized controlled trial of a nurse-delivered medication adherence intervention among HIV-positive outpatients initiating antiretroviral therapy in Beijing, China. *AIDS Behav* 15(5): 919–929.

94. Ware NC, Idoko J, Kaaya S, Biraro IA, Wyatt MA, Agbaji O, et al. 2009. Explaining adherence success in sub-Saharan Africa: An ethnographic study. *PLoS Med* 6(1): E11.

95. Lester RT, Gelmon L, Plummer FA. 2006. Cell phones: Tightening the communication gap in resource-limited antiretroviral programmes? *AIDS* 20(17): 2242–2244.

96. Hajjou M, Krech L, Lane-Barlow C, Roth L, Pribluda VS, Phanouvong S, et al. 2015. Monitoring the quality of medicines: results from Africa, Asia, and South America. *Am J Trop Med Hyg* 92(6 Suppl): 68–74. Epub 2015 Apr 20.

97. Pasma A, van't Spijker A, Hazes JM, Busschbach JJ, Luime JJ. 2013. Factors associated with adherence to pharmaceutical treatment for rheumatoid arthritis patients: A systematic review. *Semin Arthritis Rheum* 43(1): 18–28.

98. Nam SL, Fielding K, Avalos A, Dickinson D, Gaolathe T, Geissler PW. 2008. The relationship of acceptance or denial of HIV-status to antiretroviral adherence among adult HIV patients in urban Botswana. *Soc Sci Med* 67(2): 301–310.

99. Tabatabai J, Namakhoma I, Tweya H, Phiri S, Schnitzler P, Neuhann F. 2014. Understanding reasons for treatment interruption amongst patients on antiretroviral therapy--a qualitative study at the Lighthouse Clinic, Lilongwe, Malawi. *Glob Health Action* 7: 24795.

100. Campbell NL, Boustani MA, Skopelja EN, Gao S, Unverzagt FW, Murray MD. 2012. Medication adherence in older adults with cognitive impairment: A systematic evidence-based review. *Am J Geriatr Pharmacother* 10(3): 165–177.

101. Dewing S, Mathews C, Lurie M, Kagee A, Padayachee T, Lombard CJ. 2015. Predictors of poor adherence among people on antiretroviral treatment in Cape Town, South Africa: A case-control study. *AIDS Care* 27(3): 342–349.

102. Khachani I, Harmouche H, Ammouri W, Rhoufrani F, Zerouali L, Abouqal R, et al. 2012. Impact of a psychoeducative intervention on adherence to HAART among low-literacy patients in a resource-limited setting: The case of an Arab country—Morocco. *J Int Assoc Physicians AIDS Care (Chic)* 11(1): 47–56.

103. Albus C. 2010. Psychological and social factors in coronary heart disease. *Ann Med* 42(7): 487–494.

104. Herlitz J, Toth PP, Naesdal J. 2010. Low-dose aspirin therapy for cardiovascular prevention: Quantification and consequences of poor compliance or discontinuation. *Am J Cardiovasc Drugs* 10(2): 125–141.

105. Malow R, Dévieux JG, Stein JA, Rosenberg R, Jean-Gilles M, Attonito J, et al. 2013. Depression, substance abuse and other contextual predictors of adherence to antiretroviral therapy (ART) among Haitians. *AIDS Behav* 17(4): 1221–1230.

106. Blank MB, Eisenberg MM. 2013. Tailored treatment for HIV+ persons with mental illness: The intervention cascade. *J Acquir Immune Defic Syndr* 63(Suppl 1): S44–S48.

107. Mravcik V, Strada L, Štolfa J, Bencko V, Groshkova T, Reimer J, et al. 2013. Factors associated with uptake, adherence, and efficacy of hepatitis C treatment in people who inject drugs: A literature review. *Patient Prefer Adherence* 7: 1067–1075.

108. Hardon AP, Akurut D, Comoro C, Ekezie C, Irunde HF, Gerrits T, et al. 2007. Hunger, waiting time and transport costs: Time to confront challenges to ART adherence in Africa. *AIDS Care* 19(5): 658–665.

109. Tiyou A, Belachew T, Alemseged F, Biadgilign S. 2010. Predictors of adherence to antiretroviral therapy among people living with HIV/AIDS in resource-limited setting of southwest Ethiopia. *AIDS Res Ther* 7: 39.

110. McGowan CE, Fried MW. 2012. Barriers to hepatitis C treatment. *Liver Int* 32(Suppl 1): 151–156.

111. Kelly K, Posternak M, Alpert JE. 2008. Toward achieving optimal response: Understanding and managing antidepressant side effects. *Dialogues Clin Neurosci* 10(4): 409–418.

112. Murphy RA, Sunpath H, Kuritzkes DR, Venter F, Gandhi RT. 2007. Antiretroviral therapy-associated toxicities in the resource-poor world: The challenge of a limited formulary. *J Infect Dis* 196(Suppl 3): S449–S456.

113. Ammassari A, Trotta MP, Murri R, Castelli F, Narciso P, Noto P. 2002. Correlates and predictors of adherence to highly active antiretroviral therapy: Overview of published literature. *J Acquir Immune Defic Syndr* 31(Suppl 3): S123–S127.

114. Frishman WH. 2007. Importance of medication adherence in cardiovascular disease and the value of once-daily treatment regimens. *Cardiol Rev* 15(5): 257–263.

115. Valenti WM. 2004. Expanding role of conformulations in the treatment of HIV infection: Impact of fixed-dose combinations. *AIDS Read* 14(10): 541–543, 547–550.

116. Katz IT, Ryu AE, Onuegbu AG, Psaros C, Weiser SD, Bangsberg DR, et al. 2013. Impact of HIV-related stigma on treatment adherence: Systematic review and meta-synthesis. *J Int AIDS Soc* 16(3 Suppl 2): 18640.

117. Tsai JC. 2009. A comprehensive perspective on patient adherence to topical glaucoma therapy. *Ophthalmology* 116(11 Suppl): S30–S36.

118. Borris LC. 2009. Barriers to the optimal use of anticoagulants after orthopaedic surgery. *Arch Orthop Trauma Surg* 129(11): 1441–1445.

119. Lankowski AJ, Siedner MJ, Bangsberg DR, Tsai AC. 2014. Impact of geographic and transportation-related barriers on HIV outcomes in sub-Saharan Africa: A systematic review. *AIDS Behav* 18(7): 1199–1223.

120. Tuller DM, Bangsberg DR, Senkungu J, Ware NC, Emenyonu N, Weiser SD. 2010. Transportation costs impede sustained adherence and access to HAART in a clinic population in southwestern Uganda: A qualitative study. *AIDS Behav* 14(4): 778–784.

121. Tibaldi G, Salvador-Carulla L, Garcia-Gutierrez JC. 2011. From treatment adherence to advanced shared decision making: New professional strategies and attitudes in mental health care. *Curr Clin Pharmacol* 6(2): 91–99.

122. Schrijvers LH, Uitslager N, Schuurmans MJ, Fischer K. 2013. Barriers and motivators of adherence to prophylactic treatment in haemophilia: A systematic review. *Haemophilia* 19(3): 355–361.

123. Kagee A, Remien RH, Berkman A, Hoffman S, Campos L, Swartz L. 2011. Structural barriers to ART adherence in Southern Africa: Challenges and potential ways forward. *Glob Public Health* 6(1): 83–97.

124. Marzec LN, Maddox TM. 2013. Medication adherence in patients with diabetes and dyslipidemia: Associated factors and strategies for improvement. *Curr Cardiol Rep* 15(11): 418.

125. Kumarasamy N, Safren SA, Raminani SR, Pickard R, James R, Krishnan AK. 2005. Barriers and facilitators to antiretroviral medication adherence among patients with HIV in Chennai, India: A qualitative study. *AIDS Patient Care STDS* 19(8): 526–537.

126. Hoffman L, Enders J, Luo J, Segal R, Pippins J, Kimberlin C. 2003. Impact of an antidepressant management program on medication adherence. *Am J Manag Care* 9(1): 70–80.

127. Mukherjee JS, Rich ML, Socci AR, Joseph JK, Virú FA, Shin SS, et al. 2004. Programmes and principles in treatment of multidrug-resistant tuberculosis. *Lancet* 363 (9407): 474–481.

128. Haug NA, Sorensen JL. 2006. Contingency management interventions for HIV-related behaviors. *Curr HIV/AIDS Rep* 3(4): 154–159.

129. Gentry S, van-Velthoven MH, Tudor Car L, Car J. 2013. Telephone delivered interventions for reducing morbidity and mortality in people with HIV infection. *Cochrane Database Syst Rev* 5: CD009189.

130. Corotto PS, McCarey MM, Adams S, Khazanie P, Whellan DJ. 2013. Heart failure patient adherence: Epidemiology, cause, and treatment. *Heart Fail Clin* 9(1): 49–58.

131. Jaser SS, Patel N, Rothman RL, Choi L, Whittemore R. 2014. Check It! A randomized pilot of a positive psychology intervention to improve adherence in adolescents with type 1 diabetes. *Diabetes Educ* 40(5): 659–667.

132. Nachega JB, Knowlton AR, Deluca A, Schoeman JH, Watkinson L, Efron A, et al. 2006. Treatment supporter to improve adherence to antiretroviral therapy in HIV-infected South African adults. A qualitative study. *J Acquir Immune Defic Syndr* 43(Suppl 1): S127–S133.

133. Waalen J, Bruning AL, Peters MJ, Blau EM. 2009. A telephone-based intervention for increasing the use of osteoporosis medication: A randomized controlled trial. *Am J Manag Care* 15(8): E60–e70.

134. Kushel MB, Colfax G, Ragland K, Heineman A, Palacio H, Bangsberg DR. 2006. Case management is associated with improved antiretroviral adherence and CD4+ cell counts in homeless and marginally housed individuals with HIV infection. *Clin Infect Dis* 43(2): 234–242.

135. Kulik A, Desai NR, Shrank WH, Antman EM, Glynn RJ, Levin R, et al. 2013. Full prescription coverage versus usual prescription coverage after coronary artery bypass graft surgery: Analysis from the post-myocardial infarction free Rx event and economic evaluation (FREEE) randomized trial. *Circulation* 128(11 Suppl 1): S219–S225.

136. Chernew ME, Shah MR, Wegh A, Rosenberg SN, Juster IA, Rosen AB, et al. 2008. Impact of decreasing copayments on medication adherence within a disease management environment. *Health Aff (Millwood)* 27(1): 103–112.

137. Gwadry-Sridhar FH, Manias E, Lal L, Salas M, Hughes DA, Ratzki-Leewing A, et al. 2013. Impact of interventions on medication adherence and blood pressure control in patients with essential hypertension: A systematic review by the ISPOR medication adherence and persistence special interest group. *Value Health* 16(5): 863–871.

138. Schneider PJ, Murphy JE, Pedersen CA. 2008. Impact of medication packaging on adherence and treatment outcomes in older ambulatory patients. *J Am Pharm Assoc (2003)* 48(1): 58–63.

29 Mobile Electronic Health Surveys and Data Collection: History and Practical Points to Consider

Joel Selanikio

Take-Home Message

- Global health is finally beginning to catch up to the consumer world in the use of mobile technology.

Early Days of Mobile Data Collection

Before the term "mHealth" was coined to mean the use of mobile technology in the health setting, pioneers were trying to utilize the earliest of such computers to collect health data in the field. The first paper referencing this appears to be "Revolutionizing health data capture: Use of hand-held computers" by K.C. Lun et al., written 25 years ago, in 1989.

These early attempts at mobile electronic data collection were based on newly available pocket organizer computers like the Psion Organizer II XP[1] (figure 29.1), and by the late 1990s on more advanced, touchscreen devices like the Palm Pilot and the Apple Newton. Despite the limitations of these devices, numerous attempts were made to use them, and numerous articles were published extolling the benefit of this approach when compared with paper.

For all the promise of those early experiments, widespread adoption of mobile technology for data collection remained elusive and newsworthy, because both hardware and software suffered from limitations of complexity and expense—and two decades after Lun's pioneering work, the vast majority of health data in poor countries is still collected laboriously on paper.

A typical example of such data collection might be a household survey done for the purpose of determining the rate of malnutrition in a child population in, say, Southeast Asia. This would typically involve a form consisting of 30 or more questions printed on several sheets of paper. A sample of several thousand households would be selected for inclusion in the survey, and then the survey team would go to each household with a paper copy of the form and

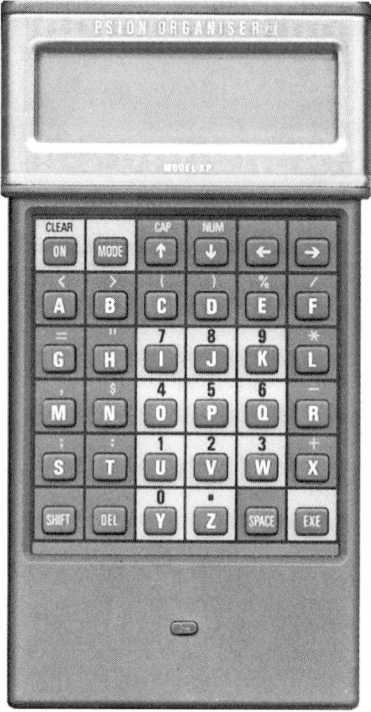

Figure 29.1
Psion Organizer II, circa 1986. Credit: Boris Cornet.

fill it out based on the information provided by the residents of the household. After collecting the thousands of completed forms, someone would be tasked with then typing all the collected information from the paper forms into a computer database—a laborious and error-prone process.

Changing Technologies Overcome Early Limitations

More recently, however, two major technological developments—the mobile phone, representing widespread, affordable computing hardware, and the Internet, representing widespread, affordable access to information—have provided the means to overcome these two limitations (table 29.1).

Now the average person in Nairobi, Kenya, has a computing device in their pocket that cost less than $50 but has orders of magnitude more computing power than NASA did when they put men on the moon in the 1960s. And though few pieces of software can rival Facebook for complexity and functionality, a 10-year-old can set up a page in minutes.

Table 29.1
Early Limitations and Their Solutions

	Limitation	Solution
Hardware	Pocket organizers never reached the level of popularity, particularly in poor countries, that would have driven the price down and allowed greater scale	The explosion of mobile phones has driven mobile computing costs down to the point that devices are now commonplace even in poor countries
Software	Software for early devices was always too complex for the nontechnologist, requiring expensive personnel to configure	The web has provided a platform for distribution of inexpensive and easy-to-use software—and lots of examples to emulate

Affordable, ubiquitous hardware and simple, self-service (i.e., configure-it-yourself, without programmers or consultants or special training) software are now—finally—revolutionizing health data collection in the field on a larger scale.

Key Points for Mobile Data Collection

Mobile data collection is finally becoming more common, after more than two decades of gestation. Increasing prosperity in developing countries, the spread of the Internet, and new business and technology models are all creating new opportunities that make it feasible for almost any organization or individual to consider this approach. Every day it seems there are more software and hardware possibilities, and this has the potential to vastly increase available data, improve data quality, and save enormous amounts of money currently spent on paper-based activities.

As described, there are currently many options for mobile electronic data collection that make it practical and affordable. Prior to implementing a mobile electronic data collection system, there are some key points for anyone contemplating this approach to keep in mind.

1. *Cost.* When determining the cost of using a system, it's important to include *all* costs in your calculations. Some systems charge per interview conducted, others per data collector. Others charge nothing for the software but require expensive programmers or other consultants in order to configure it. Sometimes, those programmers and consultants may need to be traveled to the field, another large budget item. A planning budget should compare the costs for hardware, software, personnel (trainers, programmers, consultants), travel, per diem and daily rates, data transmission costs in-country, and so on.

2. *Hardware selection.* There are now a very wide variety of mobile devices at a range of prices. Any Android or iOS device can be used with a variety of systems, and as of this writing it is possible to get a very functional Android device (including GPS capability) for as little as $75 (and that price is gradually but consistently declining). If SMS data

collection is planned, then any mobile phone at all can be used, with units available for as little as $10. Regardless of the device, it will be important to test its operation in the field, preferably by purchasing and testing only one or two, prior to buying in large numbers. It is also good practice to read online reviews, paying close attention to reports of battery life, screen quality, and durability.

3. *Preparation.* With any technology field work, it's important to plan for delays and technology issues: delays in form design, delays in training, delays in fieldwork, poor Internet connectivity, loss of electrical power, and more. Those with experience of any mobile data collection activity will know to build time into the schedule to allow some flexibility, and to always have a Plan B in case Plan A fails (e.g., even if you've planned to have your data collectors upload data from the field, train them what to do if they do not encounter an adequate cellular signal in the field).

4. *Motivation.* When thinking of using mobile devices for a preexisting paper-based data collection activity, remember that if data collectors on the ground are not collecting data on paper, it is unlikely that they will collect it using a mobile phone or tablet. Failure to collect data may reflect poor pay, lack of supervision, lack of security in the field, lack of fuel for vehicles, or many other factors—and bringing in mobile devices will not, by itself, solve any of them. Any successful data collection will need to consider the existing, and the possible, incentives and disincentives required to ensure that the data collectors will, in fact, use the technology.

Question for Discussion

- Why has the adoption of modern technologies such as the Internet and mobile been so slow within the international health and development sector, lagging far behind consumer technology in rich countries—despite the application of millions of dollars of philanthropic funding to "technology for development" projects and pilots?

Note

1. Released in 1986 with 32 kilobytes of RAM (the first iPhone, by comparison, had 8,000,000 kilobytes) and a screen consisting of two lines displaying a maximum of 16 characters each.

30 Innovations in Health Education: Digital Media and Its Capacity for Front-Line Health Worker Training

Kunal D. Patel and Tom O'Callaghan

Take-Home Messages

- Digital media can lower costs, improve efficiency, and introduce peer-to-peer learning for health worker training.
- Visuals and animation alongside text can dramatically improve training outcomes as well as overcome barriers such as disability.
- Deployment of digital training and online learning can be rapid and can provide a platform for learning surveillance.

Around the globe, we have millions of mobile devices that are delivering high-quality movie streams—instant access to high-resolution imagery—alongside a broad spectrum of growing innovation that evolves at a rapid rate. However, a lens that can focus this innovation to tackle health education in resource-limited settings has not been perfected. Therefore, what innovation we use is diffuse in its methodology and not efficient or focused. When we still have massive areas of the world where the burden of disease and mortality is upsettingly high, innovation, in particular digital media, can help perfect this lens by creating appropriate, universal educational material that can aid in health care on the front line in underdeveloped areas.

Looking back at the great wars of the twentieth century, information was paper-based, but also driven by the cinema screen. Media was used to not only push out propaganda but also health messaging. Malaria was a major concern during the wars and after, so material was created for the big screen and was successful at delivering appropriate health messaging [1]. This was film-based media, which today has been replaced by video or digital media delivery.

Coming forward to today, 90% of organizations involved in health training and education in low- and middle-income countries (LMIC) use paper-based materials, which, interestingly, have been shown to be less cost-effective than technology-driven methodologies [2]. This training is currently in place in countries where the level of primary and secondary education is poor and literacy levels vary. Even though the gross enrollment rate of women in secondary education is growing globally, the enrollment rate for women in areas such as sub-Saharan Africa is incredibly low (less than 45%). Considering that women form the majority of the front-line health workforce in LMIC, they are still not being favored compared to men for employment after primary and secondary education [3]. Combining this with a large youth skills gap, how can we train people, particularly front-line health workers, with slow, inefficient paper-based pedagogies alone? [4] We cannot—but by integrating digital media, we can create a blended and potentially interprofessional approach to health education and rapidly and efficiently train front-line health workers in "media-dark" populations. Currently, the majority of mobile health (mHealth) interventions and information and communication technologies (ICTs) focus on data collection and surveillance for front-line health workers, such as community health workers. For example, mHealth-based data collection has successfully optimized community and home-based strategies for treatment and relapse prevention among drug users living with HIV [5]. Data collection is incredibly important, but with the power of mobile technology, education can be delivered literally in the palm of your hand. SMS text messaging has been used in this regard, with some moderate success, as highlighted by the use of SMS quizzing on HIV in Uganda, but even this is limited due to network provider participation and use of incentives [6,7]. This technology must be utilized further, in combination with digital media, to allow for the following [8,9]:

• catered, fresh, and engaging content for health workers

• faster, standardized training

• lower costs per head—a potential reduction by 70% per person

• enhanced peer-to-peer and interprofessional learning—digital media can excite and be shared within the community

• increased access to evidence-based guidelines for front-line workers

• video, animation, and audio that can be viewed offline, in order to support areas with low bandwidth and connectivity.

The use of mobile technology for communication, entertainment, and education is increasing, and now the delivery of digital media–based content for health worker training is beginning to show success. For example, in Niger, deploying 3D animations on subjects such as cholera prevention and the use of neem in farming via mobile devices not only allowed individuals to overcome literacy barriers in order to access information, but also allowed for easy translation via the use of overlaid voiceovers [10].

Paper and text should not, however, be ignored completely. The majority of learners gain more from medical education that is provided as a combination of visuals and text, rather than words alone [11]. Text, in addition to digital media, can also address health issues among those with disabilities such as deafness. By adding subtitles to successful animated content that has been seen by millions worldwide, educational material to address an urgent issue becomes available and mobile for dissemination [12].

Therefore, incorporation of digital media or platforms that deliver digital media via mobile is key. It may not be necessary to develop new platforms, but rather embrace what is already being used at the school and university level. Currently, the uptake rate of such is slow, and the acknowledgment of successful technology and digital-based learning in the developing world must occur so that it can be brought to the front line. Nursing and medical schools in developed settings are already utilizing blended learning and the use of digital media. One example is the University of Edinburgh, where online video focusing on best clinical practice improved student assessment results and satisfaction ratings [13]. If this technology is delivering education successfully and is already tested, its methodology and design can be implemented on the front line in LMIC. This ultimately avoids the development of training platforms by governments and NGOs, which may not necessarily be proven, therefore reducing cost and improving deployment time.

It is not only technology in schools in the "developed world" that can be adapted for front-line health worker training, but also the model of delivery—providing digital media in an efficient learning environment. A recent model is that of the flipped classroom. Traditionally, students are taught in class and then do homework out of school. If this were "flipped"—that is, learning is done at home, via video and digital platforms, and homework is moved into the classroom—do results improve? Evidence suggests that it may—bringing digital education to the user in their home environment is improving results, especially for science, technology, engineering, and math education [14]. This model is already being adapted by medical schools and in cases such as palliative skills training, improving outcomes and student satisfaction [15,16].

Digital media permits the coverage of a wide and varied amount of subject matter. Agriculture and improved farming methods are becoming increasingly important in terms of alleviating poverty and therefore reducing health risk. Using participatory video production and mobile technology, Digital Green, based in India, has successfully improved agricultural practice and simultaneously provided a platform for learning surveillance [17,18]. By allowing end users to produce their own video content and then to disseminate them through a human-mediated technology model, the organization has progressed to addressing health in a similar fashion. By building the capacity of accredited social health activists in video production, Digital Green and their partners are now successfully screening videos on maternal and newborn health within the community. Additionally, mobile digital video use by accredited social health activists has previously been successful in motivating health workers themselves, in terms of public health knowledge delivery and uptake within their community [19].

A variety of eHealth educational initiatives exist, and many employ different strategies to help improve health education and health care worker shortages in developing countries. A few examples include:

- improved access to medical literature, such as through the World Health Organization's HINARI program (http://www.who.int/hinari/en/), which enables LMICs to gain access to 47,000 ebooks and 15,000 journals in 30 different languages.

- an increase in proprietary online textbook and resources becoming free of charge. For example, the online clinical reference tool UpToDate provides donated subscriptions to many organizations in resource-limited settings.

- targeted free training courses for medical professionals, such as that offered by the Tufts TUSK medical library.

- organizations dedicated to building and delivering innovative solutions for providers and medical training organizations, particularly at the primary care level, such as iheed (http://www.iheed.org).

- specialized software that allows low-bandwidth digital media to be transmitted, and thus permits education in low-income countries that could otherwise not be achieved, as demonstrated in the past, by the RAFT project between the University of Geneva hospitals and a hospital in Barnako, Mali.

There are, of course, barriers many will face when deploying digital media for front-line health worker training. These include access to steady bandwidth and power, which are essential for supporting ICTs. Digital media, once downloaded or pre-stored on a device, can be viewed offline, but where can the content be downloaded onto devices? Equally important, what is going to power these devices? The use of central data repositories and libraries would address this, as would increased delivery of "prepared" devices (i.e., those with content already stored on them). Groups such as the mPowering initiative, which has developed an online library of content for community health workers via the support of a public-private partnership is a modern example [20]. Nevertheless, this is not enough. Fiber and wireless infrastructure needs to improve, and the number of ICT experts needs to rise alongside improved policy and co-ordination from ministries of health, education, and information technology [21]. Additionally, in front-line health care, there needs to be more of a focus on "e-literacy" in women. With this all in place and more, digital media can flourish within a growing global mobile community.

It is important to understand that our brains are designed to recall material if an emotional link is created, which online learning and digital media such as animation and video can provide [22]. Nobel Laureate Daniel Kahneman has proven that emotion can affect our concepts and framing of consequence and risk. In other words, the emotion elicited by mobile video and animation can help health workers understand consequence and health risk within their communities. This stronger bond between screen, educational material, and trainee can therefore lead to improvement in health behaviors and knowledge.

Questions for Discussion

- Health care training is regulated in developed countries by bodies such as the Royal College of Surgeons. How can we regulate digital training in low- and middle-income countries, ensuring that nongovernmental organizations, governments, and other groups provide correct knowledge and act ethically?
- How do we address "e-literacy" issues where they are most needed?

References

1. Fedunkiw M. 2003. Malaria films: Motion pictures as a public health tool. *Am J Public Health* 93(7): 1046–1057.

2. Funes R, Hausman V, Rastegar A, Bhatia P. 2012. Preparing the next generation of community health workers: The power of technology for training. Dalberg Global Development Advisors.

3. Fiske EB. 2012. UNESCO eAtlas of gender equality in education. Paris, France: UNESCO. http://www.unesco.org/new/en/education/themes/leading-the-international -agenda/gender-and-education/resources/the-world-atlas-of-gender-equality-in -education/.

4. UNESCO. 2012. Youth and skills: Putting education to work. Paris, France: UNESCO.

5. Kirk GD, Linas BS, Westergaard RP, Piggott D, Bollinger RC, Chang LW, et al. 2013. The exposure assessment in current time study: Implementation, feasibility, and acceptability of real-time data collection in a community cohort of illicit drug users. *Aids Res Treat* 2013: 594671.

6. De Lepper AM, Eijkemans MJC, van Beijma H, Loggers JW, Tuijn CJ, Oskam L. 2013. Response patterns to interactive SMS health education quizzes at two sites in Uganda: A cohort study. *Trop Med Int Health* 18(4): 516–521.

7. Chib A, Wilkin H, Ling LX, Hoefman B, Van Biejma H. 2012. You have an important message! Evaluating the effectiveness of a text message HIV/AIDS campaign in northwest Uganda. *J Health Commun* 17(Suppl 1): 146–157.

8. Iheed. 2013. New digital media content and delivery: Revolutionizing global health education and training. mHealthEd workshop report. iheed.

9. Funes R, Hausman V, Rastegar A, Bhatia P. 2012. Preparing the next generation of community health workers: The power of technology for training. iheed.

10. Bello-Bravo J, Baoua I. 2012. Animated videos as a learning tool in developing nations: A pilot study of three animations in Maradi and surrounding areas in Niger. *EJISDC* 55(6):1–12.

11. Mayer RE. 2010. Applying the science of learning to medical education. *Med Educ* 44(6): 543–549.

12. Sukharukava Y. 2014. The three amigos: Subtitling health communication for the deaf and hard of hearing. MA thesis, School of Translation and Interpretation, University of Ottawa.

13. Holland A, Smith F, McCrossan G, Adamson E, Watt S, Penny K. 2013. Online video in clinical skills education of oral medication administration for undergraduate student nurses: A mixed methods, prospective cohort study. *Nurse Educ Today* 33(6): 663–670.

14. Love B, Hodge A, Grandgenett N, Swift AW. 2014. Student learning and perceptions in a flipped linear algebra course. *Int J Math Educ Sci Technol* 45(3): 317–324.

15. Sharma N, Lau CS, Doherty I, Harbutt D. 2015. How we flipped the medical classroom. *Med Teach* 37(4): 327–340.

16. Periyakoil VS, Basaviah P. 2013. The flipped classroom paradigm for teaching palliative care skills. *Virtual Mentor* 15(12): 1034–1037.

17. Gandhi R, Veeraraghavan R, Toyama K, Ramprasad V. 2007, *Digital Green: Participatory video for agricultural extension*. IEEE: 1–10.

18. Gonsalves J. 2013. Participatory farmer video production. http://hdl.handle .net/10568/36025

19. Association for Computing Machinery. 2010. Proc. CHI Conference on Human Factors in Computing Systems. Atlanta, GA, April 10–15. New York, NY: Association for Computing Machinery.

20. mPowering. 2014. mPowering Health Content Survey.

21. Bollinger R, Chang L, Jafari R, O'Callaghan T, Ngatia P, Settle D, et al. 2013. Leveraging information technology to bridge the health workforce gap. *Bull World Health Organ* 91(11): 890–891.

22. Moyer-Gusé E. 2008. Toward a theory of entertainment persuasion: Explaining the persuasive effects of entertainment-education messages. *Commun Theory* 18(3): 407–425.

31 Medical Devices

Vipan Nikore, Abeezer Tapia, and Juan Sebastián Osorio

Take-Home Messages

- Developing medical devices requires extensive knowledge of the local context, including specific needs and treatment paradigms.
- Integration of medical devices to innovations in global health informatics is crucial and should be considered during the early stages of the design.
- In recent years, the standard model for medical device development has become an iterative, collaborative, bottom-up approach that takes into account local medical personnel and patients.

Introduction

Even in the twenty-first century, the developing world still suffers from a myriad of preventable and controllable diseases, most of them absent from the developed world due to following proper diagnosis and well-known interventions. Medical technology can help bridge the health chasm that faces many poor nations. If medical devices have clinical benefit and are designed for the local providers and patients, there can be an improvement of standard of care for many diseases. Fortunately, global health development assistance has tripled this century, and medical technology is becoming a priority in low- and middle-income countries (LMIC) [1,2].

Traditional Medical Device Development in LMIC

Over the past several decades, there has been significant focus on medical innovation for the developed world. Traditionally, medical technological transfer has been a hand-me-down approach from developed to developing countries [3]. Unfortunately, many of these health solutions created for developed nations are not adequate for the majority of the population of developing nations. Thus, there remains a large gap in the appropriate number of medical devices to serve the tremendous unmet need that exists in emerging markets. Needs and treatment paradigms are extremely different in emerging markets—from the screening and diagnosis process, physician-patient interaction, and the accepted gold standard of care, to the motivations and expectations of local patients and cultural barriers, price points that can be paid and reimbursement process (both from private and public sector), and the different environmental elements the medical technology must address.

Until recently, approximately 95% of medical devices in LMIC were donated, and about 70–80% of these devices were nonfunctional within five years [2,4]. It is estimated that 38% of the pieces of equipment were out of service [5]. In an attempt to solve this problem, many organizations try to take technology from the developed world, strip the "bells and whistles," and provide a cheaper, less feature-rich solution for the emerging market. However, due to the dramatic patient-demographic and treatment-paradigm differences, these approaches are rarely successful in the developing world [6].

Reducing the complexity and cost, usually removing nonessential features, is known as *frugal innovation*, a term that has been generally coined for technology development in LMIC. In our case, these frugal innovations are more grassroots innovations born out of direct needs, fueled by educating the lowest strata of the society [7].

New Approaches to Medical Device Development

Devices in the developing world are currently not adapted to be rugged in harsh conditions or easily repairable. This is one of the reasons for shifting to an approach that uses bottom-up design principles, which has become a trend in recent years.

An effective approach is to conduct localized development, where one designs a medical device from scratch with the local population and medical personnel as the target audience to build the product profile around. Such an approach has shown success, but requires transitioning from a focus on sophisticated engineering solutions to a user-enabled design [3]. In this section we will discuss key concepts from innovators in the field (chapter 23 outlines the general localized development and commercialization process in more detail).

There has been an evolution from developing "appropriate technology," where the users' needs are taken into consideration [8]; to "participatory design," where innovators on the ground in the developing world are brought in for the product-design process; to, now, "co-creation," where those on the ground exchange ideas through an entire iterative development process to create a true collaborative design [3].

Tim Prestero leads the organization Design that Matters, which focuses on rapid prototyping and human-centered design. They understand that the cost of change is greater as the development process progresses, and their techniques encourage inexpensive failures and allow them to quickly test assumptions. Prototyping allows them to communicate ideas and obtain feedback from end users early. Their focus is to create devices that are hard to use incorrectly. They have developed many successful devices, such as Firefly, a newborn phototherapy device used to treat jaundice (also known as icterus, caused by high levels of bilirubin in the blood) in developing countries [9].

Some large corporations, such as Medtronic, are collaborating with health care professionals, policy makers, government agencies, patient advocacy groups, nongovernmental organizations, and other corporations to pursue innovative strategies that improve awareness, availability, and affordability of effective treatments [10].

The Consortium of Affordable Medical Technologies (CAMTech) emphasizes this co-creation approach by focusing on "people, processes, and products" [3]. CAMTech's methodology is to identify clinical challenges through clinical summits; source promising innovations through hackathons and innovation awards; and develop breakthrough medical technologies through its accelerator and physical co-creation labs in developing countries [3]. Recently, they launched the CAMTech Online Innovation Platform, an online and global network to connect innovators to experts, investors, clinical opportunities, partners, and resources.

The Little Devices Lab at MIT, directed by Jose Gomez, is extending this philosophy by having workers within the walls of hospitals and health facilities who design and maintain their own medical technology [11]. The lab has designed a do-it-yourself (DIY) methodology and toolkit called the Medical Education Design and Innovation Kit (MEDIKit), which enables physicians, nurses, and other health care workers in LMIC to create rapid prototypes of medical devices using toys and Lego-like construction blocks.

Different types of MEDIKits are designed to develop various potential devices. A modular design language helps users see the underlying logic, parts, and which physical stops keep components within safe ranges of operation [11]. Local users are able to hack and extend the modules of the kits and change functionality to create new innovations. The Little Devices Lab takes advantage of the toy and consumer electronics supply chains, which are much faster and more efficient than traditional health care supply chains.

The lab makes use of makerspaces—open spaces where anyone can make anything. These spaces are on the rise in hospitals in developing countries and invite people to explore new opportunities to create devices. Such an environment encourages an experimental workflow that leads to innovative breakthroughs.

Challenges in Medical Device Development

Many challenges to development are present in LMIC. A higher burden of disease introduces unique challenges. Lack of resources, minimal technical support, and harsher conditions [12] at the hospitals and health facilities in LMIC require devices to be rugged and easily repairable in the field. Connectivity still remains an issue, and design must assume that not everyone is online in the developing world. Regulatory roadblocks, cultural barriers, and lack of trust for local developments often make it more difficult for new players to enter the market. A recent discussion at GHDonline [13] touched on specific challenges for each of the chain of events between initial design and eventual implementation of global diagnostics, and finally agreed that a systems-wide approach is necessary to strengthening the delivery system for diagnostics.

A one-size-fit-all approach is too often used, but it is a custom design that is often required for success in LMIC. One-size-fits-all particularly fails patients with unique diseases and presentations of illness. This is another argument for the DIY approach and encouraging curiosity for how and why devices are designed for a specific disease to determine how they can be modified [14]. An example of a device trying to overcome the one-size-fits-all drawback is Diapneu, a neonatal apnea monitor developed by one of the authors and his team in Colombia [15]. This device integrates clinical and physiological information from the patient in a personalized algorithm, and its hardware is designed specifically for the neonatal population. Although the device showed to be a promising innovation, it has encountered many barriers, especially financial and cultural; thus, the importance of building trust among local collaborators and the medical community.

Examples of Success

Fortunately, there are a growing number of successful examples of devices in LMIC to point to. An inhalable vaccine-delivery technology, behavioral diagnostics for medication adherence promotion, paper microfluidic diagnostics for remote populations, and low-cost incubators for rapid tuberculosis detection have all been developed through CAMTech [3].

GlobalDiagnostiX has developed a multidisciplinary alliance with more than 35 researchers, engineers and specialists to design the first medical radiography device specifically designed for harsh tropical climatic conditions and unstable electricity networks in developing countries. They have successfully developed a device that is composed of only mechanical, solid, and stainless steel parts. It has a radiographic image sensor to withstand shocks and high temperatures. The total cost of ownership is also 10 times cheaper than other current equipment. It has an energy storage system that allows the entire system to operate for several hours without external energy [16].

Rich Fletcher, based at the MIT D-Lab and the Tata Center for Technology and Design [17], has been developing medical devices for global health with a particular focus on mobile diagnostic tools. One of his recent developments is a stethoscope that, when connected to a mobile application, is able to predict the probability of a patient having specific pulmonary diseases.

We also illustrate a successful example in depth in chapter 38 of the online supplement of this book with a case study of Embrace, a warmer designed for hypothermic infants in developing countries. The reader is also referred to the WHO Compendium of New and Emerging Health Technologies [18] and *The Lancet* Commission on Technologies for Global Health [12], a good review that includes medical devices, but reinforces the idea that technology alone is not enough, and should be accompanied by other innovations to support effective adoption and implementation.

Conclusion

Given the unique challenges of the developing world and failures of past approaches, new approaches focused on designing innovations through an iterative, collaborative, bottom-up approach are becoming the standard model for medical device development.

In fact, innovations from the developing world are beginning to trickle up to the developed world. For example, GE's Vscan Ultrasound system was originally created for the developing world but has now become commonplace in many hospitals in North America [19,20].

One must remember that creating a solution specifically designed for both high-income markets in the developed world and low-income markets in the developing world often fails. Therefore, it is important to promote and trust the innovative spirit currently percolating in LMIC [21], while continuing to foster process innovations for effective implementation and scale-up [12].

Questions for Discussion

- You have received a fellowship to be an assistant professor at a university in a developing country you have not been to before. Among your responsibilities, you will be in charge of teaching medical devices innovation to biomedical engineering students. What would be the first thing you do before starting to teach them?
- CAMTech organized a hackathon, and you participated. Your team, which consisted of engineers, clinicians, and patients, came up with a novel device for managing cardiovascular disease and was the winner of the event. Consider that during a hackathon you normally partially solve the technical challenge, and perhaps you end up with an initial draft of the business model. What would be the next step for continuing to develop the device?
- Which are the main challenges medical device development faces in the developing world? How you think collaborative design is overcoming them?

References

1. Institute for Health Metrics and Evaluation. *Financing Global Health 2010: Development Assistance and Country Spending in Economic Uncertainty.* Seattle, WA: Institute for Health Metrics and Evaluation; 2010.

2. World Health Organization. *Medical Devices: Managing the Mismatch: An Outcome of the Priority Medical Devices Project.* Geneva: World Health Organization; 2010.

3. Caldwell A, Young A, Gomez-Marquez J, Olson KR. 2011. Leaping Over the Gap: Global Health Technology 2.0. *IEEE Pulse* 2(4): 63–67.

4. Malkin RA. 2007. Design of health care technologies for the developing world. *Annu Rev Biomed Eng* 9(1): 567–587.

5. Perry L and Malkin R. 2011. Effectiveness of medical equipment donations to improve health systems: How much medical equipment is broken in the developing world? *Med Biol Eng Comput* 49(7): 719–722.

6. Prahalad CK. *Fortune at the bottom of the pyramid: Eradicating poverty through profits.* Upper Saddle River, NJ: Pearson Education; 2005: 9.

7. Mandal S. 2014. Frugal innovations for global health—perspectives for students. *IEEE Pulse* 5(1): 11–13.

8. Schumacher EF. *Small is Beautiful: Economics As If People Mattered.* New York, NY: Harper Perennial; 1973.

9. Prestero T. Design that Matters [blog]. http://www.designthatmatters.org/blog/

10. Business Civic Leadership Center. 2013. Using innovative partnerships and programs to address the global burden of noncommunicable diseases. Chamber of Commerce Foundation.

11. Gomez-Marquez, J. 2011. Design for hack in medicine: MacGyver nurses and Legos are helping us make MEDIKits for better health care. *Make Magazine* Ultimate Kit Guide. December.

12. Howitt P, Darzi A, Yang G-Z, Ashrafian H, Atun R, Barlow J, et al. 2012. Technologies for global health. *Lancet* 380 9840.: 507–535.

13. Global Health Delivery Project. 2015. Advancing care delivery: Driving demand and supply of diagnostics [expert panel]. GHDonline. http://www.ghdonline.org/global -diagnostics/discussion/driving-demand-and-supply-of-diagnostics/. Accessed November 9, 2015.

14. Gomez J. 2014. Lecture at MIT class HST 936, April 25. http://sana.mit.edu/ media/v/14.

15. Humphries C. 2012. Monitors specially designed for premature infants help detect breathing problems. *MIT Technology Review*, September/October. http://www2 .technologyreview.com/tr35/profile.aspx?TRID=1320. Accessed November 9, 2015.

16. Barraud E. 2015. Finally, X-ray imaging with the reach of developing countries. *EPFL Cooperation News*, March 17.

17. Fletcher R. Personal webpage. http://web.media.mit.edu/~fletcher/. Accessed November 9, 2015.

18. World Health Organization. 2011. New and emerging technologies. http://www.who .int/medical_devices/innovation/new_emerging_techs/en/. Accessed November 9, 2015.

19. Immelt J, Govindarajan V, Trimble C. 2009. How GE is disrupting itself. *Harv Bus Rev* 87(10): 56–65.

20. General Electric. 2014. Pocket-sized Medical Scanner with Potential to Change Healthcare Everywhere. April 18. http://newsroom.gehealthcare.com/pocket-sized -medical-scanner-with-potential-to-change-healthcare-everywhere/.

21. Kluger J. 2013. The spark of invention. *Time*, November 14. http://techland.time .com/2013/11/14/the-spark-of-invention/. Accessed November 9, 2015.

32 Image Processing in Medical Imaging

Anshuman J. Das and Ramesh Raskar

The key to diagnostic imaging becoming more accessible in low resource settings lies in an innovative combination of simple hardware and software that harnesses the power of big data. —A. J. Das

Progress in image processing in medical devices has not only made automated screening and diagnosis possible but may also lead towards predictive devices. —A. J. Das

Take-Home Messages

- Steps in image processing typically include image acquisition, image manipulation and processing, and image compression.
- Medical imaging can be classified into 2D, 3D, and 4D imaging depending on the dimensionality of the image.
- Commonly used image-processing methods include image smoothing, image registration, and image segmentation.
- Design, user experience, relationship building, and deployment strategy are key factors that determine the success of implementing an imaging technology in resource-constrained settings, and challenges encountered include cultural differences and lack of electricity and other basic resources.

Introduction

Image processing has played a very important role in medical imaging since computer tomography–based 3D imaging was demonstrated in 1972. As the technology for medical imaging improves dramatically, there is a growing need for signal- and image-processing components of medical devices. There has been rising interest in the development of new algorithms, mathematical models to mimic the human body, and applications of computer vision and machine learning for automated diagnosis [1].

Health challenges in developing countries include inadequate medical facilities, doctors, health personnel, and lack of preventive measures and awareness. In such a scenario, technology that is easily accessible can make a huge difference. For example, the mobile phone revolution has made smartphones affordable and within reach even for people even in low-resource settings. A smartphone is equipped with a powerful camera and high-resolution display, and can be easily coupled to a microscope lens to carry out microscopy of a blood sample in the field. The camera can capture images, then send them to the cloud via the Internet for processing, and a diagnosis can be made on the spot. Hence, innovative use of technology coupled with the recent advances in data analytics can save time and effort in solving global health challenges.

This chapter presents a brief overview of image processing for global health applications. It describes the various modalities of medical imaging, the need for image processing, and various tools used in image processing, along with examples in global health.

Image-Processing Pipeline

An image-processing pipeline typically consists of image acquisition, image manipulation or processing, and image compression, as shown in figure 32.1. Image acquisition is typically done using a camera or a set of detectors. Important properties of a camera during

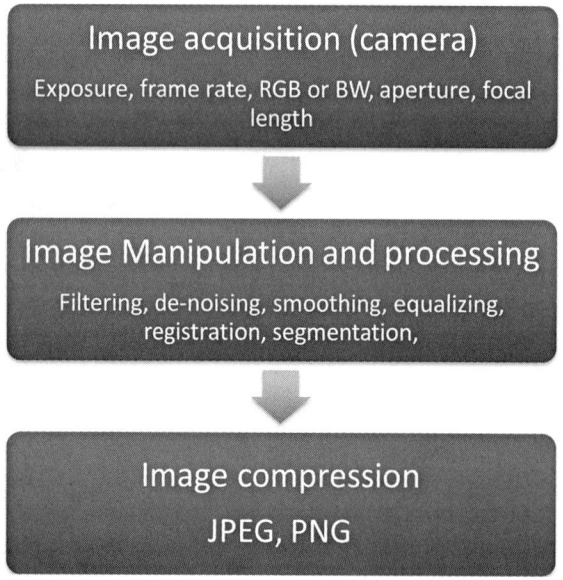

Figure 32.1
Important steps in image processing.

acquisition are exposure time, color, aperture size, frame rate, and focal length. Once the image is captured by the camera, a software code can manipulate or process the image depending upon the application. The image could be de-noised, filtered, equalized, registered, or segmented, among other manipulations. Finally, the image needs to be compressed so that it can be easily stored and shared. Compression can be lossy or lossless, and the most common compression formats are JPEG and PNG.

Imaging Modalities

Imaging for health diagnostics relies on radiation to image microscopic or macroscopic features of the human body that are relevant for clinical analysis and can be used for medical diagnosis and intervention by a clinician. Broadly, medical imaging can be classified into three categories based on the dimensionality of the image, as shown in figure 32.2.

Two-Dimensional Imaging

These modalities yield two-dimensional (2D) images of different body parts they are specialized to image. They can be as simple as using a camera to take a picture of the

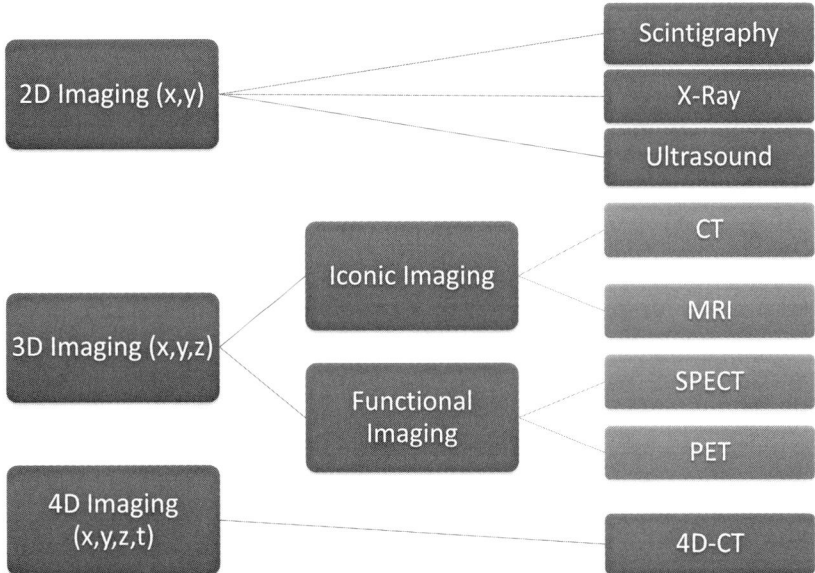

Figure 32.2
Classification of imaging modalities based on the dimensionality of the data. Adapted from [22].

region of interest or more complex, such as inserting a camera into the body. Endoscopy, colonoscopy, and otoscopy are examples of imaging modalities that involve a camera being inserted into the body to look into the nose, throat, colon, stomach, and ear.

X-Ray Imaging   X-rays are forms of high-energy electromagnetic radiation that can penetrate through bones and tissue and be used to image within the body. Different components of the body absorb X-rays to a different extent. This property can be used to create contrast between bones and tissue. X-ray imaging has been very useful to detect pneumonia, lung cancer, bowel obstruction, and kidney stones.

Ultrasonography   In this technique, high-frequency sound waves are transmitted into the body, and echoes are received as a result of sound bouncing off different parts inside the body. These echoes are processed and converted to an image. Due to the fact that sound travels with different velocities in different media, soft tissues can be distinguished from fluids. This technique is very popular in imaging the abdomen, heart, trauma and injuries, as well as tracking fetal growth in the womb.

Microscopy   This is a technique to look at microscopic objects like cells, bacteria, viruses, and other objects invisible to the naked eye. Optical microscopy can be utilized to image and diagnose cancers using fluorescence, multi-photon, lifetime, and confocal imaging modes. It can also be used to visualize abnormal cells in the case of anemia and other conditions. Electron microscopy can be used to image objects that are "nanoscopic" in nature with physical dimensions less than 100 nm. It can be used to look at internal structure of cell, tissues, and organelles.

Scintigraphy   Scintigraphy is a diagnostic test in which radioisotopes are used to image internal organs of the body. Typically a radioisotope specific to an organ in the body is ingested; then, gamma radiation emitted as a result of electron-positron annihilation is detected to form 2D images. (Annihilation is the process wherein an electron and a positron collide, resulting in gamma radiation.) This technique has been used to image lungs, bone, and the thyroid and can also be used to detect tumors.

Three-Dimensional Imaging: Anatomical Modalities

The three 2D techniques of X-ray, ultrasound, and microscopy are by far the most commonly used modalities in developing countries. They are relatively inexpensive, requiring moderate levels of operating skills. These techniques are often insufficient to arrive at a diagnosis. X-ray imaging is limited to imaging bones or chest (e.g., in the case of tuberculosis). It cannot be used to image soft tissue or fluids. Ultrasonography is useful in imaging the abdomen, but not pulmonary diseases, and generally yields low resolution images.

Hence, there is scope and need for low-cost imaging solutions that complement the above techniques in low-resource settings. Three-dimensional (3D) imaging can provide high-resolution, sometimes functional 3D images of internal organs and anatomic morphology, but they require expensive instrumentation, and higher levels of operating skills, and hence they are out of reach of many in developing countries. Various examples in this category follow.

Computed Tomography   This is a very popular imaging modality used to reconstruct the anatomical morphology of the body using X-rays. A rotating X-ray source creates different projections of the body on to a detector. Then, applying radon, these projections transform to a 3D image of the internal parts of the body. A radon transform of an image for a given set of angles is analogous to computing the projections of the image along those angles.

Magnetic Resonance Imaging   Magnetic resonance imaging (MRI) is an imaging technique that uses the property of magnetic relaxation of protons in the water molecules in the body. A pulse of radiofrequency radiation under a high magnetic field excites the protons, and subsequently they relax to the ground state. These relaxation rates are different in different tissues or surroundings. MRI has been extensively used to image soft tissue and is particular useful in imaging joints, brain, and spine.

Positron Emission Tomography   Positron emission tomography imaging harnesses the fact that a positron and an electron can annihilate to produce a pair of gamma ray photons of the same energy but traveling in opposite directions. When a patient is injected with radioisotopes that are capable of producing these gamma rays, one can image internal organs as gamma rays penetrate through tissue and bones. Further, since it is an active reaction, functional features of the region of interest can be extracted, in contrast to MRI and CT, which only provide anatomical features. For example, a molecule called fluorodeoxyglucose can be used to image glucose uptake in tissues. Fluorodeoxyglucose-based positron emission tomography has been utilized in neuroimaging and cancer metastasis.

Four-Dimensional Imaging

This imaging modality records 3D images as a function of time, hence the four dimensions. This method takes in to account the respiration of the patient and provides artifact-free images.

Need for Image Processing in Medical Imaging

Raw images produced from the modalities discussed above generally have the following characteristics: (a) low resolution; (b) noise; (c) low contrast; (d) geometric distortion; and

(e) artifacts [2]. Hence, there is a need to process images to eliminate noise and imaging artifacts.

Some image-processing methods that are commonly used in medical imaging follow.

Image Smoothing

The goal of image smoothing is to simplify an image while retaining important information. This process eliminates noise and redundant details, while at the same time preserves the useful components in an image. Common smoothing methods are Gaussian (linear), affine, and anisotropic [2]. Gaussian smoothing uses a Gaussian function to carry out blurring of an image. Anisotropic smoothing preserves significant features in an image like edges and lines by creating a scale space of a family of blurred images based on a nonlinear diffusion process.

Image Registration

Image registration is the process of aligning two or more images, or, in simpler words, stitching them together. There are many instances in medical imaging where image registration plays an important role. In tomography modalities, images are taken from different perspectives to reconstruct a 3D view of the region of interest [3]. Image registration allows the clinician to visualize a correspondence in the different sets of images.

Registration is carried out via the following steps: (1) measuring similarity between images. This can be done by using pixel intensity or features in the image. (2) A transformation is applied that maximizes similarity. Different types of registration can be applied to a set of images, depending on the rigidity of the object being imaged. A transformation can be classified as rigid if the images can be rotated or translated in order to achieve similarity or correspondence. An elastic registration, on the other hand, may be applied to human tissues and fluids where a warping or stretching needs to be carried out to achieve correspondence [3,4]. An example of nonrigid registration is in modeling cardiac function; it has been used to track heart motion in SPECT and MRI imaging [5].

Example of Image Registration in Dermatoscopy   In dermatoscopy, skin lesions are visualized and analyzed for malignancy. A lesion typically needs to satisfy certain criteria to be classified as cancerous. Physicians follow an ABCDE rule, wherein they look at asymmetry, borders (for irregularity), color uniformity, diameter, and evolution of a lesion over time. All these features can be captured in an image taken by the dermatoscope. However, comparing two images of the same lesion before and after follow-up is challenging, since there could be subtle changes in the features. Moreover, an automated analysis can minimize errors and save time. There have been several registration techniques proposed to carry out registration of dermatological images in medical conditions like psoriasis [6] and melanoma [7]. An example of image registration in dermatoscopy is shown in figure 32.3. Two lesions were compared before and after follow-up, and nine key points were determined after the registration [8].

Image Segmentation

Image segmentation is a method that provides a structured representation to an image that is not structured. It can be a visualization tool for shape analysis and automated analysis [9]. There are broadly two approaches to do segmentation: (1) a top-down approach, where the whole image is considered and then refined; and (1) a bottom-up approach, where the process begins with a point and expands to a larger region. Basically, one needs to detect boundaries in the segmented regions. Edge detection has proved to be a good starting point for segmentation. Common edge-detection techniques include approaches developed by Roberts [10], Sobel [11], Prewitt, and Canny [12]. Once the edges are detected, active contour-based methods are used to connect them to the right region boundaries. Active contours preserve the connectivity in image registration and are implemented by carrying out shrink or expansion operations iteratively on the constraints of an image.

Imaging for Global Health Applications

Most of the imaging modalities that have been mentioned are generally found in a well-equipped health care setting. These techniques use sophisticated hardware, making them expensive and bulky. Therefore, these modalities are out of reach for many people in developing countries and hence cannot be termed as truly global. Low-cost and affordable imaging solutions have emerged and are the key to mass screening, early diagnosis, detection, and prevention. Presented below are some examples of projects that use image processing and computational photography to achieve low-cost but high-quality imaging on portable platforms.

EyeNetra

A large fraction of people in developing countries can afford glasses but not expensive eye tests. Lack of proper vision impairs their lives and prevents them from leading a normal life. EyeNetra attempts to solve this problem by creating an optical clip-on device that can be attached to a smartphone to determine the refractive errors and focal range of the eye (figure 32.4). It works on the principle of Shack-Hartmann wavefront sensing, which is capable of detecting aberrations in wave fronts. A microlens array placed in front of the image sensor can create displacement of the images focused on the sensor. These displacements can be directly correlated to the wave front, which is a result of aberrations

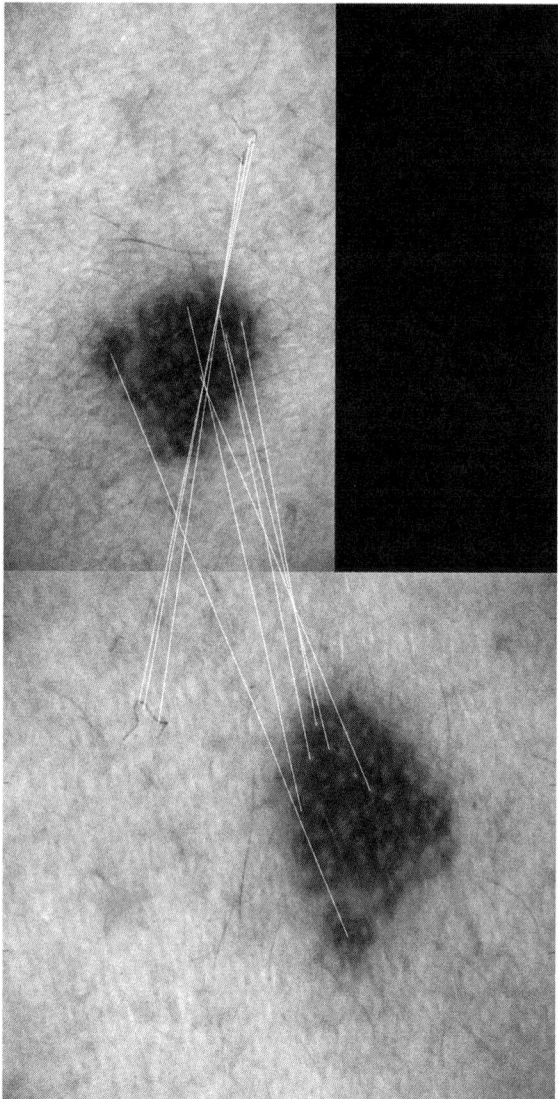

Figure 32.3
Example of image registration being carried out on a skin lesion before and after follow-up. Nine key points were determined after the process of registration. Adapted from [23].

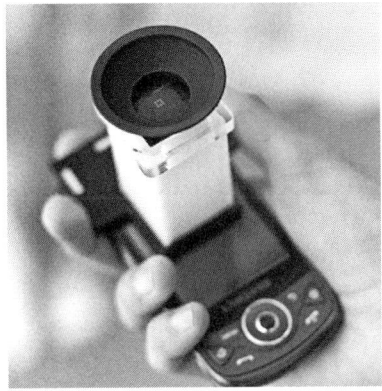

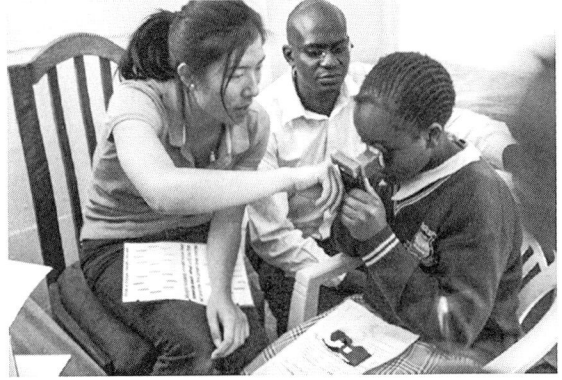

(a) Nairoby periphery – Kenya

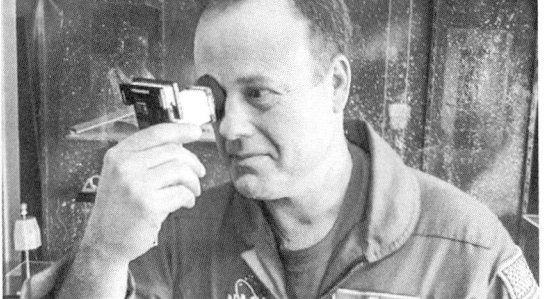

(b) Hyderabad – India

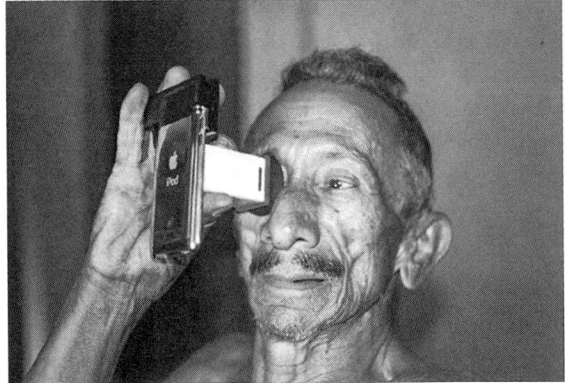

(c) Teresina periphery – Brazil

(d) NASA's Kennedy Space Center – USA

Figure 32.4
(Top) Initial prototype of EyeNetra. (Bottom) EyeNetra being tested at various sites around the world. Left photo from http://www.technologyreview.com/view/421230/cellphones-as-eye-doctors/. Image ©Andy Ryan. Right photo from http://vitor pamplona.com/deps/Pamplona_2012_thesis.pdf.

in the lens in the case of eyes. Today, EyeNetra has carried out more than 32,000 tests and is in the process of commercialization (figure 32.4). More about EyeNetra can be found at https://www.eyenetra.com/.

EyeMitra and Peekvision: Retinal Imaging on a Smartphone

Retinal imaging is a critical modality that can be used to diagnose a variety of vision-related conditions. Among them is diabetic retinopathy, which damages the retina and impairs vision in diabetic patients. EyeMitra and Peekvision are low-cost attachments on a smartphone that can look at the back of the eye and image the retina without the need of a trained expert. These devices can be utilized to quickly take pictures and perform image registration to stitch them into a single wide-field-of-view photograph that can be then sent to an expert for diagnostic opinion. EyeMitra's vision is that by taking many pictures of the retina over a long period of time, early indicators of diabetic retinopathy may be visible, leading to predictive analytics. More about EyeMitra can be found at https://deshpande.mit.edu/portfolio/project/eyemitra-feature-revealing-computational -retinal-imaging-and-predictive-analysis

Cell Phone Microscopy

Cell phone–based microscopy has become popular in the last few years, and has the potential to carry out point-of-care imaging. The simplest approach is to use a microscope objective and replace the microscope's eyepiece with a cell phone's camera. This approach suffers from the fact that high-magnification objects are bulky and very expensive and defeats the purpose of portable, low-cost microscopy. Notable contributions have been made by research groups in utilizing computational approaches to carry out cell phone microscopy.

Single Lens Off-Chip Microscopy The Camera Culture lab at the MIT Media Lab has developed computational imaging–based cell phone microscopy, as shown in figure 32.5. This technique uses an off-chip illumination arrangement using a cell phone display to make Schlieren imaging possible for microscopic samples [13]. Schlieren imaging is a technique by which density variations can be visualized in transparent media like air flow.

Holographic Lens-Free Microscopy The Ozcan group at UCLA has been pioneering lens-free holographic microscopy on a mobile phone [14,15]. They use a debayering algorithm to create monochrome images of the hologram [16]. These images are equalized with a background image, which serves as a reference for holography. A predicted hologram was created, which was iteratively improved and reconstructed to produce the microscopic image of the object, as shown in figure 32.6.

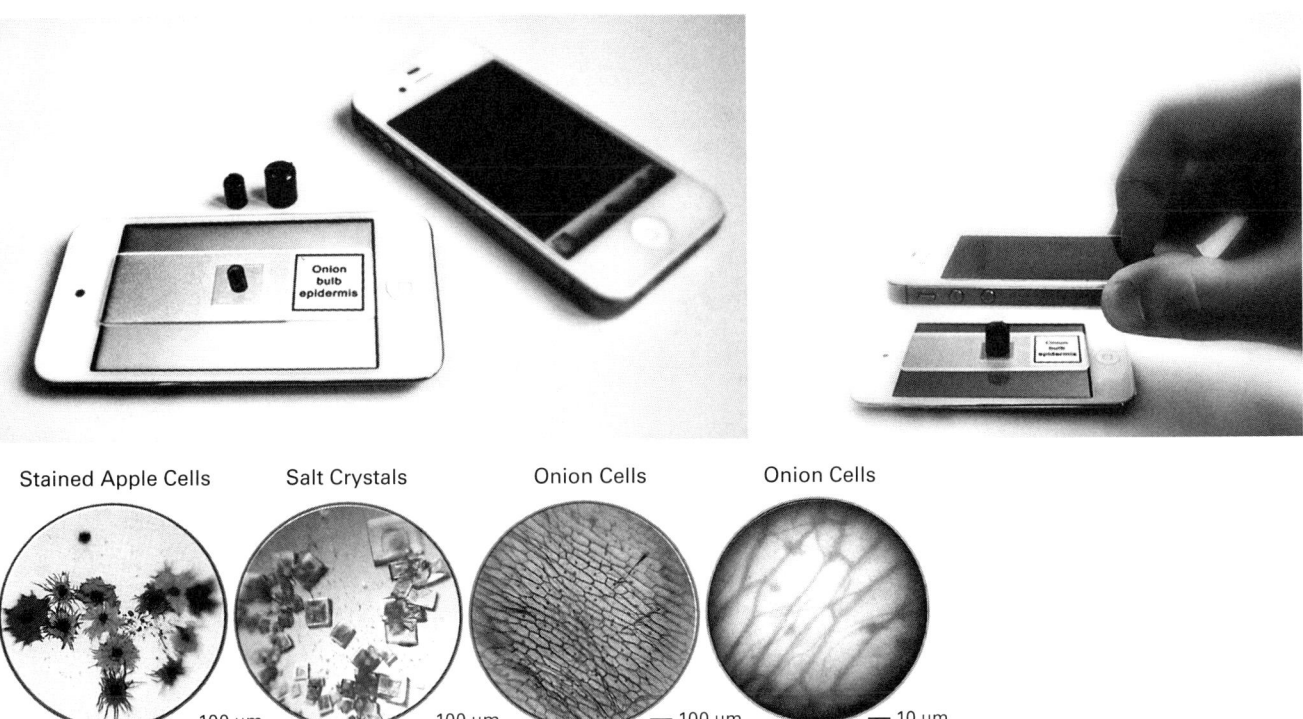

Figure 32.5
(Top) Single lens off-chip microscope prototype. (Bottom) Some images captured with the above device. Adapted from [24].

CellScope: Mobile Phone Microscopes   The Fletcher Lab at UCB has developed a host of mobile phone–based microscopes for telemedicine applications in the diagnosis of corneal abrasions, imaging the retina, and fluorescence microscopy for tuberculosis, among others [17]. Recently they showed a reverse-lens architecture for a cell phone microscope that could capture high-quality images with a wide field of view [18], as shown in figure 32.7.

Tools for Image Processing

The most common software packages used for image processing are Matlab, OpenCV, and Mathematica. Matlab contains an "image processing toolbox" that contains functions to acquire, process, and manipulate images. Mathematica and OpenCV also have a set of built-in functions to carry out image processing. Matlab and Mathematica are commercial packages, whereas OpenCV is an open-source package.

There are also open-source software tools used for basic image manipulation and visualization, such as GIMP, ImageJ, and Chimera. ImageJ and Chimera are extensively used

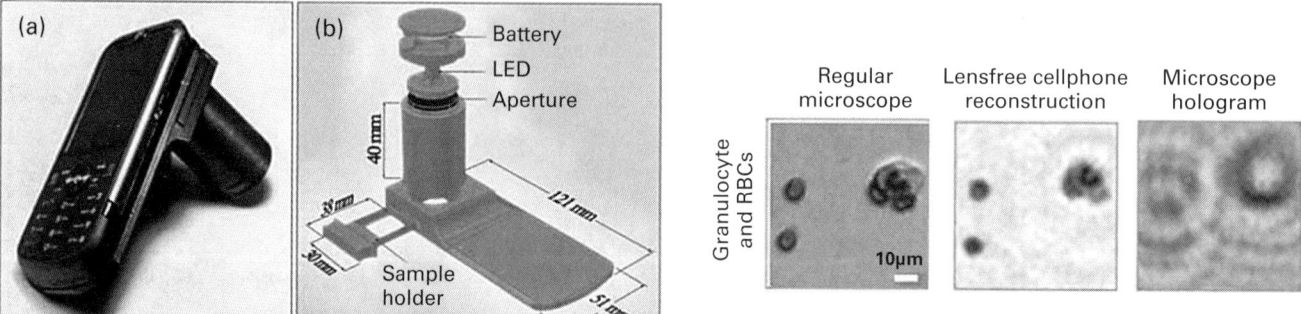

Figure 32.6
(Left) Holographic cell phone–based lens-free microscope prototype. (Right) Images of red blood cells and granulocytes captured with the device. Adapted from [25].

by life science researchers to analyze images obtained by microscopy and 3D representations of molecular structures.

Challenges in Resource-Constrained Settings

Solving the technical challenges in a device is only a part of the problem. There are other challenges that can be encountered in a resource-constrained setting, from cultural differences to lack of electricity and other basic resources. In our experience, the process of deploying a technology takes tremendous time and effort in the field. It requires building relationships with local health workers, the government, nongovernmental organizations, and hospitals. These relationships are crucial for ensuring a technology is disseminated. A device needs to not only succeed in achieving quality of measurements, but also must have a simple user interface. Design and user experience are key factors that determine the success of implementation. A complex interface may need a trained person to operate, which may not be feasible in many areas. A thorough survey of the area of interest will reveal important parameters, such as electricity and mobile phone network, occurrence of diseases, lifestyles, and cultural aspects; many of these have a role to play in the technology being deployed. For example, if the supply of electricity to the region is limited, then the device needs to rely on batteries, which would be an important design consideration. In short, the success of a technology lies not only in the technical aspects of the device but also on the deployment strategy.

Further Reading

The field of medical image processing is a vast topic. Each image-processing technique discussed in this chapter is a field in itself. There are many thorough reviews for medical

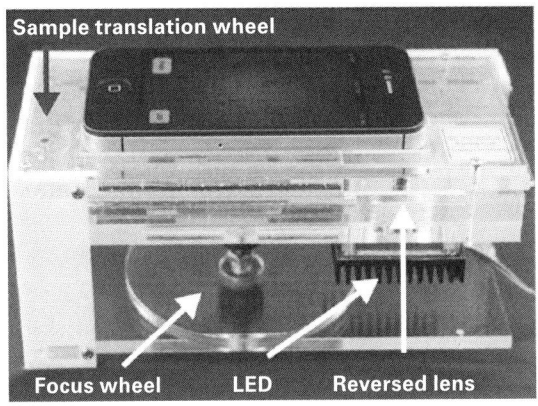

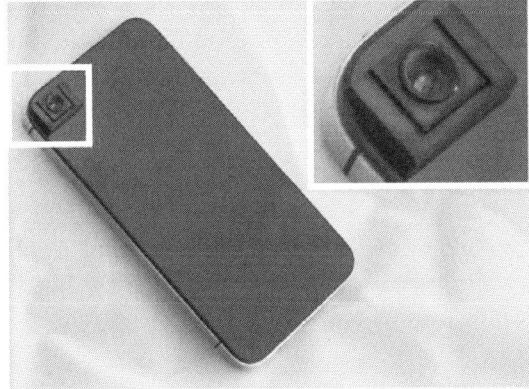

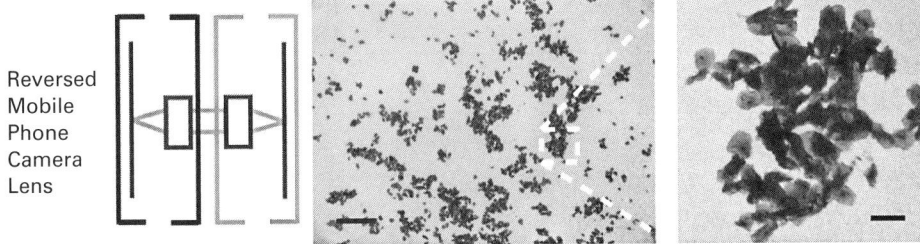

Figure 32.7
(Top) Reverse-lens cell phone microscope prototype. (Bottom) Optical architecture and images of cells captured with the device. Adapted from [26].

image processing via the various techniques. A review by Hill et al. provides a complete overview of image registration techniques [19]. A comprehensive review by Pham et al. is an important resource on medical image segmentation [20]. Methods for forward and inverse problems in optical tomography can be found in a review by Arridge [21].

Conclusion

An overview of image processing for global health applications, its need, and a few examples were presented in this chapter. In the context of global health, image processing presents promising opportunities in the area of low-cost medical diagnostics. Advances in image acquisition (cameras), registration, segmentation, and compression have taken automated screening and diagnosis closer to reality. By harnessing the power of big data, in the future these devices may be capable of predictive analysis as well. In the hands of an expert, they can assist in minimizing error and improving diagnosis. In the hands of a health worker, they can serve as a screening tool. Either way, technology can be made globally accessible by innovations in image processing.

Question for Discussion

1. How do we accelerate adoption of new medical devices and technology? Consider the benefits and risks of speedy trials, reimbursement strategies, simplifying training for clinicians, and meeting quality requirements.

References

1. Chabat F, Hansell DM, Yang GZ. 2000. Computerized decision support in medical imaging. *IEEE Eng Med Biol Mag* 19(5): 89–96. doi:10.1109/51.870235.

2. Angenent S, Pichon E, Tannenbaum A. 2006. Mathematical methods in medical image processing. *Bull Am Math Soc* 43(3): 365–396. doi:10.1090/S0273-0979-06 -01104-9.

3. Hill DLG, Batchelor PG, Holden M, Hawkes DJ. 2001. Medical image registration. *Phys Med Biol* 46(3): R1–R45. doi:10.1088/0031-9155/46/3/201.

4. Angenent S, Pichon E, Tannenbaum A. 2006. Mathematical methods in medical image processing. *Bull Am Math Soc* 43(3): 365–396. doi:10.1090/S0273-0979-06 -01104-9.

5. Rao A, Sanchez-Ortiz GI, Chandrashekara R, Lorenzo-Valdés M, Mohiaddin R, Rueckert D. Comparison of cardiac motion across subjects using non-rigid registration. In Dohi T, Kikinis R, eds. *Medical Image Computing and Computer-Assisted Intervention*. Berlin, Germany: Springer; 2002: 722–729.

6. Maletti G, Ersbøll B, Conradsen K. 2005. A combined alignment and registration scheme of lesions with psoriasis. *Inf Sci* 175(3): 141–159. http://linkinghub.elsevier.com/retrieve/pii/S0020025505000319.

7. Heng H, Bergstresser P. 2007. A new hybrid technique for dermatological image registration. Proceedings of the 7th IEEE International Conference on Bioinformatics and Bioengineering, October 14–17.

8. Anagnostopoulos CNE, Vergados DD, Mintzias P. 2013. Image registration of follow-up examinations in digital dermoscopy. IEEE 13th International Conference on Bioinformatics and Bioengineering, November 10–13.

9. Sharma N, Aggarwal LM. 2010. Automated medical image segmentation techniques. *J Med Phys* 35(1): 3–14. doi:10.4103/0971-6203.58777.

10. Roberts LG. Machine perception of three-dimensional solids. In Tippet JT, Berkowitz DA, Clapp LC, Koester CJ, Vanderburgh A, eds. *Optical and Electro-Optical Information Processing*. MIT Press, Cambridge, MA; 1965.

11. Matthews J. 2002. An introduction to edge detection: The sobel edge detector. *Generation5:* January 27.

12. Canny J. 1986. A computational approach to edge-detection. *IEEE Trans Pattern Anal Mach Intell* 8(6): 679–698.

13. Arpa A, Wetzstein G, Lanman D, Raskar R. 2012. Single lens off-chip cellphone microscopy. IEEE Computer Society Conference on Computer Vision and Pattern Recognition Workshops, June 16–21.

14. Ilhan HA, Dogar M, Ozcan M. 2014. Digital holographic microscopy and focusing methods based on image sharpness. *J Microsc* 255(3): 138–149. doi:10.1111/Jmi.12144.

15. Su TW, Ozcan A. On-chip holographic microscopy and its application for automated semen analysis. In Shaked NT, Zalevsky Z, Satterwhite LL, eds. *Biomedical optical phase microscopy and nanoscopy*. Amsterdam: Elsevier; 2013: 153–171.

16. Tseng D, Mudanyali O, Oztoprak C, Isikman SO, Sencan I, Yaglidere O, Ozcan A. 2010. Lensfree microscopy on a cellphone. *Lab Chip* 10(14): 1787–1792. doi:10.1039/C003477k.

17. Skandarajah A, Reber CD, Switz NA, Fletcher DA. 2014. Quantitative imaging with a mobile phone microscope. *PLoS One* 9(5): e96906, doi:10.1371/journal.pone.0096906.

18. Switz NA, D'Ambrosio MV, Fletcher DA. 2014. Low-cost mobile phone microscopy with a reversed mobile phone camera lens. *PLoS ONE* 9(5): e95330. doi:10.1371/journal.pone.0095330.

19. Hill DLG, Batchelor PG, Holden M, Hawkes DJ. 2001. Medical image registration. *Phys Med Biol* 46(3): R1–R45. doi:10.1088/0031-9155/46/3/201.

20. Pham, DL, Xu CY, Prince JL. 2000. Current methods in medical image segmentation. *Annu Rev Biomed Eng* 2: 315-337. doi:10.1146/annurev.bioeng.2.1.315.

21. Arridge SR. 1999. Optical tomography in medical imaging. *Inverse Probl* 15(2): R41.

22. Richter D. 2012. Current state of image processing for medical irradiation therapy. Radioelektronika, 22nd International Conference, April 17–18.

23. Anagnostopoulos CNE, Vergados DD, Mintzias P. 2013. Image registration of follow-up examinations in digital dermoscopy. IEEE 13th International Conference on Bioinformatics and Bioengineering, November 10–13.

24. Arpa A, Wetzstein G, Lanman D, Raskar R. 2012. Single lens off-chip cellphone microscopy. IEEE Computer Society Conference on Computer Vision and Pattern Recognition Workshops, June 16–21.

25. Tseng D, Mudanyali O, Oztoprak C, Isikman SO, Sencan I, Yaglidere O, et al. 2010. Lensfree microscopy on a cellphone. *Lab Chip* 10(14): 1787–1792. doi:10.1039/C003477k.

26. Switz NA, D'Ambrosio MV, and Fletcher DA. 2014. Low-cost mobile phone microscopy with a reversed mobile phone camera lens. *PLoS ONE* 9(5): e95330. doi:10.1371/journal.pone.0095330.

33 Public Health and GIS: An Introduction to Mapping

Anna Clements, Hannah Judge, and Isabel Shaw

Take-Home Messages

- Maps enable you to detect patterns and visualize indicators over space and time in ways that you cannot in spreadsheets.
- In the context of the developing world, understanding the geography of your catchment area—including the physical infrastructure—is essential for ensuring access to health services.
- Maps and geographic analysis have a powerful role to play in the monitoring and evaluation of programs, because they allow you to quantify impact and visualize project scope and scale.
- Geographic analysis requires geographic data. Identify your most pressing questions, and determine what types of data you need to reach the answers.
- The open-source community is working to make mapping more accessible. QGIS and OSM have significantly lowered the barriers to entry for organizations looking to experiment with geographic analysis.
- The way in which we think about maps has shifted significantly. Maps can now be used as dynamic visual databases and analytical tools that enable you to detect patterns and generate entirely new sets of data.

Introduction

In the United States, your zip code is a better predictor of your health than your genetic code [1]. Location is one of the most important determinants of health because your environment and socioeconomic status dictate not only the quality of the air you breathe and the food you eat, but also the hospitals and medical services you can access.

Geographic analysis can, therefore, help us understand and evaluate patterns of access and inequality, particularly when it comes to community health systems. Maps serve as compelling visual outcomes of that analysis, and continue to evolve as valuable tools for epidemiologists, program, and policy makers because of their unique ability to identify and communicate spatial trends.

One of the earliest, and most illustrious, examples of public health mapping took place in 1854, when the city of London was ravaged by a cholera epidemic. In three days, more than 100 people died on a single city block. Believing that the disease was spread through the air and not water, city authorities feared the epidemic was uncontrollable. Dr. John Snow created a map showing the distribution of every cholera-related death in the neighborhood of SoHo and used this evidence to convince the government that the Broad Street water pump was a significant source of the epidemic (figure 33.1). Not only did

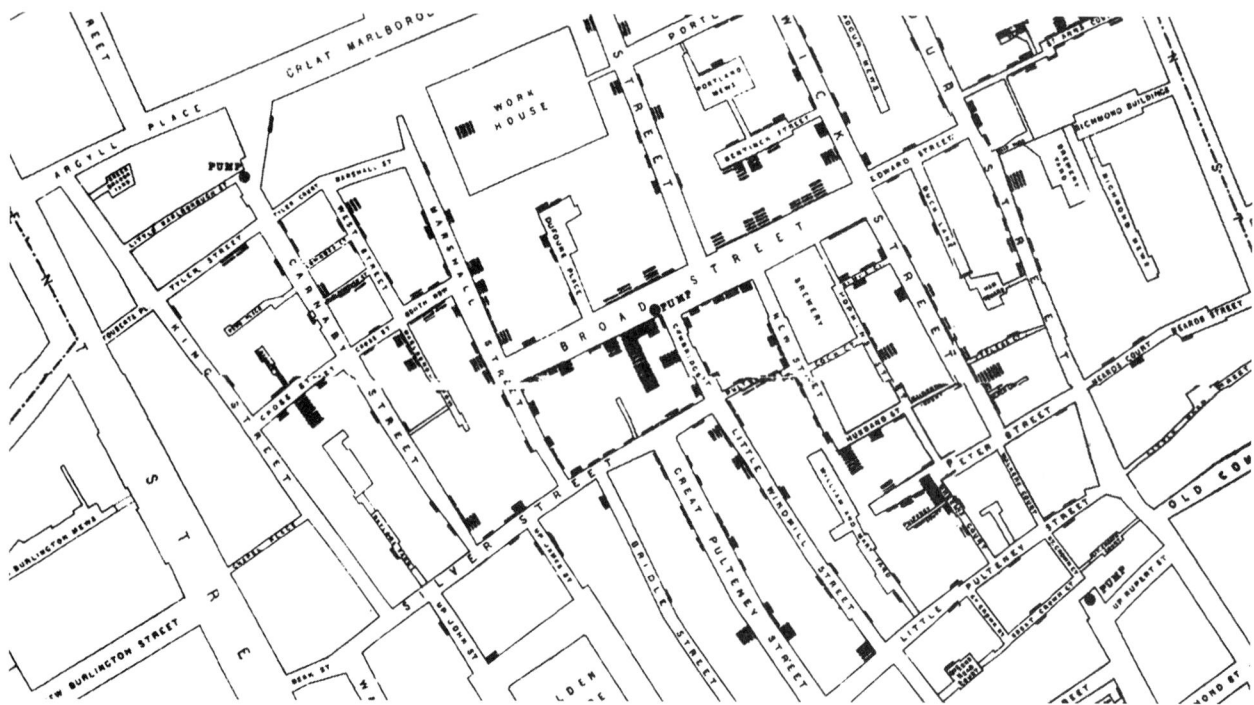

Figure 33.1
Dr. John Snow's map of cholera, 1854. From http://www.theguardian.com/news/datablog/2013/mar/15/john-snow-cholera-map. Accessed January 10, 2014.

removing the pump handle save hundreds of lives, but it also marked a significant shift in both public health policy and disease theory [2].

Current Applications

The way we think about maps is changing rapidly; gone are the days when they were used solely to help you navigate from one place to another. Maps can now serve as visual databases and dynamic tools that allow monitoring and evaluation professionals and their organizations to make real-time decisions, detect patterns, and both quantify and evaluate their impact.

In developed countries, such as the United States, health professionals have been using geographic information systems (GIS) and other complex geographic analysis tools to improve health outcomes for many years. By incorporating actionable tasks, such as tracking repeat emergency room visits, identifying food deserts, and better connecting patients with medical and social resources, analysts are leveraging geographic data to strengthen health care delivery systems.

In developing countries, however, GIS analysis is less frequently applied beyond the realm of research. This is largely due to a lack of data, in part because there is rarely the same market demand for hyperlocal spatial information in remote, developing places. These are the same places, however, in which geography plays a critical role, as physical access to primary care can be the single most determining factor in the utilization of health services, and consequently, the health of a population [3]. There is enormous potential to apply geographic analysis in these vulnerable areas in order to resolve concerns about service coverage, allocate resources effectively, and understand the distribution of phenomena across a catchment area (figure 33.2).

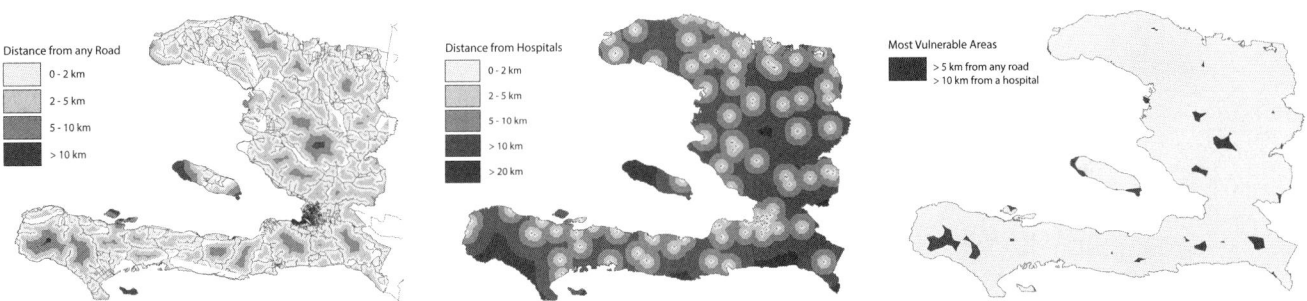

Figure 33.2
Multicriteria evaluation used to determine possible new locations for health facilities in Haiti based on distance from current roads and hospitals. December 2011.

In the context of health program implementation, the benefits of spatial analysis and visualization can be broken down into the following four categories.

1. Improved monitoring of programs, patients, and disease: detecting patterns, targeting resources more effectively.

2. Rigorous evaluation of programs: identifying gaps in coverage, quantifying impact.

3. Informed long-term planning: viewing trends over time in order to plan for the future.

4. Engagement of stakeholders: garnering support from governments, donors, local health workers, and communities.

Some specific examples of applied geographic analysis include recording distances that patients have to travel to the nearest tuberculosis directly observed treatment distribution center, quantifying a relationship between the accessibility to roads and HIV cases, informing program expansion into new communities, and evaluating and improving ambulance response times [4].

Technology and Methods

Nearly all geographic analysis relies on both global positioning systems (GPS) and GIS technologies. For the analysis that many community health organizations are interested in conducting, it is ideal to have a specific GPS point (latitude and longitude) for every household, clinic, hospital, or point of interest so that practitioners can visualize and analyze relevant programmatic data at a variety of scales. The idea, however, of embarking on a massive data collection campaign with traditional tools like pen, paper, and handheld GPS devices can be daunting.

Fortunately, the growing availability of GPS-enabled smartphones in developing countries has simplified this process significantly. With a handheld GPS, you must upload the points onto a computer and merge them into an existing database, which introduces significant potential for human error. Tools from organizations like Magpi and ODK Collect run on Android phones and allow users to build a "Location" field directly into their surveys, thereby eliminating the need for additional GPS training and data reconciliation.

Once you have collected all of the data, you can import it into a GIS and connect it with existing health and spatial data—such as administrative boundaries, population distribution, or water and road networks—to run analysis and generate maps. ArcGIS, manufactured by ESRI, is the leading proprietary GIS used to run geographic analysis by a wide range of sectors, from conservation and defense to real estate and e-commerce. Nonprofits can purchase ArcGIS at reduced rates, and receive support from ESRI. A free

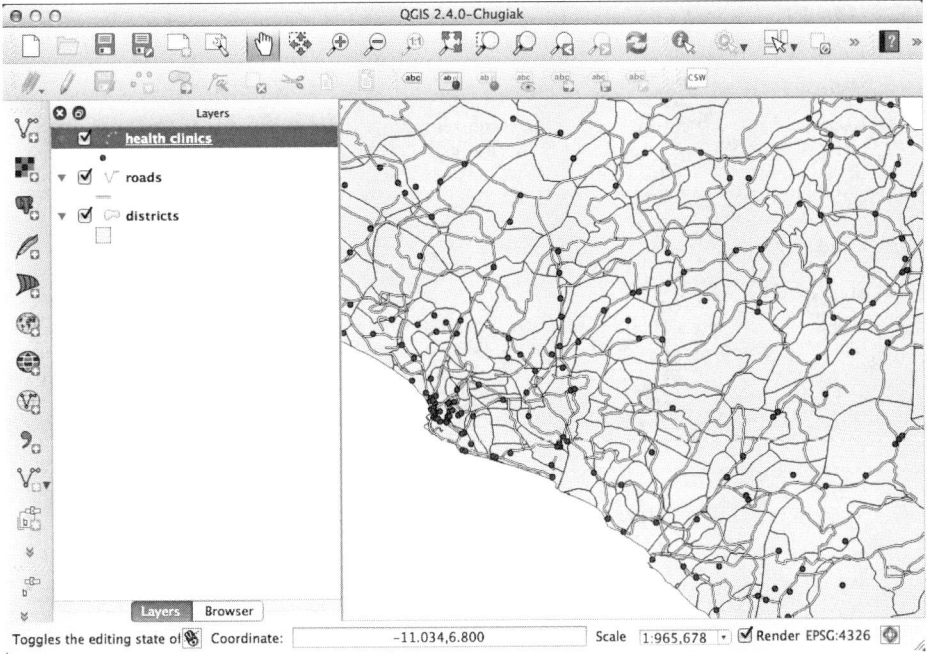

Figure 33.3
QGIS desktop software. March 2015.

and open-source alternative called QGIS is also available (figure 33.3). QGIS is a great option for organizations that have limited technical budgets or are focused on interoperability. It also has a large community of support forums and developers that are able to help with troubleshooting and development.

Table 33.1 summarizes three case studies in which the tools and methods described above were used to run specific GIS operations to achieve programmatic goals.

Despite the undisputed power of a GIS, it is important to note that organizations do not necessarily need complex software to begin thinking spatially about their work. Hand-drawn maps have proven to be incredibly valuable tools for incorporating local knowledge, enhancing community ownership, and understanding local perceptions of distance and space. As Dr. John Snow proved, visualizing pertinent health data in even the simplest ways can elicit valuable new insights that inform decision making.

Table 33.1
Case Studies in Applied GIS

Goal	Methodology	Outcome
Define an effective number of catchment areas within a community health worker (CHW) program [4]	CHWs collected locations for 10,275 homesteads in the study area. A fuzzy accessibility model based off of terrain, homestead density, and existing road networks was used to calculate average inter-homestead walking times.	By summing all walking and interview times for all homesteads, it was estimated that it would take one fieldworker in excess of 1,900 working days to complete the entire study area. Therefore, it is possible to recommend that 48 fieldworkers should be used in each 60 working day cycle.
Identify potential gaps in access to emergency obstetric care [5]	Health workers mapped C-section rates as a proportion of total expected births by cell, using population data collected by CHWs, and clinical data from health centers. Peripartum fetal mortality rates per facility-based births, as well as the rate of uterine rupture as an indication for C-section, were compared between areas of low and high C-section rates.	The lowest C-section rates were found in the more remote part of the hospital catchment area. The sector with significantly lower C-section rates had significantly higher facility-based peripartum fetal mortality and incidence of uterine rupture than the sector with the highest C-section rates.
Identify possible locations for a new clinic that will maximize accessibility for the greatest population [3]	Previous work in the region had shown that a relationship exists between decay in attendance of a specific clinic and travel time to that clinic. The reverse of this curve was used to calculate an impedance to care value. The product of the impedance value and the number of residents for each homestead were then superimposed onto a 30-m grid and filtered to calculate person-impedance per km^2.	The map identifies areas where high levels of impedance to care correspond with larger population. These areas therefore represent where a new clinic could have the greatest impact. These potential clinic sites can now be incorporated into other sociogeographical and logistic criteria to narrow down locations and make a final decision.

Obstacles and Challenges

Any new program or tool will inevitably present unforeseen challenges and obstacles, so it is important to be as intentional as possible about setting up appropriate systems from the very beginning. The complexity of GIS software demands both skilled users and quality data inputs, presenting organizations and practitioners with two significant hurdles.

The first challenge is deciding whether to train current staff or employ outside analysts. Staff members are often overworked with direct service-delivery tasks and have limited bandwidth to learn a new, complex tool. Contracting out this work, however, can be expensive and fails to build in-house capacity. And because of the continuous nature of monitoring and evaluation, initial analysis may quickly become obsolete unless the relationship with a contractor is ongoing. Consider, therefore, how frequently you want to use geographic analysis and data in your workflow. A contracted analyst may be sufficient if you wish to include insights in quarterly or annual reports, while a full-time staff member or partnership may be more appropriate if you plan to integrate the analysis into your daily or weekly strategy.

The second and, perhaps, more daunting challenge for organizations is finding or creating reliable, contextually appropriate, and updated geographic data. This could include accurate administrative boundaries, the locations of water sources, or subnational population counts, as well as any specific patient or program data. Without these foundational pieces of information, it is nearly impossible to carry out sophisticated geographic analysis.

Many organizations have already begun to lay this groundwork without realizing it. Simple data points, such as village and clinic names or patient walking distances, can be pulled out and used to visualize existing datasets. Before converting existing data or collecting anything new, however, it is essential to identify the exact questions you want to answer with your analysis and all of the data inputs you will need to reach a conclusion. It is also crucial to establish a unique ID system—whether it is an individual patient code, a community health worker name, or a clinic—that will be used to connect all of your related datasets. Rushing into an initial survey without doing long-term planning can result in inefficient or duplicate data collection efforts, messy reconciliation processes, and wasted time.

Finally, organizations must take privacy and data security into consideration from the very beginning. When working with sensitive health data, especially on the community scale, you must disassociate individuals from specific health conditions in any public-facing maps or reports. Creating user-specific access to data within an organization and aggregating data up a scale for communications materials are two simple ways to address these issues.

Crowdsourcing and Open-Source Tools

Fortunately, the open-source community is beginning to address a number of these challenges through the introduction of tools, methodologies, and open data that allow for greater collaboration and reduced costs.

The most significant of these open-source tools is OpenStreetMap (OSM). OSM is a collaborative project that aims to create a free, crowdsourced map of the world that not only harnesses the power of local knowledge, but also allows individuals and organizations to download the data for their own use. No matter where you work in the world, OSM is a great place to start before embarking on any geographic data collection effort of your own.

OpenStreetMap can also serve as an important tool in the wake of a natural disaster. After the 2010 earthquake in Haiti, for example, rescue workers were frantically trying to answer questions: who needs help, and where are they? With all central sources of information and authority devastated, the teams at OSM and their partner organization Ushahidi mobilized volunteers from around the world to fill the vacuum. By examining

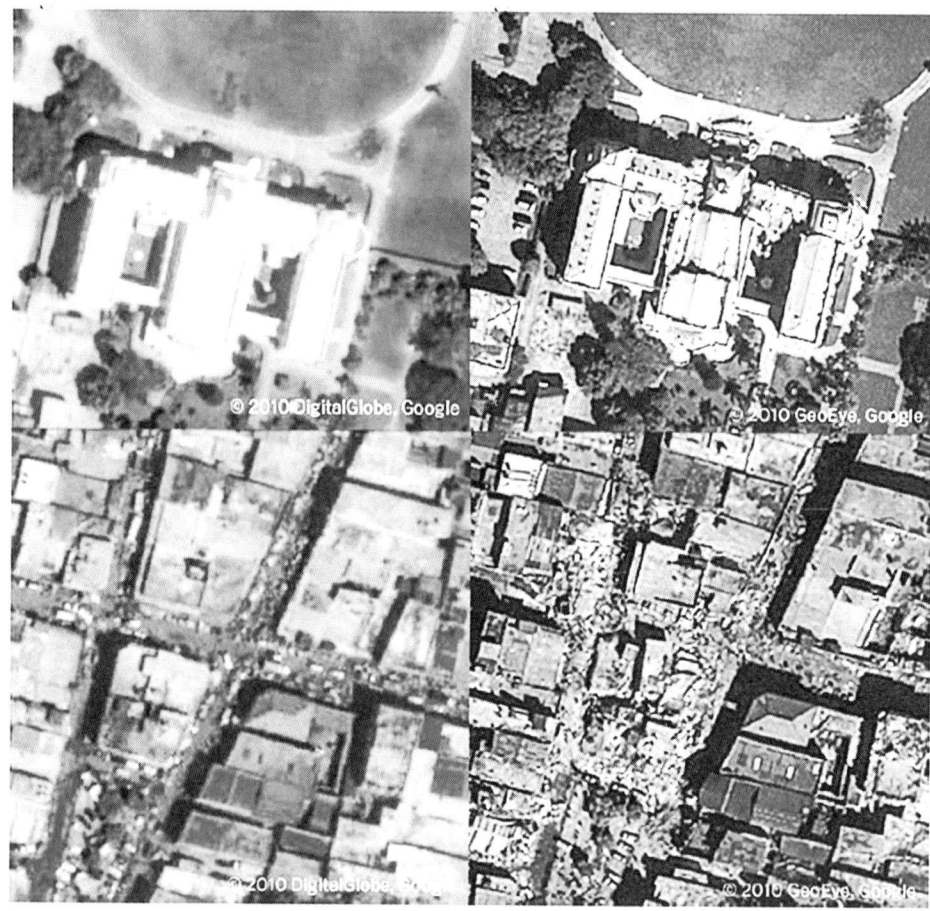

Figure 33.4
Haiti satellite imagery immediately before and after the earthquake, highlighting the improvement in resolution as well as the visible destruction. January 2010. Screenshot of Google website from Zook M, et al. 2010. Volunteered geographic information and crowdsourcing disaster relief: A case study of the Haitian earthquake. *World Med Health Policy* 2(2): 7–33.

satellite imagery and analyzing survivors' SMS, citizens were able to update the locations of passable roads, destroyed buildings, and other vital information to help direct emergency response teams on the ground (figure 33.4). This revolutionary access to locally sourced information allowed health workers to make critical decisions, focus their efforts, and save lives [6].

As the crowdsourcing movement gains momentum, the Humanitarian OpenStreetMap Team at OSM is championing efforts to build a better data infrastructure well before disaster strikes. Through a combination of on-the-ground data collection agents, partner NGOs, and remote volunteers, the team aims to improve the quality of geographic data in developing countries for a wide range of planning and development initiatives, including the delivery of basic health services.

Conclusion

Dynamic mapping tools have the potential to not only help organizations conduct more informed monitoring and evaluation of their work, but also to strengthen health systems around the world through the construction of a more robust data framework. And because public health is inextricably linked to physical infrastructure like roads or sanitation networks, being able to visualize the location—or absence of—critical services, such as public toilet blocks, water wells, or bus stops, is essential for planning and evaluation purposes on both local and national scales.

While you can compile all of this information in a spreadsheet, viewing it on a map provides a unique and actionable perspective—one that allows practitioners to visualize patterns or identify relationships between seemingly disparate factors and, ultimately, save lives. Geographic analysis is, therefore, a critical component of understanding and improving the health of a community and should be considered a necessary and irreplaceable tool among health workers.

Questions for Discussion

- What is spatial about your current work? Are there questions you ask yourself on a regular basis that may be geographic? Are there elements of your programs that depend on physical location?
- How do you envision geographic tools being integrated into the daily workflow of an organization? What challenges do you anticipate?
- How do you think we can improve the quality and quantity of geographic data in developing countries?

References

1. Williams DR. 2013. Making America healthier: What can each of us do? Lecture presented at the University of Missouri, Columbia, MO, November 16.

2. Johnson S. *The Ghost Map*. New York, NY: Penguin; 2006: 159–163.

3. Tanser F. 2006. Geographical information systems (GIS) innovations for primary health care in developing countries. *Innovations* (Spring): 110. https://www.mailman.columbia.edu/sites/default/files/pdf/tanser_2006_gis_innovations_for_phc_in_developing_countries.pdf.

4. Tanser F. 2002. The application of GIS technology to equitably distribute fieldworker workload in a large, rural South African health survey. *Trop Med Int Health* 7(1): 80.

5. Sudhof L, Amoroso C, Barebwanuwe P, Munyaneza F, Karamaga A, Zambotti G, et al. 2013. Local use of geographic information systems to improve data utilization and health services: Mapping caesarean section coverage in rural Rwanda. *Trop Med Int Health* 18(1): 18–26.

6. Zook M, Graham M, Shelton T, Gorman S. 2010. Volunteered geographic information and crowdsourcing disaster relief: A case study of the Haitian earthquake. *World Med Health Policy* 2(2): 7–33.

34 Supply-Chain Management

Justin Miranda, Jesse A. Greenspan, and Christopher Hamon

Take-Home Messages

- There are many challenges to implementing effective supply-chain management, especially in resource-limited settings.
- Supply-chain management is more than just the technology that keeps track of inventory and stock movements—it also includes the people and processes put in place to ensure the efficient and effective flow of supplies.
- An effective supply chain can lead to better quality of care for patients, cost savings for an organization, and stabilization of the public health system.
- An ineffective supply chain can have disastrous effects on a health care organization as well as the larger health care system that surrounds it.

Introduction

The main objective of a supply chain is to deliver a product from the point of origin to the point of consumption in the most effective and efficient way possible. According to the World Health Organization, supply-chain systems should "supply the right goods, in the right quantities, in the right condition, to the right place, at the right time, and at the right cost" [21].

While most supply-chain practitioners would generally agree with this statement, the specific practices adopted by organizations to satisfy this objective vary widely. Within the health care field specifically, the goal of supply-chain management is to guarantee the availability of the products needed to treat patients by maintaining an adequate supply of medications and medical supplies, preventing stock-outs, and reducing waste from expired and damaged goods. However, the practices adopted by health care organizations in the United States, for example, may vary from those organizations working in resource-limited settings in other countries due to the challenges described below, including uncertainty, fragmentation, long lead time, poor infrastructure, a lack of qualified personnel, the cost of technology, and the need for the prioritization of supply chain, good communication, qualified personnel, effective processes, and accurate data [4].

When an international health care organization's supply-chain system is functioning well, clinicians do not worry about how a health care commodity is manufactured, from which supplier it was purchased, or how it was transported from the country of origin to their facility. Nor are they concerned about how long it took for a shipment to get through customs or whether all items were received, unloaded, inspected, and put away in an efficient manner. However, when a supply-chain system is not aligned with clinical objectives and is performing poorly—for example, when a much-needed antibiotic is stocked out or when critical surgical equipment has been damaged in transit—clinicians take notice. It is under these circumstances that clinical staff become familiar with supply-chain management, or, more appropriately, with the lack of an effective and efficient supply-chain management system. Thus, clinical staff are important stakeholders in supply-chain management decisions and it is the supply-chain group's role to ensure that clinicians have the resources needed to do their jobs [19].

Technology, data collection, and electronic medical record system integration can play an important role in a well-designed supply chain and improve quality of care. However, adoption of technology without an understanding of the cost of implementation and maintenance can be detrimental. The cost of hardware, software, and operational costs, as well as the long-term support required to develop a good supply-chain management system can be expensive, and organizations should undertake a thorough cost-benefit analysis prior to implementation.

Impact of a High-Performing Supply Chain

A well-run supply-chain system can have a dramatically positive impact on a health care system. It can lead to better quality of care for patients, cost savings for the organization, and improvements in the public health system [21].

Quality of Care

When a supply-chain system is functioning well, patients get the medicines and supplies they need in a timely manner. Clinicians do not need to make do without optimal products or substitute substandard items due to stock-outs or expiry. In an efficient supply-chain system, the quality of the medications and medical supplies that are administered to patients have been thoroughly authenticated at every step of the supply chain, from regulation at the point of manufacturing, to national drug registries and customs clearance processes, order or shipment receipt processes, and the final check that a pharmacist or nurse makes on dosing, formulation, and expiration date at the point of consumption [19]. These added authentication steps reduce the risk of accidentally using medicines or supplies that are counterfeit, expired, or damaged, which enhances patient safety.

Quality of care can also be improved by data collection and integration between an electronic medical record system and a supply-chain system. This comprehensive view of the entire supply chain can be useful in understanding which products led to successful patient outcomes, projecting future programmatic and budgetary needs, protecting against corruption, and ultimately allowing for an increase in the number of patients served [19].

Cost-Effectiveness

An effective supply-chain system can also lead to cost savings for a health care organization. By accurately tracking, reviewing, and projecting an organization's supply needs, stock utilization is optimized. This optimization translates to cost savings from fewer expired medicines and supplies. It also means valuable space and money are not wasted on managing slow-moving, obsolete, or overstocked products.

When an organization is able to correctly predict which goods it will need at which times, purchasing options also open up. For example, group purchasing organizations are entities that create purchasing power for small companies by compiling their various needs into larger volumes, thus gaining access to bulk rates [16]. Using such options to save money is only possible if an organization can forecast its needs effectively.

A framework contract is an agreement between organizations and vendors that may lead to cost savings for an organization. The goal of this type of agreement is to lock in prices for specific products over a fixed term to avoid price fluctuations due to factors such as global stock shortages. In order to put a framework contract in place, an organization will need to compile a list of specific products it anticipates needing to order over the term of the agreement and provide the vendor with a sense of the volume that is likely to be ordered. Relationships with suppliers and transporters should be continuously reviewed to ensure they remain the best choice for the organization [19].

Variations in shipment costs can also be used to an organization's advantage if lead times for necessary medicines are known ahead of time. For example, it is much cheaper to ship goods via sea freight than by air. However, because sea freight takes longer to arrive at the destination port than air freight, relying on sea shipments requires more advanced planning and more accurate projections of needed goods [12].

Air transportation is very expensive and worthwhile only when used in cases of emergency such as a stock-out of a critical medicine (or when other factors such as temperature requirements necessitate shipping by air). An organization may also respond to a stock-out event by purchasing supplies in the local market, which may have higher costs and may not adhere to quality standards. Such emergency procurements, if stock-outs occur frequently, can present a large financial burden for an international health care organization [15].

Strengthened Public Health System

Ideally, international health care organizations would work with the public sector in order to support the existing supply-chain infrastructure and avoid creating parallel systems [12]. If an organization is responsible for filling in gaps in government procurement or supporting public health facilities or programs, a high-performing supply-chain system is important for the success of those efforts. Ensuring that patients are not turned away due to stock-outs also means that other facilities in the catchment area are not overburdened by an influx of patients. An effective organization or treatment program within an organization can also lead to collaboration with other health care groups. Best practices can be shared to improve national health outcomes, and consumption data can be shared to help with forecasting. In emergency situations, stock, equipment, or warehouse storage space can also be shared among organizations or with local governments.

Effective supply-chain systems will incorporate a review of all prospective vendors, including local businesses. Ideally, a health care organization will purchase at least some medicines and supplies locally, which will not only support the local economy, but also build up local capacity by creating jobs at vendor sites. For example, certain bulky or heavy items, or locally manufactured items, may be cheaper and more efficient to procure on the local market once international shipping costs and transit times are taken into account [12].

Impact of Poor Supply-Chain Management

Poor supply-chain management can cause international health care organizations to fail, seriously affecting their financial security by wasting resources and reacting to emergencies rather than accurately projecting future needs. Poor supply-chain management practices can lead to problems related to inventory availability, quality assurance, patient care, and larger systemic issues that can adversely impact the organization, including an organization's reputation with the public sector, partner organizations, and the patient population it serves [17].

Inventory availability problems occur when there is no visibility into what items are in stock, understocked, overstocked, expired, or about to expire, or when there are insufficient human resources to adequately respond to these supply-chain issues. The impact of stocked-out, understocked, and expired items is obvious—patients do not get the treatment they need. The consistent availability of medications is especially critical for complicated treatment regimens such as antiretroviral therapy for HIV/AIDS; missing doses of antiretroviral therapy can lead to increased morbidity and drug resistance, and even death [2,17].

Overstocked medicines and supplies are also an issue in that they waste valuable resources. The money and storage space wasted on unnecessary stock could have otherwise been used to purchase and store essential equipment and supplies. Storage space, because it is finite, is a valuable resource, and some medical supplies, such as oral rehydration solution used to treat dehydrated patients, take up a great deal of space. An overstock of oral rehydration solution means less space for other essential medicines [19].

Unfortunately, there are many ways the quality of medicines and medical supplies can be compromised. Medicines can be counterfeited by the supplier, tampered with during shipping, or damaged during put-away or while in storage [21]. The quality of vaccines and other cold chain medications are even harder to maintain, as their storage conditions (temperature and humidity) must meet recommended standards that are monitored and validated at every step along the supply chain [6,7]. Quality assurance is a major issue, as it is difficult to maintain staff accountability, product authentication, and close tracking in long supply chains.

Poor supply-chain management practices can have deeply detrimental effects on the budgets, programs and staffing of a health care organization as well. If an organization is frequently making emergency purchases when items become stocked out or expired, its spending on higher product prices and shipping costs may be more than its annual budget can support [9,15]. In addition, if medicines frequently stock out within a treatment program that is operated through a funding agency, the health care organization and the funding agency are susceptible to criticisms of their effectiveness, and patients' trust in the treatment program is likely to decrease [17]. If an organization has poor supply-chain management practices, the donor organization may also be unwilling to provide additional resources for further funding, or the program may be cut completely, which would require patients to find other options to continue treatment.

From clinicians to warehouse staff, burnout and turnover are common occurrences in poorly functioning supply chains. When clinicians cannot count on essential medicines being readily available from the pharmacy, there is a loss of trust in the health care organization as a whole. When staff are not provided with the training, shipping and moving equipment, storage space, and autonomy they need, there may be poor job satisfaction and high resignation rates. A smoothly operating supply chain benefits everyone [4].

Common Challenges

For international health care organizations working in resource-limited settings, implementing a successful supply-chain system is fraught with challenges. Each of these challenges is magnified in the global health context, as resources are scarce, supply-chain expertise is not well-established, and problems have a direct impact on patient care. The following are just a few of the challenges that health care organizations face when implementing supply-chain solutions.

Prioritization

Health care organizations working in resource-limited settings may not sufficiently invest in a robust supply-chain system considering other priorities and the need to allocate limited resources. For example, an organization, perhaps rightly so, may focus on direct clinical care. However, the supply chain should be seen as the backbone to the goal of providing quality health care to communities, and the demands of an effective supply chain should be prioritized in order to guarantee that clinicians will have the tools they need to treat their patients [12].

Uncertainty

Most supply-chain issues faced by health care organizations working in resource-limited settings revolve around uncertainty [5]. Uncertainty comes in many forms: supply-side shortages, delivery time variability, population growth, supply-chain disruptions due to natural disasters, political unrest, untrained staff, and many other causes [18,20]. Are roads going to be accessible to distribute drugs from the central depot this week? Is there political instability that is preventing shipments from entering a port? How much anti-malarial medication do we need during the rainy season for a catchment area whose population has seen a variable percentage growth year over year?

Even when a supply-chain system is performing at its best, the answers to these questions can be uncertain and contribute to stock-outs, missed medical treatment opportunities, sicker patients, patients who seek treatment at other facilities, or worse, patients who are lost to follow-up due to nonadherence or death.

Most stock projections are based on past consumption data. In many cases, those data are incomplete or nonexistent, which makes the output of a projection calculation unreliable. Even with good data, there is no guarantee that past consumption will predict future consumption for a given population [17]. Projecting future needs requires an understanding of complex factors including disease prevalence within a catchment area, target population growth, and spikes in consumption due to seasonality (e.g., rainy season) [12,19]. Maintaining a buffer stock is one way to mitigate risk of stock-outs amid uncertainty, but it comes at the cost of using financial resources and valuable warehouse space that could have been used for other medications and supplies, or rooms in a hospital that would have otherwise been used for patient care [15,19].

People

A lack of trained supply-chain personnel is also a significant barrier to effective supply-chain management. Thus, many organizations rely on staff who do not have supply-chain management training, such as clinical staff, to take on supply-chain responsibilities. That means that nurses, pharmacists, doctors and even administrative staff who are already busy dealing with patient care and hospital management are asked to tally up pill counts, project order quantities, complete monthly reports and perform other tasks that they are not trained or motivated to do [3,15,18]. Overlooking the need for training, managing large workloads, and improving systems easily leads to burnout, decreased motivation, and staff turnover, thereby negatively impacting the supply-chain operation [4].

It can be difficult to fill supply-chain roles with qualified personnel. Even when supply-chain management trainings do exist, they are often not high quality [3,18]. Students who are trained as supply-chain specialists, when such training opportunities are available, also may not choose to work for a nonprofit health care organization if there are more lucrative opportunities in the local private sector or abroad. In addition, employees who are certified and trained in supply-chain management while working for a nonprofit are at risk of being recruited by these other organizations with the promise of better pay. Therefore, while education and training are important, additional incentives like competitive compensation and benefits are also essential to retain staff [1].

Another major challenge when working in global settings is language. The language barrier between in-country and expatriate colleagues can be managed by a human resources department that hires locally or by expatriates who speak the local language of the country [11,13]. However, it is not feasible to ask suppliers and distributors to ensure that all packaging comes in the local language, so it may be necessary for supply-chain staff to speak multiple languages or risk missing important information on product packaging. This language barrier can be somewhat mitigated by tracking products using unique identifiers or barcoding, but implementation of these systems requires additional financial resources that must be considered.

Language is also a barrier for organizations that want to invest in training local staff because it can be difficult to find formal supply-chain management training opportunities available in languages other than English [3].

Process

In addition to having highly trained staff, it is important to have formalized and efficient processes specifically designed for an organization's supply-chain activities [4]. From put-away to picking tasks, thoughtful and coherent standard operating procedures (SOPs) are key. After SOPs are established, there needs to be comprehensive training on their use for all staff, as well as consistent enforcement of rules around accountability. A lack of

SOPs, training, or rule enforcement can lead to inventory inaccuracies, delayed distribution, and stock-outs.

SOPs should also be constantly evaluated, and redesigned if necessary according to process improvements and changes in strategy and technology [10]. Improvement initiatives around a certain SOP can put strain on another aspect of the supply chain, so any changes need to be fully thought out to prevent unanticipated errors and bottlenecks. For example, the organization's management may decide to increase the frequency of cycle counts from weekly to daily hoping to make records of onhand quantities more accurate. However, this change may necessitate, for example, adding new staff to handle the extra work or providing new technology to improve the cycle count process. If these added resources are not provided, the change could lead to employee burnout and increased error rates.

Communication

The challenge of effective communication is not specific to supply-chain management, but poor communication within the organization and with vendors and donors can have a detrimental impact on supply-chain performance. Organizations should establish clear communication between all parts of the supply chain, from procurement staff to warehouse personnel, and between the supply-chain group and other departments and managers at the organization. It is important that managers have a clear understanding of supply-chain principles and how organizational decisions, from spending cuts to changes in service delivery, impact work along the supply chain. Ideally, management would be involved throughout the entire supply-chain process, from the initial needs assessment to the delivery of goods [12].

Clear communication about supply-chain data, including stock management and distribution, is important for maintaining donor relationships [12]. Organizations embarking on new projects or seeking funding for new initiatives sometimes fail to consider supply-chain realities when developing proposals. It is imperative that supply-chain capacity and limitations be considered from the early stages of the project lifecycle to avoid challenging situations down the line. Failing to do so could result in the need to revise an already agreed-on proposal, or, more likely, taxing already scarce resources to achieve an objective or collect data in a limited amount of time.

Communication with employees is also essential to ensure that everyone shares the same mission and stays motivated to keep the supply chain running smoothly, especially when the supply chain directly impacts patient care. When employees feel accountable within the organization, they will feel comfortable making suggestions for improvement, getting involved with innovations, and buying into new practices [13].

Maintaining clear communication with external partners, such as suppliers and local ministries of health, will also improve the entire supply-chain system. For example, providing suppliers with updated demand information will help them manage their production effectively so supply-side shortages are reduced [15]. Keeping accurate documentation and communicating often with ministries of health will ease issues with international shipments and customs clearance, as well national drug regulations and tax laws [12].

Lead time

Lead time is the period between the moment when a product need is identified (i.e., through routine replenishment or a specific request) to the moment when the product is delivered and ready for consumption. International health care organizations have to deal with longer and more variable lead times than their counterparts working only in the United States, for example, due to the fact that international supply chains are more complex, products need to travel longer distances, and customs clearance times can be unpredictable [4,12,21].

The longer, more variable lead times require better planning and coordination with external partners, like suppliers. Organizations must fine-tune their needs assessments and demand projections in order to come up with realistic forecasts for medication and supply consumption. Longer lead times alone are not a problem if they are predictable and you can forecast your needs accurately—it is usually variability that causes most problems. The variability component requires an organization to keep larger amounts of buffer stock as protection against a missed delivery date or longer-than-usual customs clearance times. While needed to prevent stock-outs, unused buffer stock leads to the overstock situation described above in which money, time, and storage space are wasted on items that could have otherwise been used for other essential medications and supplies [15].

Infrastructure

Challenges related to infrastructure also lead to problems in the supply chain. Relying on spaces not designed for storage, or spaces that are too small for current or future needs, will affect an organization's ability to keep the right items in the right quantities on hand. These inadequate storage spaces also affect staff members' ability to perform their duties well, which can in turn lead to retention challenges. In addition, unstable power and internet impact the ability to collect data and transmit timely information, as well as the ability to maintain cold chains. Bad roads can lead to longer lead times and damaged products. These infrastructure challenges are especially troublesome in rural locations, where the combination of these issues creates a perfect storm of supply-chain dysfunction.

Power outages can also lead to damaged equipment, which will need to be repaired or replaced. In most cases, addressing these problems requires service from the manufacturer. As organizations do not always have this expertise in-house and the manufacturing companies usually cannot send service personnel in a timely manner, damaged equipment can go unrepaired for months or years, leading to missed diagnostic and treatment opportunities. Having access to local or regional technical support is key with respect to medical equipment. Hopefully with time, local economies will grow and diversify to be able to service these equipment failures. Until then, care must be taken when selecting and installing equipment [12].

Fragmentation

Fragmented or vertical supply chains present a challenge for international health care organizations because they require additional coordination and can result in the inefficient use of resources. Some funders or project requirements prescribe managing items for different activities separately or make stock management recommendations that fall outside of an organization's standard practices. Another reason fragmentation can occur is when organizations supplement stock with in-kind donations from partner organizations that have specific stock management or reporting requirements [4]. Fragmentation can also be caused by a mistrust of or dissatisfaction with the organization's own supply-chain system. For example, clinical and supply-chain staff who have witnessed the effects of ineffective supply chains often decide to take personal responsibility to meet their own and the organization's supply-chain needs [15].

Such fragmentation of supply-chain activities leads to stock redundancies, staffing overlaps, inefficient spending, and a lack of information sharing. For example, a single health care organization may have several projects that require a similar group of products but may not pool resources for procurement, transport, delivery, and labor. These vertical systems also require redundant storage in the same facility, wasting potentially valuable space. To minimize negative effects of fragmentation, supply chain managers should plan for new services or projects holistically and identify opportunities to gain efficiencies through coordination and centralization when donor and project requirements allow [15].

Data and Data Standards

The effectiveness of a supply-chain system is in large part dependent on the quality of available data. High-quality data allow supply-chain staff to make informed decisions on product and vendor selection and order quantity and timing; high-quality data help an organization be proactive rather than reactive and increase the efficiency of daily tasks. Unfortunately, due to the long lead times experienced by international health care organizations, low stock situations created by using poor data for planning can also take a long time to correct, highlighting the importance of high-quality data for patient care.

Data maintenance requires both a good information system and dedicated resources to monitor data quality. A good information system can be either paper or electronic, but the goal is to create access to data that are standardized through a data collection process that is as streamlined as possible. At the most basic level, the information system should outline standards for the collection of product metadata, including unique product identifier, product name, description, manufacturer, manufacturer code, temperature requirements, and package sizes. To facilitate ordering, an information system should track whether or not a product should be reordered or not. This decision can be based on feedback from the end user about the quality of a product or on the identification of formulary items, items that should always be available for the clinical services the organization is delivering, as opposed to products that the organization no longer needs or are part of a special one-time purchase.

Ordering is also made efficient by the centralization of data related to suppliers, including supplier code or identifier, lead time (for both the supplier to receive stock and transit and customs clearance time once the order is sent), and pricing. An organization may choose to give the supplier a rating or status as a "preferred" or a "secondary" partner based on factors like customer service, consistency of product availability, discounts, or human rights or environmental protection records.

To prepare accurate orders, an organization must have access to data about demand in service delivery locations, but this information is often not available [15]. A lack of accurate demand data creates uncertainty and can cause an organization to waste money and valuable storage space by over-ordering, or put patient lives at risk by under-ordering. Accurate forecasting depends on having information on patient population demographics, local prevalence of disease including the seasonality of disease, and to the organization's plans to increase or decrease the geographical service area, to start or stop treating a cadre of patients, or to add or subtract a clinical service. Collecting consumption data over time will lead to increasingly more accurate ordering [12].

Once stock arrives at a storage location, it is also important to maintain the accuracy of data about stock availability. Ensuring that physical stock (the stock available in the storage location) and theoretical stock (the stock recorded in the information management system) match is important because, when using an electronic system, this gives staff located at other sites or abroad visibility into the stock on hand at specific locations, information that is useful to consider when making ordering decisions. In addition to quantity on hand, the expiration dates and lot numbers for these quantities must be kept accurate in information management systems. Warehouse managers can use this information to ensure that products with the earliest expiration date are used first, as well as locate and quarantine specific lot numbers in the case of product recalls from the manufacturer.

Data issues that can clog the supply-chain system are numerous and can be minimized by having staff dedicated to managing data quality and standardization, including providing refresher trainings for data entry staff. Data issues that organizations should avoid are duplicate data (i.e., duplicate products or suppliers), outdated products or suppliers (i.e., products that have been discontinued or need metadata updated), and incomplete data for product or supplier metadata. However, organizations are frequently lacking staff to implement data quality improvement initiatives and even when staff time is devoted to data quality efforts, it is very time-consuming to review, correct, and merge data [10,14,21].

Technology

Technology can be a tremendous asset in a well-designed supply chain. However, adoption of technology without an understanding of the cost of implementation and maintenance can be detrimental. The impact of technology will be discussed in a separate section below.

Impact of Technology on Supply-Chain Management

Organizations of all sizes have a desire to use the latest technology in hopes that it will solve their supply-chain problems. Whether they are planning to adopt a brand new warehouse management system or implement radio-frequency identification (RFID) barcoding, these decisions should not be taken lightly. A good supply-chain management system can be expensive to implement and maintain over the first few years of ownership, which can present challenges or be unrealistic for a small nonprofit organization. If the organization is further unable to hire the right people to work with this new technology or provide the needed infrastructure, the positive effects expected may not be realized [21].

Decisions about the adoption of technology should be informed by an understanding of the true cost of implementation and maintenance. Decision makers should perform an exhaustive cost-benefit analysis to better understand what it will cost in monetary and human capital to get the system off the ground. The cost of technology adoption is often viewed myopically as the purchase and installation of software. However, a thorough cost-benefit analysis needs to include the cost of hardware and software, and operational costs, as well as long-term support [21]. Hardware and software costs include the original purchase, in addition to configuration, implementation, development, ongoing hosting, setup fees, licenses, migration from an old system, and thorough acceptance and performance testing. Operational costs include hiring the appropriate number of skilled staff to maintain the software and perform data collection, as well as providing warehouse staff with trucks, pallet movers, conveyors, and forklifts. Operational costs should also include the cost of rewriting the SOPs used to define daily activities of the warehouse and distribution network. The total cost of ownership should include long-term support costs such as maintenance and upgrades, hardware failures, scalability, and ongoing developer costs for custom features. Lastly, the more data are collected and made available, the more resources will be needed to effectively respond to the now-visible needs and demands of the supply chain. Organizations implementing new software (or any other tool that will make their inventory situation accessible and available) should anticipate this increase in work and plan on addressing it with appropriate staffing resources.

The lack of understanding around the total cost of ownership can add a huge financial and human resources burden to the organization. More challenges can arise when management fails to take proper steps to include warehouse and operations staff as stakeholders in decision making. The inclusion of end-users in making decisions about technology helps secure buy-in from those who will be most impacted by the resulting changes [2]. Staff may view changes as adding difficulty to daily tasks, so any supply-chain system changes should be coupled with training sessions and explanations of the benefits of the new system for the people doing the work [8].

This is not to say that adopting technology and information systems is not an important part of the supply-chain solution. In fact, it could be argued that technology is essential to a successful supply-chain system. However, supply-chain technology can be most beneficial when introduced after an organization establishes a sound foundation for its supply chain with qualified personnel and effective processes [6]. Then, when an organization decides to use technology to enhance its operations, the costs of implementation must be considered, as explained above. Technology is too often viewed as a panacea, especially in resource-limited settings. For example, mobile technology is booming, and yet wide-scale impact on the problems it is being used to solve has been limited. The reason has nothing to do with the efficacy of mobile technology, but rather with the cost of scaling up the technology the need for training, the need to invest in additional systems to support the influx of data, and the need to adapt innovations to different contexts [8]. Thus, it is important not to have unrealistic expectations that technology will solve problems without having to hire or train more qualified personnel and improve the processes around the technology.

Conclusion

Designing and implementing an effective supply chain is important for strengthening an international health care organization's programmatic and clinical efforts and should therefore be prioritized. An effective supply chain can lead to better quality of care for patients, cost savings for an organization, and an improved public health system. An ineffective and poorly designed supply chain can be destructive and lead to adverse events that can compromise patient safety. Technology is often thought to be an essential ingredient in creating an effective supply chain, but it is important to understand the hidden costs of implementation. An understanding of not only technology, but uncertainty, lead time, people, processes, communication, infrastructure, fragmentation, data, and data standards is key to a successful supply-chain system.

Questions for Discussion

- How does supply-chain management impact patient care?
- How does supply-chain management affect the longevity of an organization?
- How does adoption of a standard formulary (e.g., the World Health Organization Model List of Essential Medicines) impact supply-chain management?
- What factors need to be taken into consideration when performing forecasting for medical supplies and drugs to be used at a health center?
- Discuss possible solutions to each of the challenges discussed in the chapter (uncertainty, lead time, people, process, communication, infrastructure, fragmentation, technology, data, and data standards).

References

1. Garrett L. 2007. The challenge of global health. *Foreign Aff: 14–38*. Rpt in American Society of Tropical Medicine and Hygiene. http://www.astmh.org/Chalenges_of_Global_Health.htm. Accessed March 08, 2015.

2. Berger E, Jazayeri D, Sauveur M, Manasse JJ, Plancher I, Fiefe M, et al. 2007. Implementation and evaluation of a web based system for pharmacy stock management in rural Haiti. *AMIA Annu Symp Proc*: 46–50.

3. Brossette V, Silve B, Grall A, Bardy K, Pilz K, Dicko M, et al. 2010. Workforce excellence in health supply chain management: Literature review. People That Deliver, 2–3. http://peoplethatdeliver.org/sites/peoplethatdeliver.org/files/People%20that%20Deliver/files/Literature%20Review%20EN.pdf.

4. Dowling P. 2011. Healthcare supply chains in developing countries: Situational analysis. Arlington, VA: USAID Deliver Project, Task Order 4.

5. Ganeshan R, Harrison T. 1995. Introduction to supply chain management [online]. http://lcm.csa.iisc.ernet.in/scm/supply_chain_intro.html.

6. Sarley D. 2014. Supply chains for global health. Bill & Melinda Gates Foundation. http://www.impatientoptimists.org/Posts/2014/10/Supply-Chains-for-Global-Health. Accessed March 04, 2015.

7. Kaufman J, Miller R, Cheyne J. 2011. Vaccine supply chains need to be better funded and strengthened, or lives will be at risk. *Health Aff* 30: 1115.

8. Kinkade S, Verclas K. 2008. Wireless technology for social change. Washington, DC: United Nations Foundation-Vodafone Group Foundation Partnership.

9. Larson C, Burn R, Minnick-Sakal A, O'Keefe Douglas M, Kuritskye J. 2014. Strategies to reduce risks in ARV supply chains in the developing world. *Glob Health Sci Pract* 2(4): 399–400.

10. Nachtmann H, Pohl E. 2009. The state of healthcare logistics: Cost and quality improvement opportunities. Fayetteville, AR: Center for Innovation in Healthcare Logistics: 14–19.

11. Partners In Health. 2012. Unit 1: Learning about the local context. PIH Program Management Guide, 1–29. Boston, MA: Partners In Health.

12. Partners In Health. 2012. Unit 4: Managing a procurement system. PIH Program Management Guide, 1–32. Boston, MA: Partners In Health.

13. Partners In Health. 2012. Unit 5: Strengthening human resources. PIH Program Management Guide, 1–28. Boston, MA: Partners In Health.

14. Partners In Health. 2012. Unit 12: Using monitoring and evaluation for action. PIH Program Management Guide, 1–35. Boston, MA: Partners In Health.

15. Privett N, Gonsalvez D. 2014. The top ten global health supply chain issues: Perspectives from the field. *Oper Res Health Care* 3: 226–230.

16. Roark DC. 2005. Managing the healthcare supply chain. *Nurs Manage* 36(2): 36–40.

17. Schouten E, Jahn A, Ben-Smith A et al. 2011. Antiretroviral drug supply challenges in the era of scaling up ART in Malawi. *J Int AIDS Soc* 14(Suppl 1): S4.

18. Steele P. Addressing human resources in health supply chains: HR as a barrier to effective health supply chains. International Association of Public Health Logisticians. http://iaphl.org/wp-content/uploads/2016/05/HR-Supply-chains.pdf. Accessed March 04, 2015.

19. Sullivan E, Goentzel J, Weintraub R. 2012. Concept note: The global health supply chain. *Harv Bus Pub*: 1–22. https://www.ghdonline.org/cases/concept-note-the-global-health-supply-chain/.

20. Unite for Sight. Supply chains in global health. Accessed March 6, 2015. http://www.uniteforsight.org/technology-implementation/supply-chains.

21. USAID Deliver Project, Task Order 1. 2011. The logistics handbook: A practical guide for the supply chain management of health commodities. Arlington, VA: USAID Deliver Project, Task Order 1.

Contributors

Muideen Bakare, Enugu State University of Science & Technology and Federal Neuropsychiatric Hospital, Enugu, Nigeria

Mujeeb A. Basit, University of Texas Southwestern Medical School

William Bosl, University of San Francisco

Jørn Braa, University of Oslo, Norway

Elizabeth H. Bradley, Yale School of Public Health; Global Health Leadership Institute

Biyeun Buczyk, Dimagi

Leo Anthony G. Celi, MIT Critical Data, Massachusetts Institute of Technology

Connie Cheren, Partners for Care, Quality Assurance, Inc.

Anna Clements, Broad Street Maps

Gari Clifford, Emory University and Georgia Institute of Technology

Ryan Crichton, Jembi Health Systems NPC, South Africa

Bernice Dahn, Ministry of Health, Liberia

Anshuman J. Das, MIT Media Lab

Jacqueline DePasse, The Boston Consulting Group

Mosoka P. Fallah, Emergency Operation Center, Ministry of Health, Liberia

Kristin Castillo Farias, Boston Children's Hospital

Jesse Feierabend-Peters, University of Massachusetts Medical School

Mengling Feng, National University of Singapore; Institute for Infocomm Research

Tiara M. Forsyth, Harvard Medical School

Matthew P. Fox, Department of Epidemiology and Global Health, Boston University School of Public Health

Hamish S. F. Fraser, Leeds Institute of Health Sciences, University of Leeds, UK

Siedoh Freeman, Emergency Operation Center, Ministry of Health, Liberia

Mohammad Ghassemi, Institute for Medical Engineering and Science, Massachusetts Institute of Technology

Balwant Godara, eHealth Consultant and Lecturer
Tyrone Grandison, Institute for Health Metrics and Evaluation
Jesse A. Greenspan, Partners In Health
Jessica E. Haberer, Massachusetts General Hospital
Christopher Hamon, International Rescue Committee
Thomas P. Harris, Emergency Operation Center, Ministry of Health, Liberia
Andrea Ippolito, US Department of Veterans Affairs
Netty Joe, Emergency Operation Center, Ministry of Health, Liberia
Hannah Judge, Broad Street Maps
Jessica Kenney, Center for Global Health, Massachusetts General Hospital
Foster Kerrison, Commonwealth of Massachusetts, Executive Office of Health and Human Services.
Boonchai Kijsanayotin, Health Systems Research Institute, Ministry of Public Health, Thailand
Alain Labrique, Johns Hopkins Global mHealth Initiative
Jocelyn Ling, Incandescent
Diego Lopez, University of Cauca, Colombia
Alvin B. Marcelo, National Telehealth Center, University of the Philippines Manila, Philippines
David J. Meyers, Brown University
Laura J. Mintz, The MetroHealth System
Justin Miranda, OpenBoxes
Julian Mitton, Center for Global Health, Massachusetts General Hospital
Biju Mohandes, World Bank Group
Deshendran Moodley, Department of Computer Science, University of Cape Town, South Africa
Kerim Munir, Harvard Medical School
Jonathan M. Mwangi, Department of Medical Biochemistry, Mount Kenya University
Daniel Myung, Merck Sharpe & Dohme
Sunil Nair, Beth Israel Deaconess Medical Center
Vipan Nikore, MIT Critical Data, Massachusetts Institute of Technology
Linus Ndegwa, Partners for Care; Mount Kenya University, Thika, Kenya
Tolbert Nyenswah, Emergency Operation Center, Ministry of Health, Liberia
Tom O'Callaghan, Iheed, Ireland
Peter K. Olds, Brigham and Women's Hospital
Kristian R. Olson, Center for Global Health, Massachusetts General Hospital
Juan Sebastián Osorio, EIA University and CES University, Colombia
Kenneth E. Paik, MIT Critical Data, Massachusetts Institute of Technology
F. Mita Paramita, BrightFront Group
Kunal D. Patel, Iheed, Ireland

William Perry, The University of Auckland, New Zealand

William C. Philbrick, RTI International

Anban Pillay, Discipline of Computer Science, University of KwaZulu-Natal, South Africa

Arvind Raghu, Institute of Biomedical Engineering, University of Oxford, UK

Ramesh Raskar, MIT Media Lab

Kenneth J. Rothman, Department of Clinical Epidemiology, Boston University

Sundeep Sahay, University of Oslo, Norway

Raymond Francis Sarmiento, Centers for Disease Control and Prevention, Atlanta

Christopher J. Seebregts, Jembi Health Systems NPC, South Africa

Joel Selanikio, Magpi

Isabel Shaw, Broad Street Maps

Rose Shuman, BrightFront Group

Clayton Sims, Dimagi

Sagree Singh, Discipline of Computer Science, University of KwaZulu-Natal, South Africa

Tony Somers, Impact Economics LLC

Geren S. Stone, Center for Global Health, Massachusetts General Hospital

James K. Stoller, Education Institute, Cleveland Clinic

Abeezer Tapia, Harvard Business School

Lauren A. Taylor, Harvard Business School

Jonathan M. Teich, Departments of Medicine and Emergency Medicine, Brigham & Women's Hospital

Win Min Thit, Health Systems Research Institute, Ministry of Public Health, Thailand

Samuel Vaillancourt, Li Ka Shing Knowledge Institute, St. Michael's Hospital

Lavanya Vasudevan, Johns Hopkins Global mHealth Initiative

Adrian Velasquez, Newport Hospital

Susana Vieira, Instituto Superior Técnico, Universidade de Lisboa, Portugal

Karren Visser, In Collaboration with the Kenyan Medical Research Institute (KEMRI)

Eric Winkler, Sana Mobile

Rose Wyber, Nyes Institute, New Zealand

Cory Zue, Dimagi

Index